RETHINKING SUBSTANCE ABUSE

Rethinking Substance Abuse

What the Science Shows, and
What We Should Do about It

Edited by
WILLIAM R. MILLER
KATHLEEN M. CARROLL

THE GUILFORD PRESS
New York   London

© 2006 The Guilford Press
A Division of Guilford Publications, Inc.
72 Spring Street, New York, NY 10012
www.guilford.com

Printed in the United States of America

This book is printed on acid-free paper.

Last digit is print number: 9 8 7 6 5 4 3 2 1

Library of Congress Cataloging-in-Publication Data

Rethinking substance abuse : what the science shows, and what we should do
about it / edited by William R. Miller, Kathleen M. Carroll.
      p. cm.
  Includes bibliographical references and index.
  ISBN 1-57230-231-3 (alk. paper)
  1. Substance abuse. I. Miller, William R. II. Carroll, Kathleen.
  RC564.M545 2006
  362.29—dc22

                                                         2005020524

About the Editors

William R. Miller, PhD, is Distinguished Professor of Psychology and Psychiatry at the University of New Mexico. A recipient of the Jellinek Memorial Award for alcoholism research, he is fundamentally interested in the psychology of change, and has focused in particular on the development, testing, and dissemination of behavioral treatments for addictions. Dr. Miller's publications include more than 30 books and 300 articles and chapters spanning behavior therapies, motivation, self-regulation, and the interface of psychology with spirituality and religion. He is named by the Institute for Scientific Information as one of the "world's most cited scientists."

Kathleen M. Carroll, PhD, is Professor of Psychiatry at the Yale University School of Medicine. The author of over 180 journal articles and chapters, her research and clinical interests lie in the area of developing and evaluating behavioral therapies for substance use disorders, and combining therapies to maximize treatment outcome. Dr. Carroll is the past president of Division 50 (Addictions) of the American Psychological Association, and holds both Senior Scientist and MERIT awards from the National Institute on Drug Abuse, the latter being awarded to the top 1% of National Institutes of Health investigators.

Contributors

Warren K. Bickel, PhD, Department of Psychiatry and Center for Addiction Research, University of Arkansas for Medical Sciences, Little Rock, Arkansas

Robert G. Carlson, PhD, Center for Interventions, Treatment, and Addictions Research, Department of Community Health, Wright State University, Boonshoft School of Medicine, Dayton, Ohio

Kathleen M. Carroll, PhD, Department of Psychiatry, Yale University School of Medicine, New Haven, Connecticut; Department of Psychiatry, Veterans Affairs Connecticut Healthcare Center, West Haven, Connecticut

Anna Rose Childress, PhD, Addiction Treatment Research Center and Department of Psychiatry, University of Pennsylvania School of Medicine, Philadelphia, Pennsylvania

Carlo C. DiClemente, PhD, Department of Psychology, University of Maryland, Baltimore, Maryland

Robert E. Drake, MD, Departments of Psychiatry and Community and Family Medicine, New Hampshire–Dartmouth Psychiatric Research Center, Dartmouth Medical School, Hanover, New Hampshire

Elizabeth Gifford, PhD, Program Evaluation and Resource Center, Veterans Affairs Health Care System, Menlo Park, California

Deborah Hasin, PhD, Departments of Epidemiology and Psychiatry, Columbia University, New York, New York; Department of Research Assessment and Training, New York State Psychiatric Institute, New York, New York

Mark Hatzenbuehler, BA, Department of Psychology, Yale University, New Haven, Connecticut

Michie N. Hesselbrock, PhD, University of Connecticut School of Social Work, West Hartford, Connecticut

Victor M. Hesselbrock, PhD, Department of Psychiatry, University of Connecticut Health Center, Farmington, Connecticut

Harold D. Holder, PhD, Prevention Research Center, Pacific Institute for Research and Evaluation, Berkeley, California

Keith Humphreys, MD, Program Evaluation and Resource Center, Veterans Affairs Health Care System, Menlo Park, California

George F. Koob, PhD, Department of Neuropharmacology, The Scripps Research Institute, La Jolla, California

Thomas R. Kosten, MD, Department of Psychiatry, Yale University School of Medicine, New Haven, Connecticut; Department of Psychiatry, Veterans Affairs Connecticut Healthcare Center, West Haven, Connecticut

Barbara S. McCrady, PhD, Graduate School of Applied and Professional Psychology and Center of Alcohol Studies, Rutgers University, Piscataway, New Jersey

Mark McGovern, PhD, Department of Psychiatry, New Hampshire–Dartmouth Psychiatric Research Center, Dartmouth Medical School, Hanover, New Hampshire

A. Thomas McLellan, PhD, Treatment Research Institute, Philadelphia, Pennsylvania

William R. Miller, PhD, Departments of Psychology and Psychiatry, University of New Mexico, Albuquerque, New Mexico

Rudolf H. Moos, PhD, Center for Health Care Evaluation, Veterans Affairs Health Care System, Menlo Park, California; Department of Psychiatry and Behavioral Sciences, Stanford University, Stanford, California

Kim T. Mueser, PhD, Departments of Psychiatry and Community and Family Medicine, New Hampshire–Dartmouth Psychiatric Research Center, Dartmouth Medical School, Hanover, New Hampshire

Stephanie S. O'Malley, PhD, Department of Psychiatry, Yale University School of Medicine, New Haven, Connecticut

Marc N. Potenza, MD, Problem Gambling Clinic, Connecticut Mental Health Center, New Haven, Connecticut; Women and Addictions Core of Women's Health Research and Department of Psychiatry, Yale University School of Medicine, New Haven, Connecticut

Bruce J. Rounsaville, MD, Department of Psychiatry, Yale University School of Medicine, New Haven, Connecticut; Department of Psychiatry, Veterans Affairs Connecticut Healthcare Center, West Haven, Connecticut

Win Turner, PhD, Department of Psychiatry, Dartmouth Medical School, Hanover, New Hampshire

Rachel Waxman, BA, Department of Research Assessment and Training, New York State Psychiatric Institute, New York, New York

Preface

For as long as there have been written records, people have been searching for what to do about the troublesome use of psychoactive drugs. Ancient Greek remedies for excessive alcohol use included placing an eel at the bottom of the unfortunate drinker's generous goblet of red wine. Historically, problem drinkers have been whipped, dunked, shocked, poisoned with potions, chained, dialyzed, terrorized, and drugged with hallucinogens, Interferon, and all manner of psychiatric medications. More recently, the users of illicit drugs have been lectured to, fined, put to work, imprisoned, "scared straight," given "attack therapy," and sent to boot camps. In his history of Australia, *The Fatal Shore*, Robert Hughes recounts how even torture, starvation, and execution failed to deter tobacco and alcohol use among exiled prisoners.

This history would suggest that drug problems are fairly intransigent, and that attempts to modify them are doomed to failure. Yet this is not the case; even (and sometimes especially) severely drug-dependent people can show a turnabout in their drug use in response to treatment or changing circumstances. Drug problems are, in fact, quite changeable. One reason we have both devoted decades to drug treatment research is the enormous and rewarding changes that occur in people's lives when they escape from the downward spiral of drug dependence.

What is different now from even 20 years ago is that scientific research has revealed a great deal about the nature of drug problems[1] and how they can be prevented and treated. Thousands of new reports appear each year in the scientific literature, so many that it is impossible for any one person to digest them all. That's the good news.

The bad news is that very little of this science has found its way into practice. Clinicians, treatment systems, training programs, and

---

[1]Throughout this book we use "drug problems" to encompass the problematic use of alcohol, prescription medications, and illicit psychoactive drugs.

policymakers established habits of practice well before this wealth of research was available. Such habits take time to change, and it is common for there to be a substantial delay in the diffusion of innovations into practice.[2] Even the interventions being developed and tested today lag behind research advances and make use of only a small proportion of the available scientific knowledge.

With this in mind, we convened a "think tank" conference in New Mexico in 2004, bringing together leading addiction scientists to share the fruits of research in their respective areas, and to discuss possible implications for intervention. This meeting, entitled the Conference on Approaches for Combating the Troublesome Use of Substances (CACTUS), was supported in part by a grant from the Robert Wood Johnson Foundation. All of the authors of chapters in this book participated in CACTUS by preparing a scholarly summary in advance of the meeting. These were distributed to all participants, who committed to read them before arrival. Only brief summaries of each review were presented at CACTUS, where most of the time was devoted to discussion of interrelationships among research findings and to brainstorming implications for practice. The raw fruit of the brainstorming sessions can be found at casaa.unm.edu/cactus.html. The authors then revised their reviews in light of discussion of their work at CACTUS. Their final products comprise the chapters of this volume.

These chapters are unusual in several ways. First, we prohibited traditional scientific citation that interrupts the flow of text with inserted references. Instead we asked and entrusted authors to provide a summary of what is known and what is at least reasonably well supported by current research in their areas. A check on the accuracy of these summaries came through presenting them to their senior scientist peers at the CACTUS meeting, and making revisions in response to critiques. We also asked each author to derive a set of principles from the raw science that may have relevance to intervention. Finally, we asked the authors to set aside, as much as possible, brand-name treatments and familiar service models and systems, and to refrain from making specific recommendations for intervention. The chapters thus focus on principles rather than practices, from which readers can draw their own conclusions. In the final chapter of this book, we offer our own integration of the rich material summarized in these chapters, from which we derive 10 broad recommendations for how to reduce the substantial suffering and social harms associated with drug problems.

WILLIAM R. MILLER, PHD
KATHLEEN M. CARROLL, PHD

---

[2]Everett Rogers, *Diffusion of Innovations* (5th ed.). New York: Free Press, 2003.

Acknowledgments

We gratefully acknowledge the grant support of the Robert Wood Johnson Foundation, without which this conference and volume would not have occurred. Planning and practice arrangements for the meeting were capably overseen by Dee Ann Quintana and Delilah Yao. We also appreciate the superb editorial assistance of the editors and staff at The Guilford Press in the preparation of this book.

Most of all, we are grateful to those who committed 3 full days to participate actively in the CACTUS event. Including the invited speakers who contributed chapters to this volume, the following were participants in CACTUS:

Lisa T. Arciniega, PhD, University of New Mexico
Catherine Baca, MD, University of New Mexico
Jordan Bell, MS, University of New Mexico
Warren K. Bickel, PhD, University of Vermont
Jack Blaine, MD, National Institute on Drug Abuse
Jason Blankenship, PhD, University of New Mexico
Michael Bogenschutz, MD, University of New Mexico Health Sciences Center
Robert G. Carlson, PhD, Wright State University School of Medicine
Kathleen M. Carroll, PhD, VA Connecticut Healthcare System
Anna Rose Childress, PhD, University of Pennsylvania School of Medicine
Mikyta Daugherty, MS, University of New Mexico
Carlo C. DiClemente, PhD, University of Maryland–Baltimore
Bonnie Duran, DrPH, University of New Mexico
Denise Ernst, MA, MS, University of New Mexico
Sarah Feldstein, MS, University of New Mexico
Alyssa Forcehimes, MS, University of New Mexico
Jessica Goodkind, PhD, University of New Mexico Health Sciences Center
Deborah Hasin, PhD, Columbia University

Victor M. Hesselbrock, PhD, University of Connecticut Health Center
Reid K. Hester, PhD, Behavior Therapy Associates
Jenny Hettema, MS, University of New Mexico
Harold D. Holder, PhD, Prevention Research Center, Berkeley
Keith Humphreys, PhD, Stanford University School of Medicine
Wendy Johnson, MS, University of New Mexico
Jennifer Knapp, BA, University of New Mexico
George F. Koob, PhD, Scripps Research Institute
Charlene E. LeFauve, PhD, Center for Substance Abuse Treatment
A. Thomas McLellan, PhD, Treatment Research Institute
Barbara S. McCrady, PhD, Rutgers University
Jaime Milford, MS, University of New Mexico
William R. Miller, PhD, University of New Mexico
Theresa B. Moyers, PhD, University of New Mexico
Rudolf H. Moos, PhD, VA Healthcare System, Palo Alto
Kim T. Mueser, PhD, Dartmouth Psychiatric Research Center
Stephanie S. O'Malley, PhD, Yale University School of Medicine
Diane Pallas, PhD, University of New Mexico
Kristine B. Schubert, MPH, Robert Wood Johnson Foundation
Dan Squires, PhD, Brown University
Julie M. Steele, BA, University of New Mexico
Kamilla Venner, PhD, University of New Mexico
Isabel Villarreal, BA, University of New Mexico
Paula Wilbourne, PhD, VA Healthcare System, Palo Alto
Mark Willenbring, MD, National Institute on Alcohol Abuse and Alcoholism

Contents

I. Introduction

1   Defining and Addressing the Problem   3
    Kathleen M. Carroll and William R. Miller

2   The Forest and the Trees: Addiction as a Complex   8
    Self-Organizing System
    Warren K. Bickel and Marc N. Potenza

II. Biological Factors

3   The Neurobiology of Addiction: A Hedonic   25
    Calvinist View
    George F. Koob

4   What Can Human Brain Imaging Tell Us about   46
    Vulnerability to Addiction and to Relapse?
    Anna Rose Childress

5   Genetics of Substance Use Disorders   61
    Deborah Hasin, Mark Hatzenbuehler, and Rachel Waxman

III. Psychological Factors

6   Natural Change and the Troublesome Use of Substances: 81
    A Life-Course Perspective
    Carlo C. DiClemente

7   Developmental Perspectives on the Risk for Developing   97
    Substance Abuse Problems
    Victor M. Hesselbrock and Michie N. Hesselbrock

8 Comorbid Substance Use Disorders
and Psychiatric Disorders
*Kim T. Mueser, Robert E. Drake, Win Turner,
and Mark McGovern*   115

9 Motivational Factors in Addictive Behaviors   134
William R. Miller

IV. Social Factors

10 Racial and Gender Differences in Substance Abuse: 153
What Should Communities Do about Them?
Harold D. Holder

11 Family and Other Close Relationships   166
Barbara S. McCrady

12 Social Contexts and Substance Use   182
Rudolf H. Moos

13 Ethnography and Applied Substance Misuse Research: 201
Anthropological and Cross-Cultural Factors
Robert G. Carlson

V. Interventions

14 Behavioral Therapies: The Glass Would Be Half   223
Full If Only We Had a Glass
Kathleen M. Carroll and Bruce J. Rounsaville

15 Pharmacotherapy of Addictive Disorders   240
Stephanie S. O'Malley and Thomas R. Kosten

16 Religion, Spirituality, and the Troublesome Use   257
of Substances
Keith Humphreys and Elizabeth Gifford

17 What We Need Is a System: Creating a Responsive   275
and Effective Substance Abuse Treatment System
A. Thomas McLellan

18 Drawing the Scene Together: Ten Principles,   293
Ten Recommendations
William R. Miller and Kathleen M. Carroll

Index   313

Part I

Introduction

CHAPTER 1

Defining and Addressing the Problem

KATHLEEN M. CARROLL
WILLIAM R. MILLER

If There Ever Was a Time . . .

Civilizations have long wrestled with problems linked to the use of alcohol and other psychoactive substances, and have made all manner of efforts to control and restrict use of these drugs. Plato recommended complete abstinence for those younger than 18 ("Shall we not pass a law that, in the first place, no children under eighteen may touch wine at all?"). There are multiple warnings against alcohol in the Bible ("At the last it bites like a serpent, and stings like an adder. Your eyes will see strange things, and your mind utter perverse things"; Proverbs 23:32–33, NRSV). Various forms of prohibition, punishment, and condemnation, including death by stoning (Deuteronomy 21:20–21), have been tried throughout history. Most recently, we have witnessed a "war on drugs." Rarely have these efforts been informed by science or evaluated for efficacy.

Suppose we knew all that science has revealed regarding substance use problems and dependence, but had no organized systems for addressing them. Imagine if we could start from scratch to design creative ways to prevent, decrease, and treat substance use problems and disorders. What if we were to set aside all current specialist systems, brand-name treatments, and existing programs, and start from the scientific knowledge base to develop social strategies for combating these problems?

Those questions lie at the heart of this book. Our goal was to assemble the most current scientific knowledge regarding problematic use of alcohol and other drugs, and then to explore the implications of what we know for treatment and prevention. We challenged the contributors to this volume to provide a concise summary of what is known about addictions in their area of scientific expertise. Initial drafts were presented to and critiqued by the other authors at a "think tank" conference, where presentations were enriched by brainstorming and discussion. The authors then revised their summaries to create the chapters of this book. In a final chapter, we identify and integrate some common themes that emerged, and articulate a vision for more effective societal response to the troublesome use of substances.

> *Various forms of prohibition, punishment, and condemnation have been tried throughout history. Rarely have these efforts been informed by science or evaluated for efficacy.*

One unsettling consensus that emerged was the realization that the existing U.S. intervention system is in sufficiently dire straits as to constrain us very little. With drastic cuts in financial support for already starved treatment and prevention efforts, many alcohol and drug treatment programs across the United States have simply closed. Major gaps persist between what research has shown to be effective and what is actually practiced in clinical settings. Services for drug problems continue to be stigmatized, marginalized, and isolated from the rest of the health care system. Consumers have little reliable information to use in finding and selecting services, or for judging their effectiveness. Consequently it was not at all difficult to imagine starting over from scratch to envision a more compassionate, effective, and cost-efficient intervention system. If there ever was a time to reimagine strategies and systems to more effectively intervene with the problems associated with substance use, it is now. There truly is little to lose.

And Now for Something Completely Different . . .

Beyond the freedom to learn and make use of what the best science reveals regarding intervening with the problematic use of substances, the format of the meeting and this book stimulated us to think differently about a wide range of issues. That is also reflected in the format of this book, which is deliberately intended to be highly accessible to a broad audience. Instead of lengthy and highly referenced academic reviews, the chapters in this volume constitute succinct summaries of what some of the best minds in the field know about a wide range of issues associated with substance use problems. Each chapter ends with a list of "robust principles": a synthesis of what is known about each area and the logical conclusions relevant to the areas of treatment and prevention that emerge from what is known. Each chapter also includes a list of "selected readings" that highlight reviews, books, and seminal articles that summarize and integrate information on the topic covered in that chapter. Regardless of backgrounds and years of experience in the field of drug abuse, each of the authors was struck by something new in preparing his or her chapter: a long-held assumption being challenged, an insight from one perspective that could be applied to another area, a new way of thinking about old problems. All of us, editors and contributing authors alike, were confronted with our own sometimes dimly realized biases, and with the need to think in fresh and broad terms about the nature of these problems and their remedies. We hope the same will be true for you.

We asked the contributors to base their conclusions on concepts and principles for which there is sound scientific evidence. Thus this book is oriented less toward "evidence-based practices" than toward reliable science-based principles on which future interventions and services could be based.

What You Call It Matters

One of the more complex issues with which we wrestled was the use of terminology to describe the concepts and range of problems associated with the use of alcohol and other drugs. The names used to describe phenomena affect the ways in which one thinks about a problem and what to do about it. The terminology of this field is rife with overmeaning. Over the years, people with problems linked to overdrinking have been termed "drunkards," "dipsomanics," "alcoholics," "alcohol-dependent," "problem drinkers," and "alcohol abusers." Illicit drug users have been called "addicts," "dope fiends," "criminals," "drug abusers," and "drug-dependent." Each of these terms has particular connotations. Similarly, "treatment" (itself a concept carrying certain assumptions) has been variously conceived as leading to reform, rehabilitation, recovery, sobriety, relapse prevention, and harm reduction.

There is a further value to the discipline of avoiding the jargon, labels, and pejorative terms commonly used in this field. The goal was not to find politically correct euphemisms, but rather to force ourselves to think differently about the broader nature of the issues and

problems we were addressing. We chose the "troublesome use" title for
the CACTUS meeting not because it is a preferable term, but precisely
because it was unfamiliar and shook us loose from comfortable custom.
This in turn helped us to clarify some working assumptions.

Broad Perspectives

First, it became clear that we were not focusing on a particular set or
class of individuals, but rather on human behavior. Second, it became
obvious that the behavior of drug use is not isolated, but is intimately
intertwined with a range of common, long-standing human issues and
societal problems. ("Alcohol is the anesthesia by which we endure the
operation of life," said George Bernard Shaw.) In some ways, the central
issues of this field represent a microcosm of classic human dilemmas:
why we persist in patterns of behavior that clearly lead toward devastating
consequences; the tensions among our biological, individual, and social selves; whether and how to regulate our emotions; the trade-offs
of immediate gratification versus long-term personal, family, and communal welfare. The troublesome use of substances is, in this way, just
one manifestation of larger personal, social, and biological dramas.

Drug use is not isolated, but is intimately intertwined with a range of common, long-standing human issues and societal problems.

Similar underlying issues and vulnerabilities could emerge as drug dependence in one person, as sadness and isolation in another, as aggressive or criminal behavior in another, and as all of these in yet another.
We found that many of the principles and frameworks for intervention
that emerged are not necessarily specific to problems associated with
substance use, but rather apply to a broader range of human problems
that sometimes express themselves in the troublesome use of alcohol
or drugs.

The CACTUS discussions of intervention and prevention strategies also engendered stimulating dialogue about the nature of societal
values and choices, as well as personal and social regulation of behavior. For example, what should be done with the evidence that:

- Problematic drug use tends to run in families?
- High levels of stress increase vulnerability to these problems?
- Adolescent brains are less able than adult brains to self-regulate
  behavior, and also less susceptible to some of the aversive conse-
  quences of drug use?
- Involvement with religion is one of the strongest protective fac-

tors against the development of drug and alcohol problems, but not necessarily effective once those problems become established?

- Some commonly delivered prevention and treatment services have been found to be ineffective at best, or even more harmful than no intervention at all?

We were also keenly aware that, like current practices, efforts to change how to think and what to do about substance use problems can have unintended consequences.

The common concern of all the authors contributing to this volume was the desire to alleviate the enormous personal suffering and social harms related to drug use. Indeed, systems to address the troublesome use of substances should have a prominent place in any societal effort to reduce suffering and enhance human welfare. Even given the dire state of the current treatment system, there is clear optimism in the chapters of this book regarding the possibilities of reenvisioning approaches to substance use problems. Recent U.S. history contains examples of how such major change can and does occur at a societal level—for example, recent dramatic reductions in smoking and in alcohol-related driving fatalities. In both of these cases there was a convergence of greater understanding of the factors supporting these behaviors, dramatic changes in social acceptability, concerted local and national efforts to increase the cost and consequences of these behaviors, and the availability of acceptable alternatives.

> It is challenging but possible to bring about societal change in behaviors that are so pervasive, reinforcing, persistent, and costly.

It is challenging but possible to bring about societal change in behaviors that are pervasive, reinforcing, persistent, and costly. The chapters that follow summarize a wealth of scientific knowledge pertinent to and potentially applicable in addressing the troublesome use of substances. Then, in the closing chapter, we offer our integration of this knowledge and recommendations for new directions in finding better solutions.

CHAPTER 2

The Forest and the Trees

Addiction as a Complex Self-Organizing System

WARREN K. BICKEL

MARC N. POTENZA

> Another and less obvious way of unifying the chaos is to seek common elements in the diverse mental facts rather than a common agent behind them, and to explain them constructively by the various forms or arrangements of these elements as one explains houses by stones and bricks.
>
> —WILLIAM JAMES

Addiction is not well understood. At least five important questions need to be answered scientifically if we are to make substantial inroads in addressing this important public health problem. First, why does addiction continue despite the serious negative economic, health, and social consequences for the person with the disorder, his or her family, and his or her community? Second, why is addiction so difficult to treat? If addiction were easily treated with a remarkable success rate, then it is unlikely this volume would have been developed. Third, why is relapse so ubiquitous that some consider it a defining feature of addiction? Fourth, why is addiction in multiple domains (polysubstance dependence) the rule and not the exception? Fifth, why does addiction co-occur with other psychiatric disorders so frequently?

Efforts to answer these and other questions have typically referred to a singular mechanism and suggested that mechanism as being responsible for addiction. Among the many singular mechanisms that have been proposed to account for addiction are craving, mesolimbic dopaminergic neurotransmission, drug reinforcement, and sensitization. Although these approaches have been successful to varying degrees in accounting in part for at least a restricted set of phenomena related to addiction, they have provided neither a comprehensive understanding of addiction, nor have they resulted in treatments that are ubiquitously successful and produce lasting change. Perhaps these singular process approaches have such limited success because addiction is a complex multicomponent phenomenon.

Answers to the questions we have posed and perhaps to other questions may reside in a new view of addiction that also serves as the thesis of this chapter, namely, that addiction is a self-organizing complex disorder that emerges from the interaction of evolutionarily old behavioral processes and their associated brain regions. This view suggests that addiction is a disorder that develops from the interaction and resulting organization of interactions among a variety of subunits of the system. Many of these subunits developed and were passed on by natural selection because they conveyed survival advantages either alone or in combination with other units. Importantly, these subunits respond on the basis of very local and limited information. We argue that there is no centralized control by a singular process in addiction. We clarify this thesis by addressing the origins of addiction systems, the components of the addiction, and how these components may interact. Throughout this chapter, we introduce notions and terms that have been developed in behavioral economics, evolutionary psychology, and systems biology because they provide the conceptual base of our argument.

There is no centralized control by a singular process in addiction.

Origins

Its [Beirut's] origins are ancient but it burgeons with brash modernity, and it lounges upon its delectable shore. . . .
—JAMES MORRIS

In examining the origins of addiction, we should consider evolutionary contributions. Evolutionary psychology and medicine suggest that the origin of many of our contemporary behavioral and medical problems reside in and derive from our evolutionary past. Most relevant to the concerns of this chapter is the persuasive argument from evolutionary psychology that the brain should *not* be considered to function as a general-purpose computer with the ability to solve any problem. Instead, evolutionary psychology argues that specific aspects of the brain and behavior should be considered to be similar to other morphological adaptations that were preserved by natural selection. In other words, these features were selected because they solved specific adaptive problems. These specific aspects of the brain and behavior are termed "modules." *Modules* refer to physically or functionally insulated subsystems. In modular systems, control is distributed over the whole of the system without being centralized. One important consequence of these systems is that the failure of one module does not spread and result in catastrophic systemwide failure. For example, catastrophic failure would result if the central processing unit (CPU) of a computer failed. In contrast, damage to the Broca's region of the brain renders patients unable to understand speech, but leaves them still able to solve math problems, make future plans, and hear. In other cases, redundancies of modules prevent noticeable system impairment despite local damage (e.g., "silent strokes"). In these circumstances, damage to one module does not result in catastrophic failure. Moreover, modules often operate with feedback from local conditions or from their interaction with other adjacent modules.

Now consider that research on addiction has shown that drugs of dependence appear to commandeer evolutionary old portions of the brain that regulate natural reinforcers of drink, food, sex, and social interaction. Specifically, these brain areas comprise the limbic system and include the amygdala, nucleus accumbens, and prefrontal cortex (note that additional evidence suggests that the more recently evolved frontal cortical regions appear to go "off line," either functionally or structurally, during the process of addiction). Thus, the scientific literature is consistent with our premise that the constructive elements of addiction reside in our evolutionary past.

> *Drugs of dependence appear to commandeer evolutionarily old portions of the brain that regulate natural reinforcers of drink, food, sex, and social interaction.*

Combining the notions of evolutionary psychology with the scientific observations from the study of addiction suggests a new goal for the scientific study of addiction, namely, the identification of the commandeered brain/behavioral modules. Moreover, the combination of these two perspectives suggests three criteria to identify modules that may participate in addiction. First, a module and its output should be conserved across species including humans, and therefore the process should be qualitatively fixed. That is, the same functional process should be observed across species and different phenotypes including among nonaddicted individuals, although quantitative differences may exist, as might be expected with homologous processes. Second, if addiction influences the behavioral process in question, then we should expect to observe quantitative differences in this behavioral process when addicted individuals are compared with nonaddicted controls, that is, the behavioral process is quantitatively flexible. Third, if, in the process of the development of addiction, there are quantitative changes in this behavioral process (as specified above), then decreases in drug use or a change in addiction status should produce a corresponding change in the quantitative aspects of this process (again, demonstrating quantitative flexibility).

Let us consider one candidate module, delay discounting, as an exemplar, and examine whether it conforms to the proposed criteria. *Delay discounting* is a behavioral process that values delayed reinforcers less than reinforcers that are not delayed. This observation is intuitive; for example, imagine making a choice between $1,000 that would be immediately available after selection versus $1,000 that would not be available until 1 month after selection. The extent to which the immediately available money is preferred indicates how much the delayed money is discounted or valued less.

The extent of discounting can be measured precisely by using psychophysical procedures where subjects choose between an immediate and a delayed reinforcer. Although we would expect the immediate amount of money to be selected if the choice is between $1,000 available now and $1,000 available in 1 month, such information does not address the extent or magnitude of discounting. What could provide more specific knowledge regarding the extent of discounting is identifying the amount of immediately available money that the chooser values approximately the same as the delayed money. This information can be obtained by progressively decreasing the amount of the immediately available money across trials (e.g., $975, $950, $925) and keeping the delayed amount unchanged ($1,000), and then identifying the specific monetary amount that results in the chooser's switch from the immediate to the delayed amount. For example, if the chooser's preference switches when $800 is the immediately available amount, we can infer that $1,000 loses 20% of its value in 1 month. If we repeat this process at a broad range of time frames (1 day, 1 week, 1 month, 6 months, 1 year, etc.), we can construct a discounting curve.

When a discounting curve is constructed, the shape of the function takes a particular form; specifically, the curve is hyperbolic in shape and well described by Mazur's hyperbolic decay formula. Indeed, hyperbolic curves are obtained when similar procedures are arranged with several species including humans. The broad cross-species generality of this behavioral process suggests that this process is conserved evolutionarily.

Given that this behavior is conserved evolutionarily and that other research supports the conclusion that this process is mediated by evolutionarily old brain regions, then the next question is whether this process is affected by addiction. A substantial body of literature suggests that drug-dependent individuals (alcohol-, cocaine-, heroin-, tobacco-dependent) discount money substantially more than matched control normals and that the drug dependent substantially discount their drug of dependence more than an equivalent amount of money. Similarly, individuals with nondrug disorders that share core features of addiction (e.g., pathological gambling) discount rewards at excessive rates. These findings suggest that this evolutionarily conserved behavioral process is quantitatively altered in addiction.

Other studies indicate that ex-dependent drug users discount less than current users. This may suggest that this behavioral process "commandeered" during active addiction may be quantitatively altered to return to baseline when active addiction stops, although other interpretations are certainly possible. Moreover, a preliminary study conducted by one of us (WKB) indicated that discounting decreased within subjects following exposure to an intervention designed to decrease smoking among tobacco smokers.

Delay discounting meets the criteria indicating that it functions as a module as described by evolutionary psychology and that it participates in the addiction process. There are several other candidate processes, such as probability discounting, demand curves, matching law, and risk-sensitive foraging that may be similarly commandeered and for which there is supporting evidence that they would likely meet the same criteria outlined above. It is interesting to note that these modules were initially characterized in situations in which there were constraints on the availability of natural reinforcers such as the acquisition of food.

Competence and Interaction

> Help! I need somebody. Help! Not just anybody.
> Help! You know I need someone. Help!
> —JOHN LENNON AND PAUL MCCARTNEY

Modules, in and of themselves, may not be able to accomplish much. Consider a simple example using the exemplar from the prior section, discounting of delayed reinforcers. The degree of discounting may change the value of two commodities, but does not result in the acquisition and consumption of the commodity once it is selected. Other modules must interact either in parallel or in series to complete this action. Although individual modules as outlined above can respond with quantitative flexibility to changes in the environment, they are unlikely to result in novel responses to new environmental circumstances unless they interact with other modules. As such, in this section, we consider the ways these processes may interact and provide a simple example of this interaction using two modules applicable to addiction.

The interaction among modules is referred to as "protocols." According to systems biologists Marie Csete and John Doyle:

> Protocols are far more important to biologic complexity than are modules. They are complementary and intertwined, but are important to distinguish. In everyday usage, protocols are rules designed to manage relationships and processes smoothly and effectively. If modules are ingredients, parts, or components, subsystems and players, then protocols describe the corresponding recipes, architectures, rules, interfaces, etiquettes, and codes of conduct. Protocols here are rules that prescribe allowed interfaces between modules, permitting system function that could not be achieved by isolated modules. Protocols also facilitate the addition of new protocols and organization into collections of mutually supportive protocol suites. . . . A good protocol is one that supplies both robustness and evolvability.

According to this analysis, protocols are the way that modules align with each other and the mechanism by which an organism may adapt to changing circumstances.

Now consider how two modules that may be adopted in addiction may interact to further the development of addiction. One process is elasticity of demand. *Elasticity* refers to the sensitivity of consumption to price. Consumption that decreases proportionally more than the proportional increase in price is considered elastic, while consumption that decreases proportionally less than the proportional increase in price is considered inelastic. One factor that produces greater sensitivity to price (more elastic demand) is the availability of substitutes. A *substitute* is a commodity that shares features with another commodity (e.g., Pepsi vs. Coca-Cola) such that increases in the price of one commodity (Pepsi) result in increased consumption of another commodity (Coca-Cola). One source of substitution is intertemporal: instead of purchasing a more expensive commodity now, a cheaper substitute can be purchased later.

Intertemporal substitution, however, is likely influenced by how much delayed commodities are discounted (see above for a description of delay discounting). For example, if delayed commodities are radically discounted, then it is unlikely that intertemporal substitution would occur. When intertemporal substitution is unlikely, then demand for the currently available commodity will be more insensitive to price. Symmetrically, a decrease in discounting, resulting in a greater value being placed on temporally delayed events, should make consumption more sensitive to price through the process of intertemporal substitution. This interaction is a process that may result in the greater insensitivity to price or inelasticity of demand often exhibited by the drug-dependent.

Modules need to interact in order to accomplish complex activities. The number of modules that may be commandeered and interact in addiction may be considerable given that these modules are evolutionarily old and contributed to obtaining natural reinforcers such as food, water, and sex. These interactions may be the process by which addiction develops. Examination of these interactions requires methods to determine how any set of modules may interact with each other. The most useful experimental probe would be a selective intervention that would target only one module. Whether such selective interventions are available for each module remains to be determined. In the absence of such selective interventions, the next best alternative would be to perturb the system and infer the relationship among networks via the strength of correlation among them. Presumably, the more closely related the relationship among modules, the greater the correlation.

Self-Organization

> Order for free.
> —STUART KAUFFMAN

So far we have addressed how specific modules may be commandeered in addiction, and we have noted that these modules can interact and influence one another. In this section, we address the issue of how these evolutionarily old modules organize themselves into what we refer to as addiction.

Self-organization refers to a process that increases the organization of a system without being assisted or developed by an external designer. Note that this concept is in some sense the opposite of the concept of entropy. Self-organization is ubiquitous in biology and is perhaps most obvious in developing organisms.

One important consideration in the notion of self-organization is why does it occur. One important investigator in this area, Stuart Kauffman, conducted simulation studies of genetic networks and showed that he was able to predict the number of stable states of a system by specifying both the number and the strength of connections among the network elements. For example, by knowing the number of human genes and by specifying a minimal number of local inputs from each gene, Kauffman was able to obtain a reasonable approximation of the number of different tissues that should be evident in humans. These and other experiments predict that self-organization will occur in every system composed of interconnected elements. Kauffman refers to this process as "order for free."

Assuming that self-organization is an almost unavoidable consequence of multiple potential components, it is important to consider what are some of the characteristics of such systems. First, self-organizing systems are dynamic and required the lower level components continually interact in order to produce and maintain the system. This first characteristic suggests that the system would begin to disassemble if the interactions were thwarted. Second, self-organizing systems exhibit emergent properties. *Emergent properties* refer to the fact that the interacting subunits cannot be understood as the simple addition of the components. The notion of emergence may present a substantial challenge to reductive aspects of the addiction field. Third, the system may reach stability at a point that may not be optimal and in fact may be suboptimal. This characteristic suggests that optimality is not the end point of system dynamics but rather that it satisfies some minimum requirement. The fourth characteristic of a self-organizing system is that once such a system stabilizes, it is "locked in" such that changing the stability point would be difficult. To change such a system would require that additional factors and/or forces be directed at the system.

These characteristics appear quite applicable to and useful for understanding addiction. First, the notion that the components of the system must interact frequently for it to sustain itself is interesting and relevant to addiction. Interactions among modules may be instigated by ingesting the substance or engaging in use of the addictive commodity, or alternatively, by a period of abstinence. As such, the hallmark features of addiction of frequent ingestion or engagement and strenuous efforts made to obtain or participate in the addictive commodity after a brief period of abstinence may be important to supporting the system of addiction. Moreover, the disassembly of the system as a result of the lack of interaction seems applicable to recent observations by Higgins and colleagues that in-treatment abstinence predicts posttreatment abstinence independent of specific treatment received.

The second characteristic of a self-organizing system is that these systems exhibit emergent behavior. This feature arguably represents the most challenging characteristic to explain reductive and single-process approaches to addiction. Emergent behavior that is not resident in the elements of the system indicates that some aspects of addiction are irreducible and suggests that understanding these aspects of addiction can only be studied among the addicted individuals and may not be appropriately or completely modeled in simpler systems. This characteristic in particular remains to be demonstrated empirically as it pertains to addiction.

The third and fourth characteristics of self-organized systems appear quite applicable to addiction. The third characteristic is that they may stabilize at less than optimal levels. Indeed, this characteristic seems to address a hallmark component of the addiction system, that is, drug consumption or engagement in the addictive behavior continues despite negative life consequences. This process may represent the emergent behavior addressed in the prior characteristic of self-organized systems. The fourth characteristic implies that additional energy must be added to the system to alter an otherwise stable system. This aspect also seems directly applicable to addiction. Studies examining why individuals seek treatment often identify changed circumstances that involve the addition of new forces. Examples often cited for seeking treatment include involvement with the criminal justice system and loss of employment and/ or a significant relationship because of the addiction. Moreover, contingency management, one of the most effective treatments for addiction, involves the addition of a new force, a contingent reward for not engaging in the addictive behavior. A possible reason for the efficacy of this approach may reside in its ability to recommandeer modules influenced by addiction, thus resulting in system reorganization.

Ways to conceptualize the development and deconstruction of self-organized models of addiction remain a challenge. One approach to this daunting task involves using existing data about modules and their documented interactions to infer a model of the system. Such a model could determine whether some modules are more central to the process of addiction than others and suggest targets for the development of interventions. Consideration of developmental aspects within this framework seems particularly important as systems models suggest that onset of addictive behaviors (e.g., drug use, gambling during childhood/adolescence) might result in dramatically altered robust behavioral systems that at future points are relatively insensitive to our current interventions.

Development of a Multimodule
Self-Organizing System: A Proposed Model

The sciences do not try to explain, they hardly even try to interpret, they mainly make models. By a model is meant a mathematical construct, which with the addition of certain

verbal interpretations, describes observed phenomena. The justification of such a mathematical construct is solely and precisely that it is expected to work.
                                                    —JOHN VON NEUMANN

In this section, we illustrate as an example how multiple processes including those that are evolutionarily old may interact and self-organize to produce the self-organized system that we consider addiction. This is merely a proposal and may not include all the processes that may operate.

1. All other things being equal, brief intense stimuli (e.g., drugs) will be more reinforcing than long-duration, less intense stimuli as stipulated by the matching law, that is, when a drug of dependence is consumed, that drug stimulus is generally more reinforcing than other available nondrug reinforcers.

2. As a consequence of brief intense stimuli serving as a more potent reinforcer, more behavior will be allocated to the acquisition and consumption of those brief intense stimuli.

3. Increased allocation of behavior to those brief intense stimuli will tend to shorten the temporal horizon (increase the temporal discounting for reinforcers). (Note that the direct effects of drugs may exacerbate this effect.)

4. As the temporal horizon shortens, intertemporal substitution decreases. For example, if the future is sufficiently discounted so that 24 hours into the future is for all intents and purposes irrelevant, then reinforcers including drugs of dependence that may be available tomorrow at a cheaper price will not be able to substitute for current consumption.

5. Decreases in intertemporal substitution will, in turn, result in more inelastic (i.e., less sensitive to price) drug consumption. This characteristic relates to a central notion in behavioral economics that in the absence of substitution, the consumption of reinforcers will be less affected by price.

6. Shortening of the temporal horizon will also tend to diminish the reinforcing effects of stimuli that are less intense and more protracted and relatively increase the potency of brief intense drug stimuli.

7. A relative increase in the reinforcing effects of drugs of dependence and a relative decrease in the reinforcing effects of nondrug reinforcers will further increase allocation of behavior to drugs and produce a narrowing of the behavioral repertoire.

8. Narrowing of the behavioral repertoire will result in behavior being allocated to the acquisition of drugs until the minimal needs of drug consumption are met. Allocation of behavior to

other activities will only occur once the minimal needs of drug consumption are met.

9. As more behavior is allocated to the acquisition of brief intense stimuli (drugs), the likelihood of tolerance and dependence increases.

10. As tolerance develops, the amount of consumption is less likely to meet satiation levels.

11. When satiation levels are not obtainable (i.e., drug hunger), withdrawal may be experienced and risk-prone behavior will increase (e.g., risk-sensitive foraging).

12. When satiation levels are not obtainable, temporal horizons will decrease further, as will intertemporal substitution, and in turn produce less sensitivity to price, greater relative reinforcing effects of drugs, and increased tolerance. At this point, the process may be self-perpetuating, or the system may be locked into a stable, addicted state.

Answers to the Questions

> It is better to know some of the questions than all of the answers.
>
> —JAMES THURBER

In this section we revisit and attempt to answer the questions that we initially posed at the beginning of this chapter.

- *Question*: Why does addiction continue despite its serious negative economic, health, and social consequences for the person with the disorder?
- *Answer*: The processes commandeered in addiction are largely modules that address survival. As such, the temporal resolution of these processes is based on immediate events. Many of the adverse effects of addiction are only contacted later after engaging in the addictive behavior.
- *Question*: Why is addiction so difficult to treat?
- *Answer*: Perhaps many of our treatments have been developed to address only one or a few modular processes. As such, a module so affected may not influence the other aspects of the self-organized process we call addiction.
- *Question*: Why is relapse so ubiquitous?
- *Answer*: Perhaps treatments only affect or disassemble one or more modules, and the remaining system is insulated by redundancies or quickly reassembles itself.

- *Question*: Why is polyaddiction the rule and not the exception?
- *Answer*: Perhaps, across addictions, there are some modules that are shared and others that are not. By developing one addiction, a

> *Treatments [may] only affect or disassemble one or more modules, and the remaining system is insulated by redundancies or quickly reassembles itself.*

threshold level of constituents of another addiction is achieved such that incorporation of remaining modules is easily accomplished.

- *Question*: Why is addiction and co-occurrence with other psychiatric disorders so prevalent?
- *Answer*: Addiction and other psychiatric disorders may share modules. Therefore, by having one disorder, one already has several of the constituents of another disorder, placing one at increased risk for full development of the second disorder.

Conclusion

Addiction may represent an emergent property resulting from the interaction of components (modules) and may not reside in any single component part. The components of addiction may be related to evolutionarily old processes historically involved in resource acquisition and survival. A modular systems model approach to addiction may explain differences among forms of addiction—for example, perhaps not all of the same modules are involved in every form of addiction. Predisposing factors could also result from one or more modules having significant quantitative variation. Moreover, modular systems models may help us to understand the differential effectiveness of treatments. Perhaps some treatments only influence modules that are not central in the network of interactions. Lastly and most importantly, modular systems models may suggest a rational approach for the development of more effective treatments. Although much of this framework is speculative, the promise of this new approach for understanding addiction warrants further investigation and consideration by the field given its potential for generating hypotheses that may be formally tested and advancing current prevention and treatment strategies.

Robust Principles

1. Once an addiction system has been established via the interaction of multiple components, then it will be robust and insensitive to a large number of putatively corrective forces.
2. Treatment seeking by addicted individuals will occur only when

new environmental forces are applied. These forces include the intervention of the legal system, or the loss of employment, loved ones, and/or health.

3. One environmental process that produces changes is contingent positive reinforcement. The effectiveness of this treatment approach reveals much about the process of addiction. In particular, it suggests that the organizing and initiating forces of addiction reside in the intense brief immediate reinforcers of drugs, and that the application of immediate prosocial reinforcers provides an alternative organizing force.

4. An important consequence of using positive reinforcement to decrease drug use is that it stops the interaction of the components that comprise addiction.

5. Medications that are effective for the treatment of addiction such as buprenorphine, methadone, and the nicotine patch provide pharmacological effects that are similar to those effects of abused drugs. The differences between the medication and the abused drugs reside in the brevity and intensity of the stimulus. The abused drugs are brief and intense, while the medications are neither brief nor intense. This feature is important for understanding processes that organize or initiate the process of addiction.

6. The lack of effectiveness of many treatments suggests that these treatments may only influence one module or a small set of modules. Modular systems can lose components without experiencing catastrophic failure.

7. Outcomes among individuals with multiple comorbid addictions or psychiatric conditions are worse relative to those in people without complicating co-conditions. The poorer outcome could be explained by co-occurring disorders sharing modules with the primary addiction. If this were true, additional interactions could sustain the comorbid disorders.

8. In order to be effective, treatments must either influence so many modules that the result is a catastrophic failure of the addiction system, or alter the module that initiates the organization and/or maintenance of the other modules.

Acknowledgment

Preparation of this chapter was supported by Grant Nos. 5R37 DA 006526-14, RO1 DA 11692, and RO1 DA 12997 from the National Institute on Drug Abuse.

Suggested Readings

Arthur, W. B. (1989). Competing technologies, increasing returns and lock-in by historical events. *Economic Journal, 99,* 116–131.

Bickel, W. K., DeGrandpre, R. J., & Higgins, S. T. (1995). The behavioral economics of concurrent drug reinforcers: A review and reanalysis of drug self-administration research. *Psychopharmacology, 3,* 250–259.

Bickel, W. K., Odum, A. L., & Madden, G. L. (1999). Impulsivity and cigarette smoking: Delay discounting in current, never, and ex-smokers. *Psychopharmacology, 146,* 447–454.

Buchman, T. G. (2002). The community of the self. *Nature, 420,* 246–251.

Camazine, S., Deneubourg, J. L., Franks, N. R., Sneyd, J., Theraulaz, G., & Bonabeau, E. (2001). *Self-organization in biological systems.* Princeton, NJ: Princeton University Press.

Chambers, R. A., Krystal, J. H., & Self, D. W. (2001). A neurobiological basis for substance abuse comorbidity in schizophrenia. *Biological Psychiatry, 50,* 71–83.

Chambers, R. A., Taylor, J. R., & Potenza, M. N. (2003). Developmental neurocircuitry of motivation in adolescence: A critical period of addiction vulnerability. *American Journal of Psychiatry, 160*(6), 1041–1052.

Csete, M. E., & Doyle, J. C. (2002). Reverse engineering of biological complexity. *Science, 295,* 1664–1669.

Heil, S. H., Alessi, S. M., Lussier, J. P., Badger, G. J., & Higgins, S. T. (2004). An experimental test of the influence of prior cigarette smoking abstinence on future abstinence. *Nicotine and Tobacco Research, 6*(3), 471–479.

Jensen, H. (1998). *Self-organized criticality: Emergent complex behavior in physical and biological systems.* New York: Cambridge University Press.

Kirby, K. N. (1997). Bidding on the future: Evidence against normative discounting of delayed rewards. *Journal of Experimental Psychology: General, 126,* 54–70.

Mazur, J. E. (1987). An adjusting procedure for studying delayed reinforcement. In M. L. Commons, J. E. Mazur, J. A. Nevin, & H. Rachlin (Eds.), *Quantitative analysis of behavior: Vol. 5. The effect of delay and of intervening events on reinforcement value* (pp. 55–73). Hillsdale, NJ: Erlbaum.

Nesse, R. M., & Williams, G. C. (1998). Evolution and the origins of disease. *Scientific American, 29,* 86–93.

Nestler, E. J., & Landsman, D. (2001). Learning about addiction from the genome. *Nature, 409,* 834–835.

Verdejo-Garcia, A., Lopez-Torrecillas, F., Gimenez, C. O., & Perez-Garcia, M. (2004). Clinical implications and methodological challenges in the study of the neuropsychological correlates of cannabis, stimulant, and opioid abuse. *Neuropsychology Review, 14,* 1–41.

Part II

Biological Factors

CHAPTER 3

The Neurobiology of Addiction

A Hedonic Calvinist View

GEORGE F. KOOB

Animal Models of Drug Abuse and Dependence

Drug addiction, also known as substance dependence, is a chronically relapsing disorder characterized by (1) a compulsion to seek and take the drug, (2) loss of control in limiting intake, and (3) emergence of a negative emotional state (e.g., dysphoria, anxiety, irritability) when access to the drug is prevented (defined here as dependence). Clinically, the occasional but limited use of an abusable drug is distinct from escalated drug use and the emergence of chronic drug dependence. An important goal of current neurobiological research is to understand the neuropharmacological and neuroadaptive mechanisms within specific neurocircuits that mediate the transition from occasional, controlled drug use to the loss of behavioral control over drug seeking and drug taking that defines chronic addiction. Drug addiction has been conceptualized as a disorder that progresses from impulsivity to compulsivity in a collapsed cycle of addiction comprising three stages: preoccupation/anticipation, binge intoxication, and withdrawal/negative affect (Figure 3.1).

> Drug addiction has been conceptualized as a disorder that progresses from impulsivity to compulsivity.

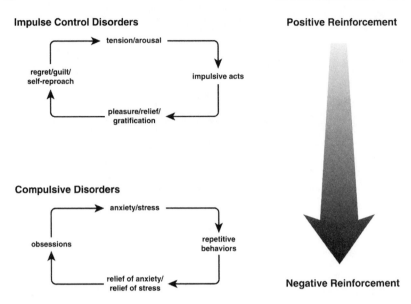

FIGURE 3.1. Diagram showing stages of impulse control disorder and compulsive disorder cycles related to the sources of reinforcement. In impulse control disorders an increasing tension and arousal occurs before the impulsive act, with pleasure, gratification, or relief during the act, and regret or guilt following the act. In compulsive disorders, there are recurrent and persistent thoughts (obsessions) that cause marked anxiety and stress, followed by repetitive behaviors (compulsions) that are aimed at preventing or reducing distress. Positive reinforcement (pleasure/ gratification) is more closely associated with impulse control disorders. Negative reinforcement (relief of anxiety or relief of stress) is more closely associated with compulsive disorders. From Koob (2004). Copyright 2004 by University of Nebraska Press. Reprinted by permission.

Different theoretical perspectives ranging from experimental psychology, to social psychology, to neurobiology can be superimposed on these three stages, which are conceptualized as feeding into each other, becoming more intense, and moving from positive to negative reinforcement. Our conceptual framework has focused on "motivational" aspects of addiction and an emphasis on the transition from drug use to addiction where emergence of a negative emotional state (e.g., dysphoria, anxiety, irritability; the "dark side") emerges when access to the drug is prevented.

Much of the recent progress in understanding the mechanisms of addiction has derived from the study of animal models of addiction on specific drugs such as opiates, stimulants, and alcohol. While no animal model of addiction fully encompasses the human condition, animal models do permit investigation of specific elements of the process of drug addiction. Such elements can be defined by models of different systems, models of psychological constructs such as positive and negative reinforcement, and models of different stages of the addiction cycle. While the predominant focus in animal studies has been on the synaptic sites (initial neurotransmitter sites) and the transductive mechanisms (how these sites convey changes in excitability) in the nervous system on which drugs of abuse act initially to produce their positive reinforcing effects, new animal models of components of the negative reinforcing effects of dependence have been developed and are beginning to be used to explore how the nervous system adapts to drug use. The present review explores the neurobiological mechanisms of addiction that are involved in various stages of the addiction cycle, but focuses on the neurochemical changes associated with the transition from drug taking to drug addiction, the motivational effects of withdrawal and protracted abstinence, and the vulnerability to relapse.

Intravenous Drug Self-Administration

Initial drug use is thought to arise from the neurochemical actions causing the positive reinforcing effects of a drug. Well-validated animal models exist for the positive reinforcing effects of drugs of abuse, and these animal models have high predictive validity. Drugs that are self-administered by animals correspond well with those that have high abuse potential, and intravenous drug self-administration is considered an animal model that is predictive of abuse potential. Intravenous self-administration of psychostimulants and opiates and oral self-administration of ethanol (alcohol) in rodents produces characteristic patterns of behavior that facilitate neuropharmacological study.

Brain Stimulation Reward

Animals will reliably self-administer electrical stimulation into certain brain areas (termed "brain stimulation reward"). Humans have described electrical stimulation in some of these areas as pleasurable. Animals will perform a variety of tasks to self-administer short electrical trains of stimulation (250 milliseconds) to many different brain areas, but the highest rates and greatest preference for stimulation follow the course of the medial forebrain bundle coursing bidirectionally from the midbrain to the basal forebrain. The study of the neuroanatomical and neurochemical substrates of intracranial self-stimulation (ICSS) has led to the hypothesis that it directly activates neuronal circuits that are activated by conventional reinforcers (e.g., food, water, sex), and that ICSS may reflect the direct electrical stimulation of the brain systems involved in motivated behavior. Drugs of abuse decrease thresholds for ICSS. Moreover, there is a good correspondence between the ability of drugs to decrease ICSS thresholds and their abuse potential.

Place Preference

Place preference, or place conditioning, is a nonoperant procedure for assessing the reinforcing efficacy of drugs using a classical or Pavlovian conditioning procedure. In a simple version of the place preference paradigm, animals experience two distinct neutral environments that are subsequently paired spatially and temporally with distinct drug or nondrug (vehicle) states. The animal is later given an opportunity to choose to enter and explore either environment. The time spent in the drug-paired environment is considered an index of the reinforcing value of the drug. Animals exhibit a conditioned preference for an environment associated with drugs that function as positive reinforcers (e.g., they spend more time in the drug-paired compared to the placebo-paired environment) and avoid the environment that induces aversive states (i.e., conditioned place aversion). This procedure permits assessment of the conditioning of drug reinforcement and can provide indirect information regarding the positive and negative reinforcing effects of drugs.

Escalation of Drug Intake

Escalation in drug self-administration can be observed in animal models of prolonged access to intravenous drug self-administration and provides a framework with which to model the transition from drug use to drug addiction. Historically, animal models of drug self-administration involved the establishment of stable behavior from day to day to allow the reliable interpretation of data provided by within-subject designs aimed at exploring the neuropharmacological and neurobiological bases of the reinforcing effects of acute cocaine. To explore the possibility that differential access to intravenous cocaine self-administration in rats may produce different patterns of drug intake, rats were allowed access to intravenous self-administration of cocaine for 1 or 6 hours per day. One-hour access (short access, or ShA) to intravenous cocaine per session produced low and stable intake as observed previously. In contrast, with 6-hour access (long access, or LgA) to cocaine, drug intake gradually escalated over days (Figure 3.2). In the escalation group, there was increased intake during the first hour of the session, sustained intake over the entire session, and an upward shift in the dose–effect function, suggesting an increase in hedonic set point. When animals were allowed access to different doses of cocaine, both the LgA

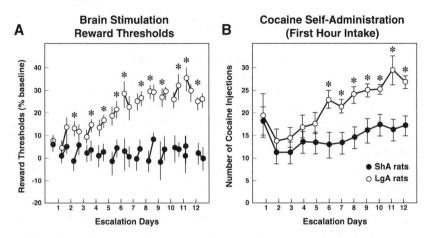

FIGURE 3.2. Relationship between elevation in ICSS reward thresholds and cocaine intake escalation. Left: Percent change from baseline ICSS thresholds. Right: Number of cocaine injections earned during the first hour of each session. *$p < .05$ compared to drug-naive and/or ShA rats, tests of simple main effects. Two groups of rats were tested, one with limited 1-hour access to intravenous cocaine self-administration (short access, or ShA) and the other with extended 6-hour access (long access, or LgA). Brain reward thresholds were measured in all rats two times per day, 3 hours and 17–22 hours after each daily self-administration session or the control procedure (drug-naive rats). From Ahmed, Kenny, Koob, and Markou (2002). Copyright 2002 by Nature Publishing Group. Reprinted by permission.

and the ShA animals titrated their cocaine intake, but the LgA rats consistently self-administered almost twice as much cocaine at any dose tested, further suggesting an upward shift in the set point for cocaine reward for the escalated animals.

Animal Models of Motivational Effects of Drug Withdrawal

The transition from occasional drug use to drug addiction has been hypothesized to require an additional source of reinforcement: the reduction of the aversive (negative) emotional state ("dark side") arising from repeated use. Here, drug taking presumably removes the dysphoria, anxiety, irritability, and other unpleasant feelings produced by drug abstinence. Other somatic physical signs, such as tremor, temperature changes, and sweating, which also reflect the state of dependence, are hypothesized to make less of a contribution to the motivation for drug seeking. One likely mechanism for the negative emotional state associated with drug abstinence may be a reduction in brain reward function.

The same animal models used to study the positive reinforcing effects of drugs of abuse can be used to measure the negative emotional state associated with drug withdrawal. Decreases in reward (i.e., increases in threshold for brain stimulation reward) have been observed in animals following withdrawal from psychomotor stimulants, opiates, ethanol, delta-9-tetrahydrocannabinol (THC), and nicotine, and are dose-related to the amount of drug that had been administered to them before withdrawal. Place aversion also has been used to measure the aversive stimulus effects of withdrawal from drugs of abuse. Here, in contrast to the place-preference conditioning discussed above, rats exposed to a particular environment while undergoing precipitated withdrawal to a drug later (24 hours to days) spend less time in the withdrawal-paired environment when subsequently presented with a choice between that environment and one or two possible unpaired environments. Place aversions have been observed in precipitated opiate, nicotine, and THC withdrawal.

Animal Models of Craving

Human studies have shown that the presentation of drugs themselves or of stimuli previously associated with drug delivery or drug withdrawal increase the likelihood of relapse as well as self-reports of craving and motivation to engage in drug taking. A condition often associated with drug craving in humans is cognitive awareness of drug availability. Discriminative stimuli therefore may have a prominent role in craving and the resumption of drug-seeking behavior in abstinent individuals. Moreover, the response-contingent conditioned stimulus, acting as a conditioned reinforcer, may contribute to the maintenance of subsequent drug-seeking behavior once it is initiated. In fact, these contingencies can be conceptualized as resembling those associated with the relapse process in humans—certain drug-related cues may provide the initial central motivational state to engage in drug-seeking behavior while others may maintain this behavior until the primary reinforcer is obtained. Stress is considered a major precipitant of relapse in humans. A recent factor analysis of Marlatt's relapse taxonomy found negative emotion, which includes many forms of stressors, to be a key factor in relapse.

Animal models have been developed that reflect all three stimuli important for relapse: ingestion of the drug itself, cues associated with the drug, and exposure to stressors (Table 3.1). Drug-induced reinstatement has been consistently demonstrated following extinction in animals with systemic or intracerebral noncontingent drug infusions. After a priming injection with the drug, the latency to reinitiate responding or the amount of responding on the previously extinguished lever is used to reflect the motivation for drug seeking. A number of animal models are available for characterizing cue-induced reinstate-

TABLE 3.1. Neurobiology of Relapse in Animal Models

Animal model	Neuropharmacological system	Brain structure
Drug-induced reinstatement	Dopamine Opioid peptides	Medial prefrontal cortex
Cue-induced reinstatement	Dopamine Opioid peptides Glutamate	Basolateral amygdala
Stress-induced reinstatement	Corticotropin-releasing factor Norepinephrine	Bed nucleus of the stria terminalis

ment where the reinforcing value imparted on formerly neutral environmental stimuli have been associated repeatedly with drug self-administration. Some of these involve conditioned reinforcement where the ability of the previously neutral, drug-paired stimulus to maintain responding in the absence of drug injections provides a measure of the conditioned reinforcing value of these stimuli. In second-order schedules, animals can be trained to work for a previously neutral stimulus that ultimately predicts drug availability. Finally, subsequent re-exposure after extinction to a cocaine-associated stimulus, but not the non-reward-associated stimulus, produces strong recovery of responding at the previously active lever in the absence of any further drug availability. Consistent with the well-established conditioned cue reactivity in human alcoholics, the motivating effects of alcohol-related stimuli are highly resistant to extinction in that they retain their efficacy in eliciting alcohol-seeking behavior over more than 1 month of repeated testing. Animal models for stress-induced reinstatement show that stressors also elicit strong recovery of extinguished drug-seeking behavior in the absence of further drug availability. Administration of acute intermittent footshock induced reinstatement of cocaine-taking behavior after prolonged extinction; this was as effective as a priming injection of drugs of abuse.

Neuropharmacology of Intoxication

A key element of drug addiction is how the brain reward system changes with the development of addiction. One must understand the neurobiological bases for acute drug reward (the "light side") to understand how these systems change with the development of addiction. A principle focus of research on the neurobiology of the positive reinforcing effects of drugs of abuse has been the origins and terminal areas of the mesocorticolimbic dopamine system. There is compelling evidence for the importance of this system in drug reward. This specific circuit has been broadened to include the many neural inputs and outputs that interact with the ventral tegmental area and the basal forebrain, and as such has been termed by some as the "mesolimbic reward system." More recently, specific components of the basal forebrain known as the "extended amygdala" have been identified with drug reward and have been the object of study (see below; Figure 3.3). As the neural circuits for the reinforcing effects of drugs of abuse have evolved, the role of neurotransmitters/neuromodulators also has evolved. Four of those systems are discussed below: the mesolimbic dopamine system, the opioid peptide system, the gamma-aminobutyric acid system, and the endocannabinoid system (Table 3.2).

Dopamine

The major components of the mesolimbic dopamine system are the ventral tegmental area (the site of dopaminergic cell bodies), the basal

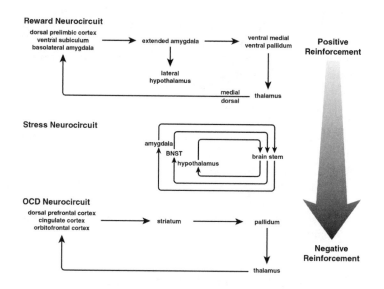

FIGURE 3.3. Three brain circuits hypothesized to be recruited at different stages of the addiction cycle as addiction moves from positive reinforcement to negative reinforcement. The top circuit refers to the brain reward system with a focus on the extended amygdala/lateral hypothalamic loop and extended amygdala/ventral pallidum loop. The middle circuit refers to the brain stress circuits in feed-forward loops. The bottom circuit refers to the obsessive–compulsive loop of the dorsal striatum/pallidum and thalamus. From Koob and Le Moal (2004). Copyright 2004 by Cambridge University Press. Reprinted by permission.

TABLE 3.2. Neurobiological Substrates for the Acute Reinforcing Effects of Drugs of Abuse

Drug of abuse	Neurotransmitter	Site
Cocaine and amphetamines	Dopamine Gamma-aminobutyric acid	Nucleus accumbens Amygdala
Opiates	Opioid peptides Dopamine Endocannabinoids	Nucleus accumbens Ventral tegmental area
Nicotine	Nicotinic acetylcholine Dopamine Gamma-aminobutyric acid Opioid peptides	Nucleus accumbens Ventral tegmental area Amygdala
Delta-9-tetrahydrocannabinol	Endocannabinoids Opioid peptides Dopamine	Nucleus accumbens Ventral tegmental area
Alcohol	Dopamine Opioid peptides Gamma-aminobutyric acid Eendocannabinoids	Nucleus accumbens Ventral tegmental area Amygdala

forebrain (the nucleus accumbens, olfactory tubercle, amygdala, and frontal and limbic cortices), and the dopaminergic connection between the ventral tegmental area and the basal forebrain. The dopamine system appears to be the critical substrate for both the psychomotor stimulant effects of amphetamine and cocaine and their reinforcing actions (Figure 3.4). Three dopamine receptor subtypes have been implicated in the reinforcing actions of cocaine as measured by intravenous self-administration and place preference: D_1, D_2, and D_3. Nicotine, another psychomotor stimulant, is a direct agonist at nicotinic acetylcholine receptors that are widely distributed throughout the brain. The nicotinic receptors mainly implicated in the reinforcing actions of nicotine again are localized to the brain mesocorticolimbic dopamine system. There also is evidence implicating dopamine in the reinforcing actions of low, non-dependence-inducing doses of alcohol. Dopamine receptor antagonists have been shown to reduce lever pressing for alcohol in nondeprived rats. Moreover, extracellular dopamine levels have been shown to increase in nondependent rats orally self-administering low doses of alcohol. However, virtually complete 6-hydroxydopamine denervation of the nucleus accumbens failed to alter voluntary responding for alcohol and opiates, suggesting that dopamine-independent neurochemical systems also contribute significantly to the mediation of alcohol's reinforcing actions.

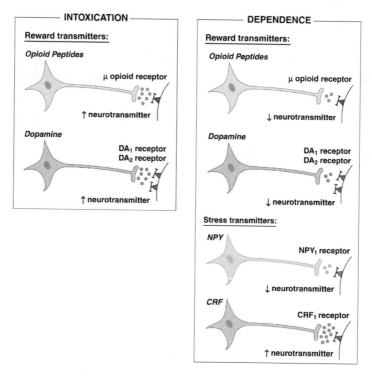

FIGURE 3.4. Comparison of the activities of neurotransmitter systems implicated in alcohol intoxication and dependence. From Roberts and Koob (2003). Copyright 2003 by Elsevier. Reprinted by permission.

Opioid Peptides

Opioid drugs of abuse bind to opioid receptors in the brain to produce most, if not all, of their psychotropic effects. Three distinct families of opioid peptides have been discovered in the mammalian brain that also bind to these receptors—enkephalins, endorphins, and dynorphins—and mechanisms for their synthesis, release, and breakdown have been identified as well as specific circuits localized to the ventral tegmental area, the extrapyramidal system, and the extended amygdala systems. Three opioid receptors were cloned that confirmed the original pharmacological designation of mu, delta, and kappa opioid receptors.

Pharmacological studies have shown that the mu opioid receptor subtype appears to be particularly important for the reinforcing actions of heroin and morphine. Knockout mice (see Genetic Targets section, below) born without the mu receptor fail to show morphine-induced analgesia or morphine-induced conditioned place preference. The sites of action for opioid antagonists to block the reinforcing effects of opioids appear to be associated with the same neural circuitry associated with psychomotor stimulant reward, specifically, neural elements in the region of the ventral tegmental area and the nucleus accumbens.

Opioid receptor antagonists also decrease alcohol self-administration. As a result, alcohol has long been hypothesized to activate opioid peptide systems. Again, the mu opioid receptor appears to be mostly responsible for the opioid contribution to the reinforcing effects of alcohol in that mice bearing knockout of the mu opioid receptor do not drink alcohol. The brain sites for such interactions are likely to be in the ventral tegmental area and the basal forebrain.

Gamma-Aminobutyric Acid

Gamma-aminobutyric acid (GABA) has long been considered a major inhibitory neurotransmitter in the mammalian brain. Alcohol and other sedatives–hypnotics, such as barbiturates and benzodiazepines, produce a characteristic euphoria, disinhibition, anxiety reduction, sedation, and hypnosis that contribute to the acute reinforcing effects associated with facilitation of the $GABA_A$ activity. The ionotropic $GABA_A$ receptor is largely postsynaptic. Benzodiazepines, barbiturates, alcohol, and neuroactive steroids act through it either via binding sites (benzodiazepines) or allosterically (barbiturates, alcohol, and neuroactive steroids). There are high concentrations of GABA and $GABA_A$ receptors throughout the brain, but the most important for drugs of abuse involve GABA-ergic neurons and receptors in the ventral tegmental area and the basal forebrain extrapyramidal and extended amygdala systems where GABA-ergic antagonists reverse many of the behavioral effects of alcohol that are associated with intoxication.

Endocannabinoids

The major psychoactive ingredient in marijuana, THC, is a drug of abuse and dependence. The initial site of THC binding is the cannabinoid CB_1 receptor, which is widely distributed throughout the brain, but is particularly concentrated in the extrapyramidal motor system of the rat. Endogenous ligands for the THC receptor include two neuromodulators (substances that modulate neurotransmission but do not fulfill all of the requirements of a neurotransmitter), an arachidonic acid derivative, arachidonoylethanolamide (called anandamide), and 2-arachidonylglycerol. Low-dose intravenous self-administration of THC has been observed in squirrel monkeys and rodents. THC and synthetic cannabinoid self-administration is blocked by the CB_1 receptor antagonist SR-141716A. Blockade of the CB_1 receptor also has been shown in animal models to modify the reinforcing effects of opiates and alcohol, which suggests a potential role of cannabinoid systems in the acute reinforcing effects of drugs of abuse. Self-administration of opiates, alcohol, and nicotine also has been attenuated by administration of CB_1 antagonists, suggesting a potential role for endogenous cannabinoids in drug reward.

Neuropharmacology of Motivational Effects of Dependence

Decreased Brain Reward Function: Addiction

All major drugs of abuse decrease reward thresholds when administered acutely. This effect has been hypothesized to reflect a facilitation of brain reward function. Similarly, withdrawal from all major drugs of abuse raises reward thresholds. Such effects have been observed with amphetamines, cocaine, opiates, alcohol, nicotine, and THC. To test the hypothesis that extended access to a drug such as cocaine is accompanied by a chronic perturbation in brain reward homeostasis, the effect of differential exposure to cocaine self-administration on brain stimulation reward thresholds was examined. Rats with prolonged access to cocaine escalated their drug intake and showed a progressive elevation in brain reward thresholds. These data provide compelling evidence for brain reward dysfunction in escalated cocaine self-administration and provide strong support for a hedonic reward dysfunction model of drug addiction (see below).

The neural substrates and neuropharmacological mechanisms for the negative motivational effects of drug withdrawal (the "dark side") may involve disruption of the same neural systems implicated in the positive reinforcing effects (the "light side") of drugs of abuse (Table 3.3). As such, these effects may reflect changes in the activity of reward neurotransmitter systems in the midbrain and forebrain implicated in the positive reinforcing effects of drugs. Examples of such changes at the neurochemical level include decreases in dopaminergic and serotonergic transmission in the nucleus accumbens during drug withdrawal as measured by *in vivo* microdialysis, increased sensitivity of opioid receptor transduction mechanisms in the nucleus accumbens during opiate withdrawal, decreased GABA-ergic and increased N-methyl-D-aspartate (NMDA) glutamatergic transmission during alcohol withdrawal, and differential regional changes in nicotine receptor function. The decreases in reward neurotransmitters have been hypothesized to contribute significantly to the negative motivational state associated

TABLE 3.3. Neurotransmitters Implicated in the Motivational Effects of Withdrawal from Drugs of Abuse

Neurotransmitter	Functional effect
↓ Dopamine	"Dysphoria"
↓ Serotonin	"Dysphoria"
↓ Gamma-aminobutyric acid	Anxiety, panic attacks
↓ Neuropeptide Y	Antistress
↑ Dynorphin	"Dysphoria"
↑ Corticotropin-releasing factor	Stress
↑ Norepinephrine	Stress

with acute drug abstinence and may trigger long-term biochemical changes that contribute to the clinical syndrome of protracted abstinence and vulnerability to relapse.

Activation of Brain Stress Systems

Different neurochemical systems involved in stress modulation also may be engaged within the neurocircuitry of the basal forebrain in an attempt to overcome the chronic presence of the perturbing drug and to restore normal function despite the presence of drugs. Corticotropin-releasing factor (CRF) is a 41-amino-acid polypeptide with a wide distribution throughout the brain but with high concentrations of cell bodies in the paraventricular nucleus of the hypothalamus, the basal forebrain, and notably the extended amygdala and brain stem. Central administration of CRF mimics the behavioral response to activation and stress in rodents. Administration of competitive CRF receptor antagonists generally has the opposite effects.

Drugs of abuse, and particularly alcohol, are powerful activators of "stress" systems, an effect that may have important implications for understanding the neurobiology of dependence and relapse. Both acute and chronic ethanol activate the hypothalamic–pituitary–adrenal axis, which appears to be the result of release of CRF in the hypothalamus to activate the classic neuroendocrine stress response. Evidence suggests that chronic ethanol also may interact with an extensive extrahypothalamic, extraneuroendocrine CRF system implicated in behavioral responses to stress. The anxiogenic-like effect of alcohol withdrawal can be reversed by administration of CRF antagonists. Increases in extracellular levels of CRF are observed in the amygdala and bed nucleus of the stria terminalis (BNST) during alcohol withdrawal. Opiate withdrawal-induced place aversion can be blocked by local administration of a CRF antagonist into the central nucleus of the amygdala.

Increases in extracellular levels of CRF in the central nucleus of the amygdala also have been observed during withdrawal from opiates, cocaine, and THC. Even more intriguing is the observation that a competitive CRF antagonist that has no effect on alcohol self-administration in nondependent rats effectively eliminates excessive drinking in dependent rats.

Neuropeptide Y (NPY) is well documented to have effects opposite to those of CRF (i.e., antistress effects). Acute withdrawal from alcohol also is associated with decreases in the levels of NPY in the brain. Intracerebroventricular administration of NPY in alcohol-preferring rats decreases alcohol self-administration. These studies suggest that decreased activity of NPY, parallel to increased activity of CRF, may provide a motivational basis for alcohol self-administration during alcohol withdrawal.

Thus, during the development of dependence, there occurs both a change in function of neurotransmitters associated with the acute reinforcing effects of drugs of abuse (the "light side": dopamine, opioid peptides, serotonin, and GABA), and a recruitment of the brain stress system neurotransmitters (the "dark side": CRF and norepinephrine) and dysregulation of the NPY brain antistress system. Again, activation of the brain stress systems may not only contribute to the negative motivational state associated with acute abstinence, but also may contribute to the vulnerability to stressors observed with protracted abstinence in humans.

The neuroanatomical entity termed the extended amygdala may represent a common anatomical substrate for acute drug reward and the negative effects of compulsive drug administration on reward function. The extended amygdala is comprised of the BNST, the central nucleus of the amygdala, and a transition zone in the medial subregion of the nucleus accumbens (shell of the nucleus accumbens). The extended amygdala receives numerous afferents from limbic structures such as the basolateral amygdala and the hippocampus, and sends efferents not only to the medial part of the ventral pallidum but also a large projection to the lateral hypothalamus, thus further defining the specific brain areas that interface classical limbic (emotional) structures with the extrapyramidal motor system.

Neuropharmacology of Relapse

Drug-Induced Reinstatement

Reinstatement of cocaine reinforcement in models of cocaine-primed reinstatement shows a role for dopaminergic systems. Most evidence suggests that dopamine agonist-induced reinstatement is mediated by dopamine D_2 receptors rather than by D_1 receptors. With opiates and alcohol, there is evidence for roles of mu opioid receptors. There also is pharmacological evidence of a glutamatergic involvement in drug-priming reinstatement. All of these neuropharmacological actions have been localized to the medial prefrontal cortex–nucleus accumbens–ventral pallidum circuit hypothesized to mediate cocaine reinstatement.

Cue-Induced Reinstatement

Neuropharmacological and neurobiological studies of cue-induced reinstatement in animals have critically implicated the basolateral amygdala and prefrontal cortex. The results from these studies are consistent with brain-imaging studies in humans that have shown that cocaine cue-induced craving is associated with activation of the amygdala and anterior cingulate cortex. The neurochemical substrates underlying conditioned effects to drugs involve dopaminergic, glutamatergic, and opioid systems in the basal forebrain.

Stress-Induced Reinstatement

There is significant evidence for a critical role of the brain stress neurotransmitter CRF. CRF antagonists and norepinephrine antagonists can block footshock-induced reinstatement of cocaine- and opiate-seeking behavior in rats. The brain site critical for the CRF role in footshock-induced reinstatement appears to be the BNST, an area rich in CRF receptors, terminals, and cell bodies.

Vulnerability to Addiction—Genetic Targets

There is strong evidence for a genetic component to alcoholism and a moderate to significant genetic component to smoking. Advances in molecular biology have led to our ability to systematically inactivate the genes that control the expression of proteins that make up receptors or neurotransmitter/neuromodulators in the central nervous system using the gene knockout approach. Knockout mice have a gene that has been inactivated by homologous recombination. A knockout mouse deficient in both alleles of a gene is homozygous for the deletion and is termed a "null mutation" (–/–). A mouse that is deficient in only one of the two alleles for the gene is termed a "heterozygote" (+/–). Transgenic knock-in mice have an extra gene introduced into their germline.

An additional copy of a normal gene is inserted into the genome of the mouse to examine the effects of overexpression of the product of that gene. While such an approach does not guarantee that these genes are the same ones that are vulnerable in the human population, they provide viable candidates for exploring the genetic basis of endophenotypes associated with addiction.

Notable positive results with gene knockout studies in mice have focused on knockout of the mu opioid receptor, which eliminates opioid, nicotine, and cannabinoid reward and alcohol drinking in mice. Opiate (morphine) reinforcement as measured by place preference or self-administration is absent in mu knockout mice. Moreover, there is no development of somatic signs of dependence to morphine in these mice. Indeed, to date all morphine effects tested, including analgesia, hyperlocomotion, respiratory depression, and inhibition of gastrointestinal transit, are abolished in mu knockout mice.

Selective deletion of the genes for expression of different dopamine receptor subtypes and the dopamine transporter have revealed significant effects to challenges with psychomotor stimulants. D_1 knockout mice show no response to D_1 agonists or antagonists and show a blunted response to the locomotor-activating effects of cocaine and amphetamine. D_1 knockout mice do not show a deficit in the acquisition of conditioned place preference for cocaine. D_1 knockout mice also are impaired in their acquisition of intravenous cocaine self-administration compared to wildtype mice. D_2 knockout mice have severe motor deficits and blunted responses to psychostimulants and opiates, but the effects on psychostimulant reward are less consistent. Dopamine transporter knockout mice are dramatically hyperactive but also show a blunted response to psychostimulants. Although developmental factors must be taken into account for the compensatory effect of deleting any one or a combination of genes, it is clear that D_1 and D_2 receptors and the dopamine transporter play important roles in the actions of psychomotor stimulants.

Allostatic View of the Neuropharmacology of Addiction

Counteradaptation

Counteradaptation hypotheses have long been proposed where the initial acute effect of the drug is opposed or counteracted by homeostatic changes in systems that mediate primary drug effects. In opponent process theory, tolerance and dependence are inextricably linked, and affective states, pleasant or aversive, were hypothesized to be opposed automatically by centrally mediated mechanisms that reduce the intensity of these affective states. The conceptual framework of opponent process counteradaptation involves an initial *a-process* (positive hedonic effect; "light side") occurring shortly after presentation of the reinforcer followed by a *b-process* (negative hedonic effect; "dark side") appearing after the a-process has terminated. The b-process is slow to decay, and gets larger with repeated exposure. In the context of drug dependence, Solomon argued that the first few self-administrations of an opiate drug promote a pattern of motivational changes where the onset of the drug effect produces a euphoria that is the a-process, followed by a decline in intensity. Then, after the drug wears off, the b-process emerges as an aversive craving state. This b-process gets larger and larger over time, in effect contributing to or producing more complete tolerance to the initial euphoric effects of the drug.

Neuroadaptation and Allostasis

More recently, opponent process theory and, to a lesser extent, sensitization theory have been expanded into the domains of the neurocircuitry and neurobiology of drug addiction from a physiological perspective. An allostatic model of the brain motivational systems has been proposed to explain the persistent changes in motivation that are associated with vulnerability to relapse in addiction. This model may generalize to other psychopathologies associated with dysregulated motivational systems. *Allostasis* from the addiction perspective has been defined as the process of maintaining apparent reward function stability through changes in brain reward and stress mechanisms. The allostatic state represents a chronic deviation of reward set point that often is not overtly observed while the individual is actively taking drugs. Thus, according to the allostatic view, not only does the b-process get larger with repeated drug taking, but the reward set point from which the a-process and b-process are anchored gradually shifts downward, creating an allostatic state. The allostatic state is fueled not only by decreased function of reward circuits per se (decreases in dopamine, opioid peptides, and GABA; "light side"), but also by the activation of brain and hormonal stress responses (increases in CRF; "dark side"). From the perspective of a given drug, it is unknown whether the hypothesized reward dysfunction is specific to that drug, common to all addictions, or a combination of both perspectives. However, from the data generated to date, and the established anatomical connections, the manifestation of this allostatic state as compulsive drug taking and loss of control over drug taking is hypothesized to be critically based on dysregulation of specific neurotransmitter functions in the extended amygdala. Decreases in the function of reward systems (GABA, dopamine, serotonin, and opioid peptides; "light side") as well as dysregulation of brain stress systems (CRF and NPY; "dark side") are hypothesized to contribute to a shift in reward set point. Thus a chronic elevation in reward thresholds is viewed as a key element in the development of addiction and is viewed as setting up other sources of self-regulation failure and persistent vulnerability to relapse (after protracted abstinence).

It is hypothesized further that the pathology of this neurocircuitry is the basis for the emotional dysfunction long associated with drug addiction and alcoholism in humans. Some of this neurocircuitry pathology persists into protracted abstinence, thereby providing a strong motivational basis for relapse. The view that drug addiction and alcoholism are the pathology that results from an allostatic mechanism that usurps the circuits established for natural rewards provides a realistic approach to identifying the neurobiological factors that produce vulnerability to addiction and relapse.

A chronic elevation in reward thresholds is a key element in the development of addiction and sets up other sources of self-regulation failure and persistent vulnerability to relapse.

A biological perspective on the brain's reward system in the context of nondrug states suggests that it may be a limited resource. A hedonic system with limited energy was conceptualized early on by Carl Jung, who regarded the psyche as a relatively closed system near that of "entropy." In an entropy situation, the system is closed and no energy from the outside can be fed into it. The term "libido" was used to describe a limited general life instinct or psychic energy. One can expend the psychic energy hedonic resource rapidly in a binge of compulsive behavior but at the risk of entering into the spiraling dysregulation of the addiction cycle, thereby triggering allostatic mechanisms and ultimately allostatic load. A more regulated "hedonic Calvinistic" approach where the brain's reward system is allowed the time and resources to return to a near homeostatic set point would prevent the development of allostatic load and the subsequent spiraling distress associated with an addiction-like cycle.

Future Directions

Based on these principles, the following questions remain as challenges to the field in the domain of the neurobiology of addiction. The future avenues of research focus on the neurobiological bases for the transition to addiction and the vulnerability to relapse.

- What neurobiological processes convey vulnerability to the transition from drug use to abuse and addiction (system, cellular, and molecular)?

- What neurobiological processes convey vulnerability for relapse (system, cellular, and molecular)?
- How do environmental and genetic factors facilitate the changes in neurobiological processes that convey vulnerability to addiction?
- How do environmental and genetic factors facilitate the changes in neurobiological processes that convey protection from addiction?
- How can the brain best "recover" to eliminate abuse and addiction and to eliminate relapse (behavioral therapies, pharmacotherapies)?

Summary and Conclusions

A conceptual structure for drug addiction focused on changes in reward function that lead to excessive drug intake provides a heuristic framework with which to identify the neurobiological and neuroadaptive mechanisms involved in the development of drug addiction. The brain reward system implicated in the development of addiction is comprised of key elements of a basal forebrain macrostructure termed the "extended amygdala" and its connections. Neuropharmacological studies in animal models of addiction have provided evidence for the decreases of specific neurochemical mechanisms in specific brain reward neurochemical systems in the extended amygdala (dopamine, opioid peptides, GABA, and endocannabinoids; "light side"). There also is recruitment of brain stress systems (CRF and norepinephrine; "dark side") and dysregulation of brain antistress systems (NPY) that provide the negative motivational state associated with drug abstinence. The changes in the reward and stress systems are hypothesized to maintain hedonic stability in an allostatic state (altered reward set point), as opposed to a homeostatic state, and as such convey the vulnerability for development of dependence and relapse in addiction. Similar neurochemical systems have been implicated in animal models of relapse, with dopamine and opioid peptide systems (and glutamate) being implicated in drug- and cue-induced relapse, possibly more in prefrontal cortical and basolateral amygdala projections to the extended amygdala than in the extended amygdala itself. The brain stress systems in the extended amygdala are directly implicated in stress-induced relapse. Genetic studies to

Changes in the reward and stress systems convey the vulnerability for development of dependence and relapse in addiction.

date in animals using knockouts of specific genes suggest roles for the genes encoding the neurochemical elements involved in the brain reward (dopamine, opioid peptide) and antistress (NPY) systems in the vulnerability to addiction. Gaps in our knowledge center on identifying the molecular changes that contribute to the neuroadaptations within specific motivationally relevant neurocircuits associated with the transition to dependence, motivational withdrawal, protracted abstinence, and vulnerability to relapse. Nevertheless, the identification of specific neurochemical systems within specific components of the brain reward and stress systems that have an important role in mediating various sources of motivation for drug-seeking behavior provides a solid foundation for bridging the molecular/cellular gap. A conceptual perspective invoking the physiological construct of allostasis provides a heuristic framework for relating these neurochemical changes to the human pathology of addiction.

Robust Principles

1. Neurotransmitters such as dopamine and opioid peptides mediate the acute reinforcing effects of drugs of abuse in a specialized basal forebrain superstructure called the "extended amygdala" (it consists of the central nucleus of the amygdala, the bed nucleus of the stria terminalis, and the transition zone in the shell of the nucleus accumbens).
2. These same "reward" neurotransmitters are dysregulated during the development of addiction (decreased dopamine and dopamine D_2 receptors).
3. Dysregulation of reward function by drugs of abuse involves decreases in the function of neurotransmitter systems that mediate the positive reinforcing effects of drugs of abuse, but also involves dysregulation of brain stress systems (increased CRF and decreased NPY).
4. Animal models of "craving" (drug-, cue-, and stress-induced reinstatement) suggest a critical involvement of the prefrontal cortex → nucleus accumbens → ventral pallidum neurocircuit and neurotransmitters such as dopamine, opioid peptides, glutamate, and CRF.
5. Genetic and environmental factors can lend vulnerability to any part of the dysregulation of neurotransmitter function associated with the brain reward and stress systems during the development of dependence.
6. Excessive drug taking per se dysregulates the brain reward system.

Acknowledgments

This chapter is publication number 16882-NP from The Scripps Research Institute. Research was supported by National Institutes of Health Grant Nos. AA06420 and AA08459 from the National Institute on Alcohol Abuse and Alcoholism, Nos. DA04043 and DA04398 from the National Institute on Drug Abuse, and No. DK26741 from the National Institute of Diabetes and Digestive and Kidney Diseases. Research also was supported by the Pearson Center for Alcoholism and Addiction Research at The Scripps Research Institute. I gratefully acknowledge the editorial and research assistance of Michael A. Arends.

Suggested Reading

Ahmed, S. H., Kenny, P. J., Koob, G. F., & Markou, A. (2002). Neurobiological evidence for hedonic allostasis associated with escalating cocaine use. *Nature Neuroscience, 5,* 625–626.

Di Chiara, G., & North, R. A. (1992). Neurobiology of opiate abuse. *Trends in Pharmacological Sciences, 13,* 185–193.

Heilig, M., Koob, G. F., Ekman, R., & Britton, K. T. (1994). Corticotropin-releasing factor and neuropeptide Y: Role in emotional integration. *Trends in Neurosciences, 17,* 80–85.

Heinrichs, S. C., & Koob, G. F. (2004). Corticotropin-releasing factor in brain: A role in activation, arousal, and affect regulation. *Journal of Pharmacology and Experimental Therapeutics, 311,* 427–440.

Koob, G. F. (2003). Neuroadaptive mechanisms of addiction: Studies on the extended amygdala. *European Neuropsychopharmacology, 13,* 442–452.

Koob, G. F. (2004). Allostatic view of motivation: Implications for psychopathology. In R. A. Bevins & M. T. Bardo (Eds.), *Nebraska Symposium on Motivation: Vol. 50. Motivational factors in the etiology of drug abuse* (pp. 1–18). Lincoln: University of Nebraska Press.

Koob, G. F., Sanna, P. P., & Bloom, F. E. (1998). Neuroscience of addiction. *Neuron, 21,* 467–476.

McFarland, K., & Kalivas, P. W. (2001). The circuitry mediating cocaine-induced reinstatement of drug-seeking behavior. *Journal of Neuroscience, 21,* 8655–8663.

Roberts, A. J., & Koob, G. F. (2004). Alcohol: Ethanol antagonists/amethystic agents. In G. Adelman & B. H. Smith (Eds.), *Encyclopedia of neuroscience* (3rd ed.) [CD-ROM]. New York: Elsevier.

Shaham, Y., Shalev, U., Lu, L., De Wit, H., & Stewart, J. (2003). The reinstatement model of drug relapse: History, methodology and major findings. *Psychopharmacology, 168,* 3–20.

Shippenberg, T. S., & Koob, G. F. (2002). Recent advances in animal models of drug addiction and alcoholism. In K. L. Davis, D. Charney, J. T. Coyle, & C. Nemeroff (Eds.), *Neuropsychopharmacology: The fifth generation of progress* (pp. 1381–1397). Philadelphia: Lippincott Williams & Wilkins.

CHAPTER 4

What Can Human Brain Imaging Tell Us about Vulnerability to Addiction and to Relapse?

ANNA ROSE CHILDRESS

For most of human history, the addictions were regarded as everything but medical disorders. They were variously viewed as evidence of demonic possession, moral/spiritual weakness, or willful misbehavior. The harsh judgments about addiction etiology are colored both by the extraordinary pain that these disorders inflict and by their seeming volitional nature: the addicted individual "chooses" to take drugs or alcohol, despite repeated and painful negative consequences.

This "choice" puzzles and angers the family and friends of the addicted individual. They recognize that most people use substances without becoming addicted, and that many of those with substance problems simply stop on their own, without professional help. These observations often lead to even harsher judgments of those who remain entrenched: if some people can stop drug or alcohol use after making a simple commitment to do so, those who continue must be *choosing* not to stop. A common lay assumption is that people are similarly equipped for managing their impulses toward drugs or alcohol.

The emerging brain data clearly suggest that we are not "all created equal" when it comes to our ability to manage (to "STOP!") our impulses toward immediate reward and to weigh the future consequences of our choices—processes critical to maintaining commitment and motivation for abstinence (or any long-term goal). We are also not "all created equal" in the response of our brain's ancient reward (GO!) circuitry to drugs of abuse and to the signals for them. These "GO!" differences are linked to drug "liking," and may represent a complementary source of addiction and relapse vulnerability.

Individual differences in the brain's "GO!" and "STOP!" systems promise to help us understand—at a fundamental level—the extraordinary heterogeneities we encounter in the arena of human substance use.

> We are not "all created equal" in the response of our brain's ancient reward (GO!) circuitry to drugs of abuse.

We will eventually know why one individual is able to "take or leave" a drug that completely devastates the life of another. Brain findings may also help us understand the heterogeneities of addiction treatment outcome. For example, the brains of individuals who can stop drug use with little or no formal intervention are likely to be very different from the brains of those who—despite suffering equally profound negative consequences of their substance use—seem unable to achieve even a single week of continuous abstinence.

Discovering the biological constraints under which our patients struggle will hopefully guide development of treatment and prevention strategies that are matched to individual profiles of brain strengths and vulnerabilities. Neuroimaging tools can play a critical role in characterizing these strengths and vulnerabilities, in developing new (behavioral and pharmacological) interventions, and—eventually—in reshaping the nosology of these much maligned and poorly understood disorders, the addictions.

Aim and Disclaim

This chapter uses a "GO!"–"STOP!" framework to discuss several brain differences in addicted individuals, to generate novel suggestions for treatment and for prevention, and to identify the many gaps in our current research knowledge. In this framework, the vulnerability to relapse, and to addiction itself, may lie in the function (and dysfunction) of two critical brain systems: (1) the ancient brain "GO!" system, which underlies the powerful motivation for natural rewards such as food and sex, and (2) the brain's inhibitory or "STOP!" systems, which are responsible for "putting on the brakes," for deciding when pursuit of a desired reward would be a danger or a disadvantage in the long term.

This broad-brush "GO!"–"STOP!" framework reflects my own attempt to integrate findings in a rapidly expanding research area, as

well as my clinically driven hypotheses about the critical brain vulnerabilities that may predispose individuals to addiction and relapse. I see
these biological vulnerabilities as complementary to, and interactive
with, the other well-documented environmental sources of addiction
vulnerability (e.g., peers, drug availability).

Recognizing the biological contributions to addiction vulnerability
is sometimes viewed as reducing the patients' role and responsibility in
managing the disorder. On the contrary: our addiction patients' compliance with a well-managed and well-matched treatment regimen will
always impact treatment outcome, as it clearly does in so many other
chronic disorders (e.g., asthma, hypertension, diabetes). Recognizing
our addicted patients' biological constraints does not reduce their responsibility for pursuing and complying with treatment, but knowledge
of these constraints will hopefully lead to treatments that are well
matched both to their strengths and to their vulnerabilities.

Starting at Birth: Heredity May Create Brain Differences That Increase Addiction Vulnerability

Some differences in the brain's "GO!" and "STOP!" systems are likely
the result of heredity. Hereditary factors are known to play a significant role in determining addiction vulnerability. The role of heredity is
usually estimated by comparing the rates of addiction for identical
twins (who share the same genes) as compared to fraternal twins (who
share only half the same genes). Complex genetic models can also help
determine the role of shared and unshared environmental factors, and
their interaction with the inherited vulnerability.

The patterns of heritability in the addictions show that they—like
most psychiatric disorders—are unfortunately not determined by a "single gene," but are likely "polygenic," the result of several genes that in
combination can increase the probability of addiction. In addition, some
genetic factors are associated with abuse of one specific drug class (e.g.,
opiates), but not others. Adding to this complexity, the genetic factors
that shape "initial drug use" seem to be independent of those that govern
the transitions from "use" to "addiction" and from abstinence to relapse
(the return to drug use after a period of being drug-free).

In the face of this complexity, a recent finding is particularly wel-
come. Genetic models applied to a large sample of Vietnam-era twins
have pointed to a common (though as yet unidentified) genetic vulnerability to addiction that is shared across many substance classes. We do
not, at this point, know the specific brain differences that underlie
these "shared genetic vulnerabilities." However, we eventually may be
able to link observed brain differences—for example, poorly developed

"STOP!" circuitry—to specific genetic factors shared across many addictions. This will offer a great leap forward in our understanding of not just one addiction, but of many.

Adolescence: A Period of Developmental Imbalance in the Brain's "GO!" and "STOP!" Circuitry

Genetic vulnerabilities to addiction may interact with a critical period of developmental vulnerability: adolescence. In normal adolescence, changes in the brain's "GO!" system are powerfully evident, with hormonal changes readying the system's response to rewards (e.g., sexual opportunity) that will ensure the all-important (from an evolutionary standpoint) attempt to reproduce. In contrast, the brain's "STOP!" circuitry is not yet fully developed in adolescence: the frontal lobes, so critical for good decision making, are now known to continue to mature well into the 20s. This asymmetry—a fully developed "GO!" system and a vulnerable, not yet fully developed "STOP!" system—likely account for several familiar phenomena of normal adolescence: the new pull of sexual rewards, increased risk taking, and decision making weighted in the moment rather than in the future.

> In normal adolescence, changes in the "GO!" system are powerfully evident. In contrast, the brain's "STOP" circuitry is not yet fully developed.

The developmental imbalance between the brain's "GO!" and "STOP!" systems in adolescence may represent a critical period of vulnerability for exposure to powerfully rewarding drugs of abuse. The adolescent brain is able to respond to rewards, including powerful drug rewards, but the brain's systems for governing the pursuit of these rewards, and for weighing the potential negative consequences of this pursuit, are often lagging behind.

Despite the normal "developmental imbalance" in the brain's "GO!" and "STOP!" systems, most adolescents who drink, smoke, or use illicit drugs do not become addicted. However, this imbalance is a sensitive biological backdrop against which even small additional alterations in the system—by virtue of heredity, environment (including drug exposure), or their interaction—may "tilt the scales" toward addiction.

Brain-imaging studies in adolescents are scarce, but they will be critical for characterizing the "normal" developmental imbalance of the "GO!" and "STOP!" systems, as well as for identifying specific brain markers of addiction vulnerability. Studies in adolescents will also inform the interpretation of existing brain "differences" in addicted adults. Which of these observed differences in adults predated—and perhaps even predisposed—the drug use? And which brain differences in the addicted adult brain are the *result* of many years of exposure to the drug of abuse? Imaging studies at only one time-point in adulthood have trouble answering this important "the chicken or the egg?" question. Imaging studies in adolescents who are at risk for drug use but have *not* yet begun to use the drug will be critical in teasing apart which brain differences are the potential causes of addiction and which are its consequences.

Brain Imaging Can Be Used to "See" Inside the Addicted Brain

How can we identify the brain differences that may be associated with addiction vulnerability? Addiction has a very long human history, but our ability to "see" any brain differences important for addiction vulnerability is relatively recent. Within the past two decades, human brain-imaging techniques have revolutionized the field of psychiatric and neurological research, allowing us to visualize both the structure and the function of living human brains. Imaging research has now begun to identify differences in the "GO!" and "STOP!" brain systems of addicted individuals that may be critical in addiction vulnerability.

Brain Imaging Shows Differences in the "GO!" System of Addicted Individuals

The brain's "GO!" circuitry is comprised of an ancient network of interconnected structures whose evolutionary function is to ensure pursuit of the natural rewards necessary for daily survival (food) and for survival of the species (sex). For survival, it is not sufficient simply to appreciate the natural rewards whenever they happen to occur: it is critical to learn which cues in the environment signal the essential rewards, so that these rewards can be accessed again and again. The learned signals for reward—the sight of a desired food or a reproductive partner—have a powerful "pull" or incentive value.

Drugs of abuse are known to act through the brain's circuitry for natural rewards, but they activate the system in a much stronger, supranormal way. This supranormal activation likely accounts for their powerful subjective effects (which, in the case of cocaine and heroin are likened to "orgasm, but much stronger") and for the strong pull of drug cues.

Though many chemical messenger systems are involved in the brain circuitry for reward and for reward signals, the neurotransmitter *dopamine* has been the focus of most research attention in human brain-imaging studies. This focus is due, in part, to the large number of animal studies that implicate dopamine in natural and drug rewards, and in the signals for these rewards. The dopamine focus is also due to a current research limitation: there are several dopamine-related tracers available for human brain-imaging research, but very few are available for the other transmitter systems.

Most drugs of abuse acutely increase the level of dopamine in brain regions critical for reward. This allows more dopamine to "lock on" to specialized dopamine receptors, increasing transmission of the dopamine message. The increased message may be associated with an increase in positive mood, energy, arousal, or motor activity—all functions that have been linked to brain dopamine.

Low D_2 Dopamine Receptors

In terms of addiction vulnerability, one might expect that individuals with more dopamine receptors would potentially experience a greater (positive) drug effect and might therefore be *more likely* to become addicted. Brain-imaging research suggests the opposite may be true. Cocaine-addicted adults with long histories of addiction had *low numbers of dopamine (type "D_2") receptors* in the striatum (a critical way station in the reward circuitry), as compared with controls who had no history of any substance abuse.

CONSEQUENCE OR CAUSE?

For some years, the finding of low D_2 dopamine receptors in cocaine patients was regarded as a possible *consequence* of their cocaine use. This interpretation was based on knowledge (from animal studies) that the increased flood of dopamine caused by cocaine or other drugs of abuse can often trigger adaptive, or compensatory, responses in the brain. In the case of "too much" dopamine message, reductions in dopamine synthesis, in dopamine release, or in numbers of dopamine receptors could help reduce the transmission of the message and help bring the dopamine system back into balance (i.e., homeostasis).

Dramatic recent findings suggest that *low D_2 receptors may also predate drug use, and may constitute a vulnerability factor in their own right.* In a study of normal controls without addiction, those individuals who "liked" an infusion of the stimulant methylphenidate had D_2 receptor levels (again, in the striatum) that were as low as those in cocaine patients addicted for many years! In the same study, individuals with a higher, "normal" level of D_2 receptors experienced the stimulant as "too much" and downright unpleasant. The study suggests that a higher level of D_2 dopamine receptors may actually be protective against "liking" the effects of a powerful stimulant.

This potential protective effect of higher dopamine D_2 receptors—and the interaction of environmental experience with this effect—was dramatically demonstrated in recent imaging studies with nonhuman primates given the opportunity to self-administer cocaine. Individually housed male monkeys were imaged, and some were then group-housed, allowing dominance hierarchies to be established. "Alpha male" monkeys, who had achieved dominance in the group-housing situation, showed a significant *increase* in dopamine D_2 receptors in the striatum, and *did not find cocaine initially appealing*. But the subordinate monkeys, who had low D_2 dopamine receptors, avidly self-administered cocaine.

SUMMARY

These imaging findings suggest that a genetically determined trait, the initial level of D_2 dopamine receptors in the striatal portion of the "GO!" system, may be one vulnerability factor for drug liking, drug taking, and eventual addiction. *These findings equally demonstrate the critical role of the environment in determining whether or not a genetic vulnerability is expressed . . . or even in reshaping the trait itself!* For example, the human control subjects with low D_2 receptors (those who had "drug liking" in the methylphenidate study) had survived adolescence and early adulthood without developing addiction. And the "mastery" experiences of the alpha male monkeys apparently reshaped a biological risk factor for addiction into one of protection!

PREVENTION/TREATMENT IMPLICATIONS

For those at risk, a prevention/treatment implication of these findings is that the D_2 receptor levels might be "reset" to a more protective level. Teaching social/behavioral coping tools to increase mastery and control over stressors could help turn a vulnerable (with low D_2 dopamine receptors) individual into one who is more like the alpha monkey: ready to take on challenges and challengers, and less compelled by cocaine. Alternatively, a medication could be used to "reset" the "GO!" system to a more protective level. Agents that occupy the dopamine D_2 receptors but block their action should—over time—lead to a compensatory increase in the D_2 receptors. Unfortunately, chronic administration of dopamine-blocking drugs (e.g., the familiar antipsychotics chlorpromazine/Thorazine and haloperidol/Haldol) have side effects, including tics and Parkinson-like motor effects, which make them undesirable for long-term treatment. Medications that reduce the activity of the dopamine system, but do not completely block it, would be better tolerated. GABA (gamma-aminobutyric acid) agents would have this "kinder and gentler" reducing effect on brain dopamine—potentially resulting in a gradual (compensatory) increase in D_2 dopamine receptors. Consistent with this prediction, one GABA-ergic medication, the $GABA_B$ agonist baclofen, has shown some early promise in the treatment of cocaine, alcohol, and opiate dependence (trials addressing nicotine dependence are just beginning). Whether $GABA_B$ agonists could also have a prophylactic effect in those at risk for addiction has not yet been tested, but this benefit would be predicted by the adult brain-imaging findings with D_2 dopamine receptors.

The Brain's Response to Drugs of Abuse, and to Drug "GO!" Cues

As previously described, most drugs of abuse increase dopamine levels in critical parts of the "GO!" circuitry. Animal research shows that the learned signals, or "cues," for these drugs (as well as for natural rewards) also increase dopamine release in these same brain regions. In humans, drug cues trigger strong craving and arousal, and may precede relapse. The brain response to drugs, and to their signals, thus represent two additional sources of potential addiction vulnerability in the "GO!" system.

THE BRAIN'S RESPONSE TO DRUGS OF ABUSE

Research in animals has shown that the brain's response to drugs of abuse (as measured by brain dopamine release, or by behavioral activation to the drug) can "sensitize" or increase with repeated exposures to the drug. This might lead to the prediction that chronic drug use in humans would similarly lead to an increased brain response, as compared to those who have not previously used the drug. Contrary to this expectation, imaging studies in chronic cocaine users have shown that the brain's dopamine response to administration of a stimulant is actually *lower* than the response of nondrug users.

Consequence or Cause? Though this lower brain response can be interpreted as evidence for "tolerance" (a reduced response to a drug as a consequence of repeated administrations), we do not yet know whether the response is indeed an effect of cocaine exposure, or whether it—as with lower D_2 receptors—may have also been present *prior* to chronic cocaine use. How could a lower brain response to rewards be a risk factor? One possibility is that a lower brain dopamine response to natural rewards would mean that these rewards are insufficiently engaging, while the powerful, supranormal stimulation by drugs of abuse is experienced as "just right." Some theories of sensation seeking and thrill seeking take this view: for sensation seekers, the arousal produced by natural rewards may be low, and thus high-intensity, high-arousal experiences are pursued and experienced as pleasurable. In contrast, for those with a normal response to natural rewards, high-intensity (often higher risk) experiences (e.g., parachuting, bungee jumping, mountain climbing) could be experienced as overwhelming and unpleasant.

Prevention/Treatment Implications. Research studies in adolescents will actually be critical in interpreting the adult finding of a lower brain response to a stimulant in chronic cocaine users. If a blunted brain response to reward appears to be a preexisting feature in adolescents at risk for later addiction, early prevention might encourage the pursuit of highly stimulating nondrug activities that are prosocial—for example, volunteering with paramedics or firefighters, or in a hospital emergency room. (This approach is sometimes followed with drug abusers in recovery to offer them high-arousal reward alternatives to drug taking.) In the future (as discussed previously in the "low D_2 dopamine receptor" Prevention/Treatment Implications section), it may also be possible to effect a pharmacological "reset" of the "GO!" circuitry in those at risk. The goal would be to enhance the brain response to natural rewards in those for whom it is blunted . . . with the "reset" simultaneously causing drugs of abuse to be experienced as overstimulating/aversive.

THE BRAIN'S RESPONSE TO DRUG "GO!" CUES

As previously described, animal research has shown activation of the brain's reward circuitry both by drugs of abuse and by the cues signaling these drugs. Both the drug and the cues for the drug lead to dopamine increases at important nodes in the reward circuitry.

In humans, cues regularly associated with drug use (e.g., the sight of a drug-using friend, a drug dealer, a drug-using location, or drug paraphernalia) can trigger profound motivation, or "GO!," for the drug of choice, potentially leading to use/relapse. Brain-imaging studies of this "GO!" state in addicted adults have shown activation of several way stations in the motivational/reward circuitry, including those linked to attention, affect, autonomic arousal, and the rapid valencing of incoming stimuli as "good" or "bad." There is also similarity in the brain regions activated by the "GO!" for cues for cocaine, heroin, or cigarettes, likely reflecting a common motivational circuitry. This circuitry normally manages the motivation for natural rewards, as demonstrated by human brain-imaging studies using food (chocolate) or sexual stimuli.

Addicted adults often report the "GO!" state for drugs as much stronger than that for natural rewards. If adolescents at risk also form stronger "GO!" states for drugs of abuse than for natural rewards, this could be a vulnerability to future addiction. A very recent functional magnetic resonance imaging study in adolescents with alcohol use disorder indeed found that the brain's response (which included regions in the reward circuitry) to visual cues of their preferred alcohol beverage was larger than the response to pictures of a nonalcohol beverage.

Prevention/Treatment Implications. Preventing the formation of cue-triggered drug "GO!" states would involve minimizing brain exposure to the drug and/or minimizing the brain impact of exposures that do occur through experimentation. The latter option could potentially involve a protective medication in those at highest risk for addiction. (This is not as futuristic as it sounds: a maintenance medication that modulates the dopamine system could minimize the impact of the drug on the brain, including the ability of the drug to support the learned incentive properties of the cues that signal it.)

For adults and for adolescents, the pull of drug "GO!" cues is an important treatment target because of the potential link to relapse. Both behavioral and medication interventions are being tested. Behavioral treatments involve the teaching of active "anticraving" strategies for coping with the cue-induced craving; these may include alternative responses, distraction, aversive imagery, mastery imagery, cognitive techniques, and—particularly—a focus on the negative consequences of acting on the drug "GO!".

For most substance abuse patients, the behavioral techniques are difficult to apply when they are already in the throes of a full-blown craving episode. Medications that help bring the powerful "GO!" into a more manageable range are much needed. The GABA$_B$ agonist medication baclofen has shown promise in blunting the response to cocaine and heroin cues in animals, and it also blunts the craving and brain activation by cocaine cues in humans. Other candidate medications for reducing the brain's response to drug cues would include the recent dopaminergic "partial agonists." These "Goldilocks" agents act to keep the dopamine system within "just right" homeostatic bounds: when the activity of the system is too high (e.g., following administration of the drug of abuse or exposure to the cues for it), these drugs could act to reduce dopamine activity. But if the activity of the system falls too low (as might occur during drug withdrawal), the agents can act to increase activity, providing a sensitive moment-to-moment modulation of the system. Most dopamine partial agonists are not yet approved for human use, and they have not yet been tried in the substance abuse treatment setting.

Brain Imaging Also Indicates Deficits in the "STOP!" Circuitry of Addicted Adults

Individual differences in the brain's "GO!" circuitry, and in the powerful "GO!" states to drug cues, may be important contributors to adolescent addiction vulnerability. However, there are now growing indications that defects in the brain's "STOP!" circuitry may be an equally critical, and complementary, source of addiction vulnerability.

The brain's frontal regions usually exert a modulatory, or "braking," function on the downstream "GO!"regions. Intact frontal regions are critical for good decision making, for allowing the individual to weigh the promise of immediate reward against other competing rewards, and—particularly relevant for addiction—for deciding against the (often delayed) negative consequences of pursuing the immediate (drug) reward.

In children, the brain's frontal functions are not yet developed—young children tend to have difficulty in inhibiting impulses toward a reward, in delaying gratification, and in making decisions that go beyond the moment. These abilities develop further in adolescence, but the brain's frontal lobes—and their associated functions—continue maturing into young adulthood.

There appear to be striking individual differences in the effectiveness of the brain's "STOP!" circuitry, with addicted adults showing a variety of deficits. Addicted adults often do poorly in tests of long-term strategy and decision making and show deficits in neuropsychological tests for ability to inhibit an overtrained or prepotent response. Brain-imaging data in chronic cocaine users shows both functional and structural defects in the frontal regions. Functionally, there is evidence of lower activity (both blood flow and glucose metabolism are reduced) in these critical frontal regions of cocaine patients as compared to nonusers. Structurally, there is evidence for less concentrated gray matter (i.e., fewer nerve cells) in the frontal regions of cocaine patients, and chronic alcoholics show a similar finding. These differences in the brain's "STOP!" circuitry can help explain why substance abusers find it so difficult to inhibit or manage the pull of drug "GO!" cues.

> *There appear to be striking individual differences in the effectiveness of the brain's "STOP!" circuitry, with addicted adults showing a variety of deficits.*

Cause or Consequence?

As with some of the previously discussed findings, it is not possible to tell from a one-time imaging study with addicted adults whether an observed brain difference predated the long history of drug use, or whether it may also reflect the impact of long-term drug exposure. Studies with primates do show that chronic exposure to stimulants can undermine frontal inhibitory functions, which may help explain—in part—the poor frontal function in some human cocaine users. But the primate findings do not preclude the possibility that individuals with poorer frontal function may be at early risk for making poor choices regarding drug experimentation or other risky behaviors. Such adolescents would be very poorly equipped for handling the "GO!" of drugs and drug cues.

Consistent with this latter notion, childhood psychiatric disorders such as attention-deficit/hyperactivity disorder (ADHD)—especially when accompanied by conduct disorder—are risk factors for adolescent substance abuse. A recent study of Colorado twins found that a latent trait represented by symptom counts from ADHD and conduct disorder, along with substance abuse experimentation and novelty seeking, had an extraordinarily high heritability of .84. Even children who fail to meet the full clinical criteria for ADHD or conduct disorder may share a biological vulnerability (e.g., "disinhibition"; poor frontal function) that would increase the risk for managing the pull of rewarding drugs and their associated cues.

Prevention/Treatment Implications

Early screening for frontal deficits could play an important role in selecting children who may need extra behavioral or medication supports. Stimulant medications have played an important role in treating children with ADHD, and proper treatment with these medications is associated with a *reduced risk* of later substance use problems. This is an important point, as there had been concern that early exposure to stimulant medications could be associated with increased risk of later substance abuse. For parents who remain concerned about this possibility, the new availability of a nonstimulant medication such as atomoxetine (Strattera) offers an appealing option. This medication is effective in bolstering frontal function (increasing the neurotransmitters necessary for attention, impulse control, inhibition, etc.), but does not increase dopamine in the striatal portions of the reward circuitry associated with euphoria and abuse liability. Such a medication could offer significant support to adolescents—and adults—with poor frontal function who may be at particular risk for substance abuse (whether or not they meet formal diagnostic criteria for ADHD). Atomoxetine has not yet been tested in addicted adults with poor frontal function, but they might be expected to show significant clinical benefit.

Robust Principles

1. The high heritability of addictions suggests that brain differences may be important in the vulnerability to these disorders.
2. Brain-imaging techniques offer the unique opportunity to "see" and to characterize brain differences in adults and in adolescents that may be associated with addiction vulnerability.
3. Individual differences in the brain's "GO!" and "STOP!" systems may represent biological constraints under which many patients struggle, and may help explain the heterogeneity of addiction treatment outcomes. We used the framework of the brain's "GO!" and "STOP!" systems for discussing some of the brain-imaging findings in addicted adults, and their implications for novel treatment and prevention strategies.
4. With regard to the brain "GO!" system, cocaine-addicted adults show lower levels of D_2 dopamine receptors and a blunted response to stimulant administration, as compared to controls. Addicted adults (cocaine, heroin, alcohol, and nicotine) and adolescents with alcohol problems have shown differential activation of the brain's reward circuitry by drug cues.
5. With regard to the "STOP!" circuitry, cocaine-addicted adults have defects in the brain's frontal regions, including less blood flow, lower metabolism, and less dense gray matter (a brain difference shared by alcoholics). These defects may help explain the addicted individual's struggle to modulate the powerful "GO!" of rewarding drugs and drug cues.
6. Frontal defects may put adolescents at increased risk for substance abuse—even relatively mild defects may add to the developmental vulnerability of an immature "STOP!" system. This hypothesis is consistent with the fact that (untreated) clinical disorders with known frontal defects (e.g., ADHD, conduct disorder) can increase the risk for adolescent substance use.
7. In several of the current "one-point-in-time" imaging studies in addicted adults, it is difficult to know whether the findings predated (and possibly predisposed) the drug use and/or are a consequence of drug exposure—these two possibilities are not mutually exclusive. Longitudinal studies in adolescents *prior to drug use* hold the

key not only to interpreting the adult brain-imaging findings, but to our clearest understanding of human addiction vulnerability.

8. Recognizing our patients' brain vulnerabilities—and their strengths—will enable development of interventions that are novel, highly targeted, and ever more effective.

Suggested Readings

Addolorato, G., Caputo,, F., Capristo, E., Colombo, G., Gessa, G. L., & Gasbarrini, G. (2000). Ability of baclofen in reducing alcohol craving and intake: II—Preliminary clinical evidence. *Alcoholism: Clinical and Experimental Research, 24*(1), 67–71.

Brebner, K., Childress, A. R., & Roberts, D. C. (2002). A potential role for GABA(B) agonists in the treatment of psychostimulant addiction. *Alcohol and Alcoholism, 37*(5), 478–484.

Childress, A. R., Franklin, T. R., Listerud, J., Acton, P. D., & O'Brien, C. P. (2002). Neuroimaging of cocaine craving states: Cessation, stimulant administration, and drug cue paradigms. In K. L. Davis, D. Charney, J. T. Coyle, &, C. Nemeroff (Eds.), *Neuropsychopharmacology: The fifth generation of progress* (pp. 1575–1590). Philadelphia: Lippincott Williams & Wilkins.

Childress, A. R., Hole, A. V., et al. (1991). *The Coping with Craving Program: Active tools for reducing the craving/arousal to drug related cues.* Unpublished manual, Philadelphia.

Childress, A. R., Mozley, P. D., McElgin, W., Fitzgerald, J., Reivich, M., & O'Brien, C. P. (1999). Limbic activation during cue-induced cocaine craving. *American Journal of Psychiatry 156*(1), 11–18.

Childress, A. R., & O'Brien, C. P. (2000). Dopamine receptor partial agonists could address the duality of cocaine craving. *Trends in Pharmacological Sciences, 21*(1), 6–9.

Di Ciano, P., & Everitt, B. J. (2003). The GABA(B) receptor agonist baclofen attenuates cocaine- and heroin-seeking behavior by rats. *Neuropsychopharmacology, 28*(3), 510–518.

Franklin, T. R., Acton, P. D., Maldjian, J. A., Gray, J. D., Croft, J. E., Dackis, C. A., et al. (2002). Decreased gray matter concentration in the insular, orbitofrontal, cingulate, and temporal cortices of cocaine patients. *Biological Psychiatry, 51*(2), 134–142.

Jentsch, J. D., Olausson, P., De La Garza, R. II, & Taylor, J. R. (2002). Impairments of reversal learning and response perseveration after repeated, intermittent cocaine administrations to monkeys. *Neuropsychopharmacology, 26*(2), 183–190.

Lingford-Hughes, A. R., Acton, P. D., Gacinovic, S., Suckling, J., Busatto, G. F., Boddington, S. J., et al. (1998). Reduced levels of GABA-benzodiazepine receptor in alcohol dependency in the absence of grey matter atrophy. *British Journal of Psychiatry, 173*, 116–122.

Morgan, D., Grant, K. A., Gage, H. D., Mach, R. H., Kaplan, J. R., Prioleau, O., et al. (2002). Social dominance in monkeys: Dopamine D_2 receptors and co-caine self-administration. *Nature Neuroscience, 5*(2), 169–174.

Petry, N. M. (2001). Substance abuse, pathological gambling, and impulsiveness. *Drug and Alcohol Dependence, 63*(1), 29–38.

Shoptaw, S., Yang, X., Rotheram-Fuller, E. J., Hsieh, Y.-C. M., Kintaudi, P. C., Charuvastra, V. C., et al. (2003). Randomized placebo-controlled trial of baclofen for cocaine dependence: Preliminary effects for individuals with chronic patterns of cocaine use. *Journal of Clinical Psychiatry, 64*(12), 1440–1448.

Tsuang, M. T., Bar, J. L., Harley, R. M., & Lyons, M. J. (2001). The Harvard Twin Study of Substance Abuse: What we have learned. *Harvard Review of Psychiatry, 9*(6), 267–279.

Tsuang, M. T., Lyons, M. J., Harley, R. M., Xian, H., Eisen, S., Goldberg, J., et al. (1999). Genetic and environmental influences on transitions in drug use. *Behavior Genetics, 29*(6), 473–479.

Volkow, N. D., Fowler, J. S., & Wang, G, J. (2004). The addicted human brain viewed in the light of imaging studies: Brain circuits and treatment strate-gies. *Neuropharmacology, 47*(Suppl. 1), 3–13.

Volkow, N. D., Fowler, J. S., Wang, G, J., & Swanson, J. M. (2004). Dopamine in drug abuse and addiction: Results from imaging studies and treatment im-plications. *Molecular Psychiatry, 9*(6), 557–569.

Weiss, F., Maldonado-Vlaar, C. S., Parsons, L. H., Kerr, T. M., Smith, D. L., & Ben-Shahar, O. (2000). Control of cocaine-seeking behavior by drug-associated stimuli in rats: Effects on recovery of extinguished operant-responding and extracellular dopamine levels in amygdala and nucleus accumbens. *Proceedings of the National Academy of Sciences USA, 97*(8), 4321–4326.

Wilens, T. E., Faraone, S. V., Biederman, J., & Gunawardene, S. (2003). Does stim-ulant therapy of attention-deficit/hyperactivity disorder beget later sub-stance abuse?: A meta-analytic review of the literature. *Pediatrics, 111*(1), 179–185.

Wise, R. A. (2004). Dopamine, learning and motivation. *Nature Reviews Neurosci-ence, 5*(6), 483–494.

Young, S. E., Stallings, M. C., Corley, R. P., Krauter, K. S., & Hewitt, J. K. (2000). Genetic and environmental influences on behavioral disinhibition. *American Journal of Medical Genetics, 96*(5), 684–695.

Zuckerman, M., & Kuhlman, D. M. (2000). Personality and risk-taking: Common biosocial factors. *Journal of Personality, 68*(6), 999–1029.

CHAPTER 5

Genetics of Substance Use Disorders

DEBORAH HASIN
MARK HATZENBUEHLER
RACHEL WAXMAN

When the faces of sisters and brothers in a family resemble those of their parents, physical inheritance has clearly played a role in the clustering of physical characteristics within the family. Similarly, alcohol and drug dependence cluster within families. Is the familial clustering of alcohol and drug dependence also caused by physical or genetic inheritance? What is the role of environmental factors in such familial clustering? These can include such factors as abusive or neglectful parenting, negative peer influences, or alcohol or drug availability. In this chapter, we discuss human studies of the genetics of alcohol and drug dependence, its interplay with environmental factors, and some potential implications for treatment and prevention. While much of this research has focused on the etiology (i.e., causes) of these disorders, genetics are increasingly considered to be a way to refine certain types of treatment.

We start by defining some basic ideas and terms used in genetic research, and then briefly review the literature. We next discuss some current ideas, findings, work now underway, and the applicability of this research to treatment. We end with some more speculative thoughts about how this area might be extended. Some of the ideas and terminology are presented not only to inform the material that follows, but to stimulate thinking about this area of substance abuse research and what it tells us about the conditions being treated.

Terminology and Concepts

DNA

All the genetic information needed to sustain life is encoded in a long, thread-like molecule called deoxyribonucleic acid (DNA). DNA makes it possible to transmit genetic information from one generation to the next. During fertilization, DNA from the egg and the sperm combines so that the developing offspring inherits genetic material from each parent.

Chromosomes

The DNA of most organisms is packaged into structures called "chromosomes" that can be visualized as rod-shaped. Chromosomes vary in size and shape and occur in matched pairs inside the nucleus of almost every cell of the body. Humans have 23 pairs of chromosomes. Fertilization involves a fusing of chromosomes from the egg and sperm cells to result in a full set of chromosomes for the offspring that contains an equal share of genetic material from each parent. Genes have specific locations on these chromosomes. In finding genes responsible for disease risk, often a first step is to identify an area of a particular chromosome where the gene or genes is/are likely to be located. This area is then subjected to further, more detailed study and mapping.

Proteins and the Genetic Code

Proteins are the basic structural and functional molecules of living things. They not only contribute to an organism's basic form but also fulfill a myriad of functional roles. Examples of nonstructural proteins include hormones, immune system components, and enzymes. Enzymes initiate and facilitate almost all of the countless chemical reactions that sustain life. Proteins that perform the same function in the body can differ somewhat in their form, which affects how they work to some degree. The form of a protein that a person has is determined in a complex process by the genes found in the DNA.

Allele

An allele is the specific form of the gene that determines the form of the resulting protein. Many genes come in two forms, which can be noted as A and a. These alternative forms are also sometimes called "polymorphisms."

Polymorphism

A polymorphism is the particular form of the gene that determines the form of the protein. Many genes come in two forms, which can be noted as A and a, but some come in more than two forms. This is also sometimes called an "allele."

Genotype

Since each person has pairs of chromosomes, they have two copies of each gene, one from his or her mother and one from his or her father. The two copies together are called the "genotype." This can be AA, Aa, or aa.

Phenotype

A phenotype is the observable manifestation of a genotype, including the physical and behavioral characteristics of the organism, for example, its size and shape, its metabolic activities, and its pattern of movement. Height, skin color, and hair color are examples of continuous traits that are at least partly genetically determined. In genetics studies of substance disorders, phenotypes that have been often studied include dependence (yes/no), use of the substance (yes/no, or some indicator of maximum use), and particular symptoms of withdrawal. A continuous phenotype increasingly used in alcohol genetics studies is severity of alcohol dependence, indicated by the number of DSM-IV alcohol-dependence symptoms.

Protective Genetic Effect

A protective genetic effect results when any form of a gene or allele causally reduces the risk of having a disorder. For substance use disorders, this could include forms of genes or alleles that cause substance use to be subjectively unpleasant. Such unpleasant experiences should reduce the likelihood of repeated use that can lead to addiction. This is the opposite of *genetic vulnerability*. Genetic vulnerability causally increases the risk of having the disorder. This could be via a process that makes the substance use much more pleasant than it is for other people, or via a genetically determined deficiency in a neurochemical process that is corrected by the substance, leading to self-medication.

Endophenotypes

Endophenotypes are mentioned increasingly in genetics research. In contrast to the clinical phenotypes described immediately above, these are more biologically based measures. In order to be effective tools, endophenotypes must meet certain criteria, including association with a candidate gene or gene region, high heritability, and association with the disorder being studied. In the substance abuse area, these have included measurements of electrical brain activity, such as electroencephalographs (EEGs), brain oscillations, and event-related potentials (ERPs). ERPs are changes in the ongoing electrical brain activity that occur when a person responds to a stimulus, which can be visual or auditory. ERPs can be measured reliably, are highly heritable, and are related to a spectrum of disorders (attention-deficit/hyperactivity disorder [ADHD], conduct disorder, substance abuse disorder) that are often highly correlated. Interest in endophenotypes is strong because their biological nature is assumed to be closer to the genetic basis of the disorders than the clinical phenotypes. At present, the endophenotypes that have been identified for alcohol and drug use disorders are promising, but because they are related to other conditions as well (conduct disorder, ADHD), they lack specificity. Identification of an alcohol- or drug-specific endophenotype would not only facilitate genetics research, it would probably signal a substantial increase in understanding of the biological aspects of the disorders.

Phenocopy

A phenocopy is a trait or condition caused by nongenetic factors that resembles a genetically-caused condition.

Pharmacodynamics

Pharmacodynamics is the study of the biochemical and physiological effects of drugs and their mechanisms of action. Many drugs produce pharmacological responses by interacting with (binding to) specific proteins on or within cells. In studying the genetics of alcohol and drug disorders, researchers have often focused on the interactions of the abused substances with aspects of the neurotransmitter system in the brain, the chemical system of communication between nerve cells. These neural pathways are involved in memory, motivation, and emotional state, and may influence, for example, the level of pleasure or other reward an individual experiences in response to a substance, or relief of an unpleasant state. Genetic influences on neurotransmitter forms and functioning are complex. Thus identifying specific genes involved in these processes has been difficult, in part because findings in one study do not always replicate when studied by a different group.

Pharmacokinetics

Pharmacokinetics is the study of how the body processes a substance. This includes rates of metabolism and excretion. In the area of abused substances, this has been most studied for alcohol, which is largely metabolized in the liver in a two-step process involving two liver enzymes. Certain genetic influences on this process are among the best understood and most replicated in the genetics of substance abuse.

Incomplete Penetrance

When the effect of some genes does not occur unless some environmental factors are present, it is referred to as *incompletely penetrant*. For example, a person with a gene for diabetes may never get the disease unless he becomes greatly overweight, persistently stressed psychologically, or does not get enough sleep on a regular basis. The problem of incomplete penetrance complicates the genetic study of alcohol and drug disorders, as environmental factors also must be present for the disorder to emerge (at a minimum, availability of the substance).

Environmental Influences

Environmental influences can consist of a wide variety of factors, ranging from micro to macro in scope, with some levels nested within larger levels. These include prenatal influences (e.g., maternal smoking, drinking, illness, nutrition); early parenting (especially abusive parenting); peer influences, such as early teen social networks; and school, group affiliation, neighborhood, and post–high school environment (a college fraternity being one example). Stressful or traumatic events are also environmental. However, care must be taken in examining some of these, especially in the context of a genetics study or a gene–environment interaction study, as some events are correlated with the same factors that predict alcohol and drug problems, for example, risk-taking personality and traumatic experiences such as combat exposure. Larger social effects include local alcohol and drug control policies (including alcohol outlet or drug availability, enforcement of underage drinking and DWI laws). Large-scale social factors include cultural and religious factors, and state and federal policies (e.g., alcohol taxation, federal laws outlawing drug sales).

Mendelian Trait/Disease

A Mendelian trait or disease is a trait or condition whose presence or absence is entirely determined by a single gene.

Complex Trait/Disease/Disorder

A complex trait, disease, or disorder is a trait or condition whose presence or absence is determined by a combination of more than one gene, and potentially by environmental factors as well.

Family Study

A family study determines if a disorder is clustered within families. No DNA is obtained and specific genes are not studied.

Adoption Study

An adoption study determines if the presence or absence of a disorder in an adopted individual is more strongly related to the presence or absence of the disorder in his biological or adoptive parents. No DNA is obtained and specific genes are not studied.

Twin Study

A twin study determines if pairs of identical twins are more concordant for a disorder than pairs of nonidentical twins or siblings. Twins are informative for genetic studies because identical twins have identical genes, while nonidentical twins share only half their genes, on average. Due to this difference, a condition with a highly genetic basis should be concordant more often in identical than in nonidentical twins. Data from twin studies can also show the "heritability" of a disorder, meaning the proportion of variance in its occurrence accounted for by general genetic factors. Twin studies can also be used to study the influence of specific or general environmental factors. Until recently, no DNA was obtained and specific genes were not studied, but DNA is being built into newer twin studies for later testing.

Linkage Study

A linkage study design includes families, usually those that include several members with the disorder. In linkage studies, probands (index cases in a family, often patients) and their relatives are interviewed and tested for phenotypes and endophenotypes, and DNA is also collected for genotyping. All these sources of information are submitted to linkage analysis. Linkage analyses can identify a broad chromosomal region that is likely to contain a gene contributing to a disorder or behavior. The entire genetic material (i.e., the genome, the 23 chromosomes) is searched and tested for associations between gene markers and the expression of the disorder or a related behavior. The purpose of a linkage study is to narrow down the area of the genome in which to search for genes involved in the disorder. Researchers analyze whether specific alleles of those markers are more commonly found in people with the disorder or behavior than in people without it. The markers themselves are chosen randomly except that they are distributed evenly across the genome. Even though the genetic markers themselves may not be involved in causing dependence, this type of study is useful because markers that are closer to each other on the genome are more likely to be transmitted together than markers that are further away. Therefore, a marker in a specific location on a chromosome with a strong association with the disorder being studied may signal that a more intensive search of this area may pay off by identifying a specific gene or set of closely located genes that are involved in vulnerability to the disorder.

Genetic Association Studies

Association analyses aim to pinpoint the gene or genes that influence the risk for having a given trait or disorder. One of the most commonly employed experimental designs to identify genes contributing to a disease is that of candidate gene analysis, which seeks to test the association between a particular allele of the candidate gene and a specific outcome. The specific areas searched on different chromosomes for such genes may be guided by the results of linkage studies, as described above, or targeted because researchers have some information about the gene's function that might be related to the disease. In this design, many genes, or single nucleotide polymorphisms (snps) within genes, are tested for their association with the trait or disorder being studied. Often, a set of genes that are located very closely together on a chromosome are found to always be transmitted together as a group (known as a haplotype); in these cases, the relationship of haplotypes to the disorder is studied as well. Different types of samples are studied in genetic association studies. These include samples of population groups of unrelated individuals where the disorder frequency is not known in advance; samples consisting of cases and controls where the frequency of a given allele or genotype is compared in individuals with (cases) and without (controls) the disorder; and the family association study in which sibling pairs or parent/offspring trios are studied, a design that can control for certain types of population-based confounding.

Gene–Environment Interaction Study

Twin studies, as described above, focus on both genetic and environmental factors. However, the genetic association study can be modified to examine the interaction of a specific gene (or genes) and a specific environmental effect. In such studies, the interplay between genetic and environmental causes is tested statistically. If gene effects differ by whether an environmental factor is present or absent, then a statistical gene–environment interaction has been identified. One version of this would be a particular gene or allele that only caused a disorder in the presence of an environmental "catalyst." An example of this was shown in a study of why stressful experiences lead to depression in some people but not in others. A polymorphism influencing the neurotransmitter serotonin moderated the influence of stressful life events on depression. Individuals with one or two copies of one form of the gene exhibited more depressive symptoms, diagnosed depression, and suicidality in response to stressful life events than individuals with only the other form of the gene. This epidemiological study was the first clear example in psychiatry to show that an individual's response to an environmental factor is affected by his or her genetic makeup. No studies of this type have been published in the alcohol or drug fields, but one is currently underway. Future studies may also address the issue of gene–environment interaction in the context of multiple genetic and environmental effects.

Findings on Alcohol and Drug Use Disorders

Adoption Studies on Alcohol and Drug Dependence

By the early 1980s, many studies showed that alcoholism clustered within families. However, the simple family study design does not clarify whether clustering is due to shared genes, shared environments, or some combination of both. Because it was important to begin to clarify the relative contribution of genetic and environmental influences to the risk for alcoholism, a series of adoption studies were conducted. By studying adult adoptees separated from their biological parents at a very early age, as well as their adoptive and biological parents, genetic and environmental influences could be separated. These were mainly conducted in Scandinavian countries, where population registers and adoption records were more readily available for research than in the United States.

In the Scandinavian alcohol adoption studies, investigators characterized adoptees and their adoptive and biological parents for the presence or absence of alcoholism. They then tested whether the correlation or association between child and parental alcoholism was stronger for biological or adoptive parents. The studies showed that alcoholism in the biological parents was a strong predictor of alcoholism in the adopted children, even though they had been separated from their biological parents very early. Alcoholism in the adoptive parents was not strongly related to alcoholism in the adoptees, and when it was, the alcoholism tended to be a milder version. This was one of the first clear pieces of evidence that genetic factors were at work, but did not specify the *level* of genetic contribution (slight, moderate, or strong).

Fewer adoption studies have been conducted of drug use disorders, but one study of U.S. adoptees also revealed that both genetic and environmental influences were involved. In particular, alcohol abuse/dependence or antisocial personality disorder in a biological parent genetically predisposed subjects (adoptees) to drug abuse or dependence.

Twin Studies on Alcohol and Drug Dependence

Twin studies take advantage of the fact that identical twins (monozygotic, or MZ, twins) have *all* their genes in common—they are identical genetically. In contrast, fraternal twins (dizygotic, or DZ, twins) have an average of only half their genes in common. The level of twin-pair concordance for a disorder or trait can be compared between identical and fraternal twins (*concordance* here means that both twins either have or do not have the disorder). Significantly higher MZ than DZ twin-pair concordance indicates genetic heritability. This can be quantified, with 100% heritability indicating that a disorder is entirely genetic, to 50% heritability, meaning substantial contributions from both genetic and environmental factors, to near 0%, indicating that genetic factors are not involved in the disorder or trait. A large number of twin studies have been conducted for alcohol and drug use disorders. In general, adult twin studies of alcohol dependence show a heritability of 50–60%. Results of twin studies for drug use disorders show a greater range of heritabilities, perhaps because the phenotypes (the observable conditions being studied) are more varied in these studies, ranging from drug use to heavy use to abuse to dependence. However, among the twin studies that addressed drug dependence, the heritabilities were similar to those found for alcohol dependence. These studies suggest that environmental factors may play a larger role in initiation and continuation of use past an experimental level, while genetic factors take precedence among individuals who move from use to dependence.

Many different kinds of genes could theoretically contribute to the development of drug use disorders. Some genes may influence reactions to a specific drug, for example, by making use of a particular chemical more or less pleasurable. These genes would affect heritability estimates for only a single class of drug. Other genes might predispose a person to rely excessively on any psychoactive drugs. These genes would influence the development of dependence on multiple drugs, and would therefore contribute to shared heritability. When discussing the genetics of a particular drug, it is useful to know how much of the heritability is common, or shared by all drugs, and how much is unique to the drug in question.

Environmental factors may play a larger role in initiation and continuation of use past an experimental level, while genetic factors take precedence among individuals who move from use to dependence.

Some twin studies have investigated the amount of genetic variance that dependence on individual substances, such as cannabis or cocaine, shares with dependence on other drugs. Some studies have shown a high level of shared genetic variance between substances. However, other research suggests that dependence on different classes of drugs should not be considered genetically interchangeable. Furthermore, different drug classes can be influenced to different degrees by the shared vulnerability factor.

Given the very consistent predominance of males in the prevalence of alcohol and drug disorders, questions have been raised about genetic determinants of this gender difference. Thus far, a genetic explanation has not been found. A review of family and twin studies found that there are no gender differences in the genetic influence on alcoholism; comparable results for drug studies are not yet available and may differ by individual substance.

Linkage Studies on Alcohol and Drug Dependence

The purpose of linkage studies is to identify the areas on specific chromosomes likely to harbor genes causing disorders. Their design usually requires many probands (a *proband* is an index case within a family, often a patient in treatment) with relatives available for assessment and DNA analysis. Some of these studies have required multiple affected relatives per family to increase the likelihood that cases would have a genetic basis and thus be informative for a genetic study. Linkage studies were not possible before the development of efficient methods to genotype large numbers of genes from large numbers of individuals, but they can be done now if sufficient resources are available. Published linkage studies have included U.S. participants with European or African background (including studies focused on adolescents) as well as Native Americans. One of these is a large-scale study of individuals with European or African background begun in 1989 known as the Collaborative Study on the Genetics of Alcoholism (COGA). Other linkage studies focused on alcohol have begun more recently and are still in the data collection phase. Linkage studies focused on drug use disorders have also been conducted with participants whose background was European or African. Linkage results on alcohol dependence or related phenotypes (including phenotypes consisting of comorbidity, such as alcohol dependence and major depression or alcohol dependence and habitual smoking) have been found on several chromosomes, including 1, 2, 4, 7, 8, 15, and 16. Habitual smoking or a high rate of smoking has also been linked to areas on several chromosomes (11, 4, 7, 9, 14, 17), including some locations previously associated with alcohol dependence or certain anxiety disorders.

One trait investigated via linkage is low level of response (LR) to alcohol, or the need for a higher number of drinks for an effect. Studies indicate that this is a genetically influenced characteristic associated with an enhanced risk for alcohol use disorders. The LR phenotype has been reported in several groups at high risk for alcohol use disorders, including children of alcoholics, Native Americans, and Koreans, whereas the opposite, a high LR, has been noted for at least one group with relatively low levels of alcohol use disorders: Jewish subjects. A low LR is hypothesized to contribute to a transition from lighter to heavier drinking in individuals living in a relatively heavy-drinking environment. In the COGA study, several chromosomal areas, including 10, 11, and 22, seem to relate to the low LR to alcohol as a risk factor for alcohol dependence. However, further work is needed to confirm these suggestive findings.

For various other substances of abuse, animal research has linked drug response to the chromosomal region that codes for the mu opioid receptor, the primary receptor that binds to morphine. Findings on this linkage in humans await the results of studies now underway.

Association Studies

Protective Genes: Alcohol-Metabolizing Genes

One area of interest for genetics research has been genes involved in the metabolism of substances. As noted above, pharmacokinetics

involves the metabolism of substances in the body. Alcohol is metabolized in the liver through a two-step process involving liver enzymes
(alcohol dehydrogenase [ADH] and aldehyde dehydrogenase [ALDH]).
Each enzyme has different forms with different activity levels that are
determined genetically. ADH converts alcohol to acetaldehyde, a
highly toxic substance. If the process goes smoothly, the acetaldehyde is
quickly converted to acetate by ALDH and transported out of the liver.
If too much acetaldehyde is produced that is not converted to acetate,
then flushing and other unpleasant effects can occur. The forms of the
enzymes that give rise to an efficient process actually constitute risk
for heavy drinking and alcohol dependence, since individuals with
these genetically determined enzymes can drink without enduring
subjectively unpleasant experiences. Genes that contribute to an "inefficient" process of alcohol metabolism serve a protective effect. Most
individuals with European background have the genes that give rise to
an efficient process. Variants of the alcohol-metabolizing genes that
give rise to an inefficient process have been found in other ethnic
groups, largely by comparing alcoholic cases with nonalcoholic controls. Many such studies have been conducted in Asian groups, in
which the nonalcoholics were more likely to have genes coding for the
"inefficient" forms of the liver enzymes ADH_2 and $ALDH_2$. Recently,
Jewish groups have also been studied, since the protective form of
ADH_2 is relatively prevalent in this ethnic group. Most of these studies
found that ADH_2 is protective against heavy drinking and/or symptoms of alcohol dependence, although exposure to a culture where
heavy drinking is common may overcome the protective effects of the
gene.

   Research on other substances is not yet as conclusive as the work
on alcohol-metabolizing genes. One area of promise is the process of
nicotine metabolism. Cytochrome P450 (CYP) 2A6 catalyzes nicotine
C-oxidation, leading to cotinine formation, a major metabolic pathway
of nicotine in humans. Genetic polymorphisms in the human CYP2A6
gene are currently under intensive investigation.

Genes Involved in Neurotransmitters

The second major area of interest concerns the genes involved in
neural pathways that are most likely to affect substance-related behaviors. Genetic polymorphisms affecting the dopamine, serotonin, and
GABA neurotransmitters have received a great deal of attention in
the substance field because of the role of these neurotransmitters in
processes related to substance abuse. Genetic association studies of
these polymorphisms have often made use of the data from family

linkage studies, with fine mapping (genotyping of many genes within a delimited area on a chromosome) used to study particular areas suggested by linkage results or other considerations. Other studies have compared alcohol- or drug-dependent patients with controls. Results on dopamine and serotonin have been somewhat inconsistent; despite many papers, these areas are not yet considered conclusive. However, research on GABA receptor genes and alcohol dependence has been more encouraging. GABA is the brain's chief inhibitory neurotransmitter, and alcohol enhances GABA activity. $GABA_A$ receptors mediate important effects of alcohol, including anxiolysis, sedation, disruption of motor coordination, tolerance, and also EEG in the beta band. A number of leads from previous research in humans and animals suggested that GABA receptor genes might be implicated in the risk for alcohol dependence. The COGA study recently found a very strong relationship between alcohol dependence and $GABR_{A2}$ receptor genes on chromosome 4. These results have since been replicated in an independent case–control sample, providing compelling evidence that $GABR_{A2}$ is a key gene affecting the risk for alcoholism.

Genetic association studies for substances other than alcohol have not yet reached conclusive findings. Areas studied include dopamine receptor genes, various genes involved with serotonin, mu opioid receptor genes, cannabinoid receptor genes, and nicotinic receptor genes. A few generalizations can be drawn. First, the genetic contribution to substance use disorders is complex and involves multiple physiological pathways. Second, as suggested by twin and family studies, some genes probably have effects on reward pathways that lead to dependence on a range of drugs, while other genes exert their influence primarily by affecting the response to a particular class of drug. Finally, genes do not work in isolation. Specific genes that predispose members of one ethnic group to a drug disorder may not affect members of a genetically distinct group in the same way. Instead, the effect of a gene can be modified by interactions with other genes not taken into account in a particular study. Of course, environmental factors not taken into account in the genetics studies can also cause inconsistencies between findings. Therefore, genetic association studies are tackling an extremely complex and difficult task. They promise to provide important information in understanding the physiological aspects of drug abuse and dependence, but this promise will take more work to fulfill.

The genetic contribution to substance use disorders is complex and involves multiple physiological pathways.

Pharmacogenetics

In medicine, it is important to prescribe dosages of prescription drugs that are safe and effective. However, people vary in how they respond to the same amount of a medication. The result is that some people need higher doses than others, and some experience adverse effects from any amount of a particular medication or if the medication is given in a dose that is too high for them. Consequently, doctors use trial and error within recommended guidelines to determine dosages. This can delay positive response or cause adverse effects.

Pharmacogenetics is a field of research whose purpose is to overcome these clinical difficulties. It directly studies the genetic causes of variability in drug response. The techniques are similar to those used in the genetic polymorphism studies discussed earlier, but the applications are different. In pharmacological research, the phenotype is response to a prescribed drug, not the presence or absence of a disorder. In pharmacogenetics, candidate genes are examined for their influence on drug response. When polymorphisms are found, statistical methods are used to determine whether particular genetic sequences correspond to distinct patient characteristics. Eventually, for many drugs, pharmacogenetics should take much of the guesswork out of prescription, and clinicians should be able to recommend a drug or a drug dose for a particular patient based on his or her genetic profile in the genes relevant to the drug response.

Eventually, clinicians should be able to recommend a drug or a drug dose for a particular patient based on his or her genetic profile.

The use of medications as treatment for alcohol and drug dependence is a developing area. Basing their work on neuroscience findings, scientists are developing medications that potentially could target both acute responses to alcohol or other substances and neuroadaptations that can accompany chronic use. Potential medications may target specific receptor types, the series of chemical reactions set off by receptor activation, or the production of critical protein enzymes involved in these processes within cells. These are some of the medications currently being used or tested:

• *Naltrexone* binds with receptors for endogenous opioids, naturally occurring opiate-like substances that stimulate pleasurable feelings and suppress pain. Animal studies suggest that opiate antagonists like naltrexone block some of alcohol's rewarding effects. Clinical studies have reported that alcohol-dependent patients given naltrexone have better drinking outcomes than patients given a placebo.

- *Acamprosate* is thought to affect activity of the neurotransmitter glutamate. In clinical studies of alcoholics in Europe, patients given acamprosate experienced better outcomes than patients given placebo.
- *Ondansetron* reduces the activity of a serotonin receptor (5-HT_3) on which alcohol is known to act and has been shown to reduce the desire to drink in humans. A clinical trial demonstrated that ondansetron was most effective in reducing drinking in early-onset (alcohol dependent before age 25) alcoholics.

Other drugs are at earlier phases of investigation. These include *baclofen*, which activates a $GABA_B$ receptor, and *gabapentin*. Other medications that affect GABA can have side effects such as convulsions, so they are not safe. Alcohol is involved in *N*-methyl--aspartate (NMDA) receptors, and *memantine*, a drug that reduces NMDA receptor function, has potential as an anticraving drug and in treating alcohol dependence. Clinical trials to establish its efficacy are being contemplated. More recently, *topiramate*, which acts on a class of glutamate receptors (AMPA–kainate receptors), decreases glutamate activity while increasing GABA activity. A recent study reported that alcohol-dependent patients on topiramate had better outcome than patients taking a placebo.

Genetic differences between individuals may affect their responses to all these medications, a possibility that has been gaining attention. At a recent meeting on gene–environment interaction held by the National Institute on Alcohol Abuse and Alcoholism, DNA availability for many participants of randomized medication clinical trials was recognized. This DNA has seldom been analyzed for its effects on treatment response, but is a potential repository of useful information that may soon be mined to provide pharmacogenetic information.

The field of genetics is usually considered in connection with pharmacological treatments for alcohol and drug use disorders, but it has potential for other aspects of treatment and prevention as well. Most people with many alcohol- or drug-addicted relatives know that they are at risk for such addiction themselves, but the information is fairly amorphous. If genetic tests were available that provided information closer to certainty about an individual's risk for alcohol or drug dependence given use of the substances, this would provide a much clearer basis for individual decisions about substance use.

In the field of alcohol, we remain without guidelines concerning who really must stop drinking in order to recover from DSM-IV alcohol dependence, and who can recover stably from dependence even while drinking moderately. While many guidelines exist on *how* to cut down or stop in terms of psychological (e.g., motivation, cognitive planning) and environmental changes (new peer groups, avoidance of cues for bingeing), these do not address the question of abstinence versus controlled drinking. It is possible that the integration of biological findings with recommendations for change attempts may make such recommendations more informative. As an example, the recently replicated findings on $GABA_A$ receptor polymorphisms as strong predictors of risk for alcohol dependence may extend to predicting longitudinal course of dependence once it is established. If so, a test for these genetic factors and its results might be integrated into psychological and environmental recommendations. If tests were available that could be conducted in nonspecialist settings that could provide accurate information to alcohol-dependent individuals about their likelihood of recovery from alcohol dependence if they continue to drink at all, then these individuals could make much more informed decisions about the important matter of stopping entirely or attempting to moderate drinking.

The field of genetics research has much to contribute to understanding the etiology and treatment of alcohol and drug use disorders. As our understanding of the human genome and its components grows, more information should become available that can be applied to the substance abuse area. At the same time, environmental effects (including the psychosocial environment provided by nonpharmacological interventions) must be taken into account to fully understand and treat these disorders. It is hoped that the rapid advances currently taking place will result in considerable progress in the substance abuse area in the future.

Robust Principles

1. Genetic knowledge and methods have improved.
2. No one gene or environmental factor will explain risk for onset or chronicity.
3. Choice of phenotype can affect genetic results and may differ in relevance to different contexts.
4. Variation in strong unmeasured environmental factors between genetic studies may produce inconsistent genetic results.
5. Genetic variation may influence response to psychosocial treatment as well as medication.

Suggested Readings

Bierut, L. J., Dinwiddie, S. H., Begleiter, H., Crowe, R., Hesselbrock, V., Nurnberger, J. I., Jr., et al. (1998). Familial transmission of substance dependence: Alcohol, marijuana, cocaine, and habitual smoking: A report from the

Collaborative Study on the Genetics of Alcoholism. *Archives of General Psychiatry, 55*, 982–988.

Cadoret, R., Yates, W. R., Troughton, E., Woodworth, G., & Stewart, M. A. (1995). Adoption study demonstrating two genetic pathways to drug abuse. *Archives of General Psychiatry, 52*, 42–52.

Caspi, A., Sugden, K., Moffit, T. E., Taylor, A., Craig, I. W., Harrington, H., et al. Influence of life stress on depression: moderation by a polymorphism in the 5-HTT gene. *Science, 301*, 386–389.

Edenberg, H. J., Dick, D. M., Xuei, X., Tian, H., Almasy, L., Bauer, L., et al. (2004). Variations in GABRA2, encoding the alpha 2 subunit of the GABA(A) receptor, are associated with alcohol dependence and with brain oscillations. *American Journal of Human Genetics, 74*, 705–714.

Foroud, T., & Li, T.-K. (1999). Genetics of alcoholism: A review of recent studies in human and animal models. *American Journal of Addictions, 8*, 261–278.

Gelernter, J., Kranzler, H. R., & Cubells, J. (1999). Genetics of two mu opioid receptor gene (OPRM1) exon I polymorphisms: Population studies and allele frequencies in alcohol- and drug-dependent subjects. *Molecular Psychiatry, 4*, 476–483.

Hasin, D., Aharonovich, E., Liu, X., Maman, Z., Matseoane, K., Carr, L. G., et al. (2002). Alcohol dependence symptoms and alcohol dehydrogenase 2 polymorphism: Israeli Ashkenazis, Sephardics and recent Russian immigrants. *Alcoholism: Clinical and Experimental Research, 26*, 1315–1321.

Heath, A. C. (1995). Genetic influences on drinking behavior in humans. In H. Begleiter & B. Kissin (Eds.), *The genetics of alcoholism* (pp. 82–121). New York: Oxford University Press.

Higuchi, S., Matsushita, S., Murayama, M., Takagi, T., & Hayashida, M. (1995). Alcohol and aldehyde dehydrogenase polymorphisms and the risk for alcoholism. *American Journal of Psychiatry, 152*, 1219–1221.

Kendler, K. S., Jacobson, K. C., Prescott, C. A., & Neale, M. C. (2003). Specificity of genetic and environmental risk factors for use and abuse/dependence of cannabis, cocaine, hallucinogens, sedatives, stimulants, and opiates in male twins. *American Journal of Psychiatry, 160*, 687–695.

Roses, A. D. (2001). Pharmacogenetics. *Human Molecular Genetics, 10*, 2261–2267.

Schuckit, M. A., Smith, T. L., & Kalmijn, J. (2004). The search for genes contributing to the low level of response to alcohol: Patterns of findings across studies. *Alcoholism: Clinical and Experimental Research, 28*, 1449–1458.

Tsuang, M. T., Lyons, M. J., Meyer, J. M., Doyle, T., Eisen, S. A., Goldberg, J., et al. (1998). Co-occurrence of abuse of different drugs in men: the role of drug-specific and shared vulnerabilities. *Archives of General Psychiatry, 55*, 967–972.

Part III

Psychological Factors

Natural Change and the Troublesome Use of Substances

A *Life-Course Perspective*

CARLO C. DiCLEMENTE

Recovery from the troublesome use of substances is essentially the story of each individual's personal journey into abuse or dependence and the path he or she takes finding a way out. If the path into recovery does not pass through a formal treatment or intervention program, recovery is called "natural change," "spontaneous recovery," or "unaided recovery." However, the reality is that this path is seldom natural, spontaneous, or unaided, so the term I consider most descriptive is "self-change," a change directed by the individual him- or herself. Every recovery from abuse or dependence on a substance takes courage, critical decisions, and effort, and often involves supportive networks and environmental pressures that aid in moving the process forward. Recovery, whether aided or unaided, is not best represented by a single, common, developmental trajectory that one clearly could label *the* natural path to recovery. In fact, as we learn more and more about the process of change involved in substance abuse and recovery, natural change (understood as the individual's struggle to manage and overcome substance abuse) is not the opposite of treatment or intervention-aided change but is the foundation and the process underlying *all* recovery.

The life course of a problematic pattern of substance use has multiple potential entry and exit points. Not everyone who experiments with or begins to use a legal or illegal substance continues toward problematic use or develops a pattern of abuse. Moreover, individuals who do develop problematic patterns do so at different ages and at times in the course of their lives and at different rates of initiation. Many factors seem to moderate the development of the full-blown syndrome of dependence on substances and help to create exits from initial engagement and problematic use. Various intrapersonal, interpersonal, and environmental factors protect from or hasten problematic involvement. Although there is no single pathway, there are common, naturally occurring changes in the trajectory of development of abuse and dependence. In fact, trajectories or pathways for problem development differ by gender, age, and social setting. The age at which an individual begins the problematic use, genetic influences, family attitudes and behaviors related to use of substances, relationship skills and social networks, ethnic and cultural values—all these and more play a role in critical decision points of entry into or exiting from substance abuse.

Once a pattern of problematic use develops, multiple events, consequences, and opportunities can disrupt this problematic pattern. Some patterns, like college binge drinking, are transitional in nature for many individuals and appear to be linked closely to setting. Some use and abuse patterns are changed in response to significant life events, like quitting smoking when smokers decide to have a family or individuals beginning serious alcohol abuse in late life. Other patterns are incredibly stable and end in death after individuals have spent years drinking or drugging and have experienced many important losses and other negative consequences. However, for most individuals the patterns of abusive use of substances contain multiple attempts either to quit using completely or to bring the substance use under better self-control. There does seem to be a role for teachable moments and for incremental learning about how to successfully change from multiple attempts and failures. A life-course perspective is needed to understand natural change and the process of self-change.

In general, individuals are less likely to develop problematic patterns of use and better able to change the course of their problematic engagement in substance use early in their abuse career if they have fewer complicating life problems and more resources (educational, economic, social, and personal) and have opportunities for alternative sources of reinforcement. One explanation is that these individuals develop a weaker attachment to the substance in that for them substance use does not serve as many emotional, psychological, or social needs. However, the complicating factor with this explanation, making it a bit circular, is that more frequent and heavy use of substances, especially illegal substances, increases the probability of multiple problems and depleted resources. There also seem to be factors, like comorbidity with psychological and psychiatric disorders, that can make a difference in one's ability to change the pattern at an early point in its development. Co-occurring disorders create a complicated, interrelated problem matrix that can become very difficult to change.

In any case, there seem to be some differences between individuals who develop a less intense pattern of use compared with those who have more severe patterns of problematic, dependent use of substances in their ability to engage in self-directed change and to respond to consequences or brief motivational interventions (see Miller, Chapter 9, this volume). Natural changers seem to learn from consequences, see the discrepancies between their current actions and their values and goals, and shift decisional considerations as a result of these consequences and considerations. Brief interventions and teachable moments seem to activate or facilitate this natural change process so that the individual decides to modify his or her substance use. However, it is interesting to note that the change or modification that is made by self-changers in many cases is not complete abstinence but a less intense and/or nonproblematic use of the substance. This is particularly true for alcohol use but can also be seen with nicotine and other drugs of abuse.

The path leading to recovery or resolution from problematic use of substances involves the accomplishment of a series of tasks that have been identified in a sequence of stages of change (see Table 6.1). These stages represent states that individuals are in and highlight what the individual would need to do to move forward in the process of making and sustaining change of the problematic use of a substance. Substance users have to become *concerned* about the need to change, become *convinced* that the benefits of change outweigh the costs provoking a decision to change, *create* and *commit* to a viable and effective plan of action, *carry out* the plan by taking the actions needed to make the change, and *consolidate* the change into a lifestyle that can sustain the change. These tasks parallel the five identified stages of change that have been assessed in both self-change and treatment-assisted recovery. Adequately accomplishing these tasks is necessary to produce change. The evidence indicates that these tasks are important in recovery for self-changers as well as for those attending treatment in overcoming their substance abuse and dependence.

TABLE 6.1. Tasks and Stages of Change

Tasks needed to move forward	Stage of change
Concerned about the need	Precontemplation
Convinced and decision to change	Contemplation
Create and commit to a viable plan	Preparation
Carry out the plan	Action
Consolidate the change	Maintenance

Natural Change and the Onset of Problematic Use

The entire process of becoming addicted and developing problematic and sustained patterns of substance abuse can be described as a process of change involving a similar set of stages of change. However, the current chapter focuses on natural change and on the events and factors that would interrupt continued problematic engagement and dissuade individuals from continuing down the path toward more severe abuse and dependence. I will concentrate on what contributes to either early or later exits from problematic use of substances that involve self-change.

Although early use in adolescence predicts later significant problematic use of licit and illicit substances, it is not simply any use that predicts problems. The timing of when individuals begin to use is substance-specific. Cigarette smoking begins earlier than drinking alcohol. Use of both of these legal substances typically begins earlier than use of cocaine and heroin. But timing isn't everything. Sometimes early onset of use is followed by limited adolescent use of licit and illicit drugs and seems related to social risk factors in normally socialized adolescents. However, early onset followed by persistent and extensive use beyond adolescence is related to more intrapersonal factors (e.g., impulsivity) and a more problematic adolescence. There is also little evidence that simply beginning to smoke or drink alcohol is a gateway for illicit drug use. However, there is an association best described as a moderate correlation between onset of use of licit drugs and the problematic and persistent use of illicit drugs and marijuana. It is the early onset of illicit drug use and the escalation of that use that is more strongly associated with both abuse of and dependence on both alcohol and illicit drugs in later life.

Some adolescents, especially those with fewer serious personal and social problems, seem to be able to engage in problematic use during adolescence but not continue their problematic use later in their 20s. There is a type of adolescent experimentation and circumscribed use that is more time-limited, indicating that some adolescents experience problematic use of substances and then change and modify this use as they move into early adulthood. This self-change involves either a recognition that this substance use does not fit with their other values and goals and/or an association of the problematic use with a developmental period of adolescence. The natural change appears related to maturation in individuals who have the capacity, personal history, and enriched or less problematic environments that foster and support exiting from problematic use of substances early in one's life.

Ethnicity and culture also can make a difference in the progression toward persistent and serious problems with substance use. Not only do many studies show that African American and often Hispanic adolescents experiment with and begin to use nicotine, alcohol, marijuana, and other drugs less frequently than Caucasians, but they seem to have more random types of progression patterns. Powerful cultural and community forces appear to influence and make less predictable the likelihood of progression to problematic use. Clearly, some of these ethnic adolescents have experiences that change the course of the progression. However, late adolescence and early adulthood offers another risk period for these youth that indicates that they may be less protected. It is unclear whether protection provided earlier breaks down or if economic and social problems increase and make resisting problematic use more difficult.

Gender is another interesting factor in the natural change related to the initiation and continuation of problematic use of substances. Males begin using most substances earlier and more significantly than females. However, this is not always true over time and for specific substances. Smoking cigarettes, for example, seems to have become more of an equal opportunity behavior during the past 10 years. There is also an effect, called "telescoping," that seems to happen with women in relation to their progression to abuse of and dependence on alcohol and other drugs. They seem to accumulate consequences and develop greater dependence in a shorter span of time and often have a more difficult time quitting the substance. Thus rates of progression may influence the ability to change and reduce the probability of natural change. Gender and social expectations concerning gender may create greater stigmatization for females, which also seems to interfere with natural change and may hinder early exiting and provide risk for progression to more serious dependence.

Another complicating factor in the progression of substance abuse that interferes with natural change in this progression is the presence of psychological and emotional problems. Depression, anxiety, and other psychiatric disorders often manifest themselves in adolescence and early adulthood. As these become linked to the substance use, there seems to be a greater likelihood of developing a more significant and more durable problem with the substances and of having greater difficulty changing abuse and dependence on the substances. These individuals may also be more immune to shifts in social norms to change and more vulnerable to social pressure to continue problematic use. Individuals with chronic mental illness, for example, are smoking in much greater numbers than the general population and are having greater difficulty quitting. Since many smokers quit unaided, it seems that this group of chronically mentally ill smokers in particular, and psychiatric comorbidity and complications in general, make natural change of troublesome use of substances less likely.

Social stigma also appears to be involved in the process of self-change. It is often given as a reason for not seeking help and may contribute to the greater isolation of groups and networks of substance users. Thus the sense that the problematic use is viewed as abnormal and part of a stigmatized identity can create a barrier for change and encourage an overidentification with peers that makes change more difficult. This process may prolong the careers of some substance abusers. On the other hand, the avoidance of being stigmatized as a substance abuser, alcoholic, drug addict, or smoker can promote the self-change process in those who begin to realize the need for change but want to avoid the labels associated with coming to a treatment program identified with these stigmatized groups. Individuals who are more concerned about stigma may also be more responsive to brief interventions that may simply tip the decisional balance and promote some modification of the behavior since these often do not use any labels, target reduction, or moderation, and focus on problem behaviors not trait descriptions.

Substance Abuse Careers

Not only are there significant differences in how individuals progress to substance abuse and dependence and whether they get out early in the progression of problematic use, there are also very big differences in the lifetime careers of alcohol and substance abusers. Some seem able to maintain a pattern of abuse or binge use over long periods without moving on to severe dependence. Others continue frequent or daily use for many consecutive years. Still others have a variable pattern and show periods of dependence and periods of abstinence mixed with periods of nonabusive use. Natural change seems part of this process, as are interventions and treatment.

Early adulthood appears to be a period that promotes change of problematic patterns of abuse. Change is associated with the adoption of social roles that require more responsible behavior and early adult transitions related to marriage, family, and work. Clearly there are social forces and interpersonal influences that can promote problematic use or problem resolution. This seems particularly true for individuals with binge and partying types of patterns of abuse. Shifting social networks that accompany marriage, having children, and taking on more financial responsibilities support the self-change process. Consequences also seem to take on greater relevance and impact. When someone is single and young, a citation given by the police for driving under the influence has less of an impact than one given to a newly married male with a young child. Role transitions and shifting value systems promote self-change of problematic drinking and drug use. However, these changes often represent a modification of the substance use to sporadic or self-regulated use and not total abstinence forever.

Adoption of problematic use of substances in early, middle, or late adulthood appears to pose different problems and may have different genetic roots from the problematic use that begins in early adolescence. The path into problematic use later in life (after adolescence) seems more related to environmental events. Later life problematic use can be more time-delimited, responding to shifts in these environmental events. Some spouses, for example, develop what is characterized as "defensive drinking" when they begin dating and living with a heavy drinker. Sometimes acknowledging homosexual or lesbian sexual orientation and seeking sexual partners is associated with excessive drinking or use of some types of drugs. These patterns can change, often without the aid of formal treatment, as the stressful events and the enabling situations recede or are resolved and as the individual realizes the problematic aspects of this use and decides to change his or her substance use pattern.

Problematic use that continues from adolescence or young adulthood and persists into middle adulthood seems more difficult to change and less likely to be responsive to self-change. These long-standing patterns of abuse, most often meeting the definition of dependence, are difficult to change since they have persisted despite the presence of some natural consequences and continued even after there were developmental transitions that could have fostered change. Problematic use becomes an integral part of the individual's life and functioning. These are the people most typically seen in treatment programs and have become the modal or prototypic description of the alcoholic or drug abuser. However, it does seem that even in this drug-dependent population there are individuals who have been able to achieve stable recovery without the aid of treatment. The differences between treatment seekers and those who have been able to self-change without treatment are not dramatic or consistent in studies of self-change.

Several longitudinal studies of chronic alcoholics and drug abusers demonstrate that some make significant changes that include abstinence from substances for a significant period with or without treatment and then go back to problematic use. There are also chronic
substance abusers who have achieved complete abstinence that is sustained to the end of their lives without returning to drinking or drug
use of any kind. Most longitudinal studies of these individuals have
been of those who have significant treatment experiences and engaged
in mutual support groups like Alcoholics Anonymous to achieve abstinence. However, several studies of self-change have included individuals with long histories of abuse who have been able to achieve complete
abstinence even without the aid of any treatment or organized support
groups. Moreover, episodes of treatment do not necessarily eliminate
self-change attempts for individuals with severe substance dependence.
Often after a relapse posttreatment, abstinence is reinstated by a turning to mutual help programs like Alcoholics Anonymous rather than
returning to treatment programs. It is clear that for severe or chronic
alcohol or substance abusers self-change is more difficult but not impossible and that placing natural or self-change in opposition to treatment-assisted change is not appropriate.

Natural Change and the Process
of Intentional Behavior Change

Although few longitudinal studies have examined the course and process of natural or self-change, the ones that we do have indicate that
change of substance abuse patterns occurs slowly over a number of
years. Change, particularly self-change, does seem to represent a cumulative process, with an increasing number of individuals in the
group of people who are being followed being able to successfully
change and maintain their changes over many months and years. Resolution or recovery is rather stable after a time of false starts and
failed attempts. It is sometimes a painstakingly slow process. In smoking cessation, for example, the rate of unaided quitting in a year cal-
culated over a decade ago was estimated to be about 5–6% of current
smokers. However, this rate could vary significantly depending on the
composition of the samples of smokers who were followed and could
be increased by minimal interventions and by environmental pressures or policies. There are also important differences in various
subpopulations. Caucasian smokers of less means often demonstrated
less quitting, for example. Similar findings for other subgroups have
been seen with other drugs of abuse.

Following a group of self-changers over time demonstrates that there are variable patterns of change in natural recovery. Some individuals seem to get stuck at certain points in the process of change. Individuals in precontemplation can remain uninterested in change for years. Interestingly, individuals who are seriously considering change can also spend a lot of time considering but not deciding to take action. Beginning the process of unaided recovery requires that the individuals experience consequences or pressures that finally become convincing enough for them to seriously consider the need to change and then to make the decision to do something. Even after they have decided to make a change, there is movement back and forth as well as failed attempts to change that may last a day, a week, or many months. Some, of course, are able to be successful in making and sustaining the change. If you follow over time a group of individuals with problematic substance use, it seems that there is an understandable process but no single linear path through that process.

Attempts to talk to successful natural self-changers have given us a view of what they think has contributed to their change. Most often self-changers describe contemplation and decision-making elements as one of the most important aspects of their success, although they do not necessarily identify a different set of considerations from those identified by those who have been unable to resolve their problematic substance abuse. They also talk about the strategies they used to successfully change that include changing living and social environments, avoiding problematic people and places, resolving other problems, and gaining new sources of support and rewarding experiences. These interviews clearly indicate that both a decisional process and a series of behavioral changes are part of the natural recovery process of change occurring over time.

On the other hand, those who have not been successful at change do not seem to be very different in terms of their substance use habit, though sometimes they report a more intensive or extensive pattern of substance abuse. Unsuccessful changers seem to be more ambivalent about the change, have not been able to solve associated problems, and by definition have not been successful at making the decision and the changes needed to make the change stick. However, since these interviews are retrospective, unsuccessful changers are simply those who have been unsuccessful up to this point in their lives and may, if interviewed later, become successful self-changers. In general, it seems as though greater complications and additional problems can make natural resolution more difficult but not impossible to achieve. The differences between successes and failures in terms of self-change appear to be related to the successful accomplishment of the process rather than to individual differences either in the type of person or any unique patterns of substance abuse involved.

One other important revelation from the studies of self-changers is that although the current recovery is attributed to natural or self-change, some of these individuals had received some assistance from health care or addiction services. In fact, in some studies many of these natural changers had had previous "unsuccessful" experiences with some treatment or mutual help interventions. Even when individuals who had used these formal types of interventions are eliminated, the remaining group of self-changers often point to the influence of health care professionals like physicians or some other occurrence that is indirectly associated with more formal interventions, like contact with a recovering friend who went to treatment.

Natural recovery is not the opposite of assisted recovery and the two are intertwined in interesting and, as yet, not completely understood ways. Studies of self-change do not describe a process of change that seems to differ in any significant way from treatment-assisted change. The main differences seem to be that in treatment more professionals are involved, more formal strategies and skill building are employed, and greater support from providers and mutual help support systems are available. Another difference that seems to be very important for some self-changers is that by not accessing treatment they are able to avoid the stigmatization of being labeled a substance abuser, a drug addict, or an alcoholic. This sense of stigma associated with treatment seems most relevant for alcohol and illegal drug use, since treatments for nicotine addiction are more accessible without the stigma of being labeled an addict. However, most smokers prefer to quit their nicotine addiction on their own without formal treatment, many even without minimal interventions. For them, however, there may be something akin to stigma since they indicate that they are unwilling to ask for help and prefer to do it on their own. Asking for help is difficult and seems to undermine self-esteem for some people. Thus stigma and protecting self-esteem may be other important factors that contribute to self-change in contrast to treatment seeking.

Natural recovery is not the opposite of assisted recovery and the two are intertwined in interesting and, as yet, not completely understood ways.

For many individuals natural change and treatment-assisted change are complementary and not mutually exclusive. Examining individuals who enter treatment indicates that many of them have completed some of the tasks of recovery before entering treatment. Many are already convinced that they have a problem with their substance use but have not made a firm decision about whether to address or what to do about this problem. Others have made the decision and are seeking help to figure out how to successfully change. Still others have already made the change and are seeking support and skills to keep abstinent. However, there are still a significant number who are merely seeking relief from discomfort or external pressures and not recovery as they turn to professionals for help. In effect, treatment begins at whatever point in the process of self-change that the individual seeking treatment has achieved when he or she walks through the door or picks up the telephone. Intervention and treatments have the task of supporting and consolidating what has already been accomplished and assisting the individual to move forward in the recovery process. However, if the individual is stuck in the precontemplation stage of recovery on entry to treatment and providers are unable to move that person forward, treatment will fail because self-change is static. Treatment builds on self-change and has a reciprocal relationship with natural recovery. It is never treatment *or* self-change but treatment *and* self-change.

The process of change represented by the stages of change and the tasks identified in each of the stages are an interesting and informative way to describe both the process of natural recovery and the process of change involved in treatment-assisted change. In this perspective, treatment is an adjunct to self-change rather than the other way around. Studies have shown that there are certain indicators taken prior to the individuals entering treatment that are important to successful outcomes regardless of the type of treatment. These indicators are typically related to the process of change and represent the tasks outlined by the stages of change. Individual motivation for change and motivation for treatment prior to entering treatment have been identified as important predictors not only of participation in treatment but of long-term outcomes. Individuals' personal evaluations of their decisional considerations and reasons for change, their personal evaluations of self-efficacy to abstain from or moderate substance use, and their levels of temptation or craving to use on entering treatment also have been associated with recovery outcomes. In addition, it seems that the changes or gains made in the first couple of weeks of treatment are critical for long-term success. Clearly what the client brings to treatment in terms of motivation, decision making, confidence, and commitment are critical to what happens in the first weeks of treatment and ultimately to successful recovery.

Treatment appears to enhance and support the process of change but continues to rely on self-change and natural recovery as well. Successful clients in treatment tend to participate more fully in the treatment, do the assigned homework between sessions, make use of ancillary services and supports, and generally engage in specific coping processes of change in their lives more than the failures. Moreover, maintenance of change tasks extend well beyond the scope of most treatments so continued change is the province of the individual substance abuser, hopefully using some the skills and lessons learned in treatment but implementing them either on his or her own or with some mutual help for support. Natural change and the process of self-change is the larger context for recovery. Treatment is a time-limited, circumscribed experience or series of experiences that interacts with and hopefully enhances the self-change process on the road to recovery. This perspective can also help us to understand the role of brief, opportunistic interventions in the career of substance abusers. Brief interventions that take advantage of naturally occurring events or that provide short encounters with information, feedback, or advice interact also with the process of self-change and can promote that process. Brief interventions, especially those that are connected with other meaningful events or negative consequences in an individual's life, can increase concern, promote decision making, support commitment to take action, and offer some plan or behavioral actions that can help the individuals accomplish some important tasks of self-change. The success of brief interventions for substance abuse problems can only be understood in the context of a self-change process since the intervention is so brief in many cases that it could not reasonably be considered to be responsible for all the coping activities and change processes needed to make changes in substance use.

Treatment is a time-limited, circumscribed experience that interacts with and hopefully enhances the self-change process on the road to recovery.

Minimal interventions and guided self-change interventions are also based on the premise that individuals, given some guidance, can successfully resolve their substance use problems. This premise is at the heart of all self-help approaches. One problem with employing self-help approaches for substance users in the past was the belief, now discredited, that substance users could not change without the aid of treatment. This belief was fostered by the reality of recurring relapses and the definition of substance dependence currently being used in diagnostic systems. Failure at self-change is viewed as one of the defining characteristics of dependence. One of the diagnostic criteria for dependence is that the individual has tried unsuccessfully to stop using the substance. Often successful self-changers would be viewed as not dependent and having a less serious substance abuse problem precisely because they were able to change on their own. However, most self-changers also report multiple unsuccessful quit attempts. The studies of self-change do not support the contention that only individuals diagnosed as substance abusers can use self-change and those dependent on substances cannot. In fact, brief interventions, guided self-change, and mutual help programs have been successful for individuals with serious and significant substance use problems as well as those with less severe problems.

Studies of self-change do not support the contention that only individuals diagnosed as substance abusers can use self-change and those dependent on substances cannot.

An important distinction needs to be made between modifications to substance use that are intrinsically motivated and clearly use the process of intentional behavior change and modifications that are largely extrinsically motivated. Negative consequences and contingencies as well as some positive contingencies can promote modifications of substance use. Individuals on probation for drinking or drug infractions often suspend their substance use for the duration of the probation without the intention of making any sustained change in their use. Problem drinkers who have experienced a serious negative consequence, like a visit to a trauma center or emergency room, often change their pattern of use dramatically for a period of time and then resume their prior level of drinking. Pregnant women smokers will stop smoking for the duration of the pregnancy only to begin again postpartum. Drug abusers will stop using drugs when rewarded for clean urines and return to use if artificial external rewards are not replaced with meaningful ones in the natural environment (see Carroll & Rounsaville, Chapter 14, this volume). Sometimes these events, rewards, and experiences serve as interventions to spur the process of self-change. However, at other times they may simply serve to motivate a temporary suspension of the behavior that does not engage the intentional process of change and the self-change involved in natural recovery.

The process of intentional behavior change outlined in the transtheoretical model of change was explored initially by examining self-change of nicotine addiction and has been refined by looking at both minimal and more intensive interventions with other substances of abuse. The change process is delineated by a specific set of tasks identified by the stages, change activities called "processes of change," and the context and markers of change like decisional considerations, temptation, and self-efficacy. The model provides a structure with which to understand and explore the natural change phenomenon and relate it to the recovery process experienced and described in treatment-assisted successful change of substance abuse. Although we have learned a lot about this process in prior research, there continue to be a number of intriguing questions particularly related to self-change and the interaction between self-change and both brief interventions and longer treatment programs that require continued exploration. However, the past 20 years of research on natural change, the change process, and the model have discredited the following myths: (1) that substance abusers do not or cannot change; (2) that substance abusers cannot change on their own; (3) that substance abusers are impervious to consequences and contingencies; and (4) that we cannot understand the process of recovery for problematic use of substances. The challenge for the next 20 years is to better understand and integrate more fully the phenomenon of self-change with interventions and treatment efforts, policy initiatives, and societal views of substance abuse.

Conclusion

Natural change or self-change is a fundamental process in combating troublesome use of substances. A broad perspective on this natural change process offers hope for substance abusers, questions current assumptions and prejudices about substance abusers, and challenges providers and policymakers to thoughtfully integrate their interventions to complement and promote natural change and recovery.

There are many interesting questions that need to be answered in order to continue developing our understanding of natural or self-change. How and when do consequences teach the individuals and provoke appropriate concern and decision making? Do brief interventions work better for individuals at different stages of the change process? Does prior success or failure in self-change determine the success or failure of natural or treatment-assisted recovery? Can the natural change process be accelerated? Are the nonabstinent natural change outcomes as stable as the abstinent ones? How can legal mandates and extrinsic contingencies promote the self-change process and create sustained change of substance abuse? These and other questions need to be answered in order to provide guidance both in guiding self-change and in the development of brief interventions to promote change.

Robust Principles

1. Successful self-change of substance abuse without formal intervention or treatment does occur for every type of abusable substance.
2. Although self-change is more likely to occur with less extensive or less intensive patterns of substance abuse and for individuals who have experienced some important negative consequences, it is not limited only to abusers or to specific subgroups identified by demographics or substance abuse history.
3. Natural recovery is not a process that differs from treatment-assisted

recovery. There is a similar intentional process of change that involves concern, decisional considerations, commitment and planning, and taking effective action that are responsible for recovery produced by self-changers as well as by treatment-assisted successful changers.

4. Environmental considerations, developmental transitions, associated problems, access to resources, and resolution of associated problems seem particularly important for promoting or hindering self-change.

5. Natural change outcomes are often not as absolute as treatment outcomes in terms of abstinence and often include moderation and self-modulated substance use outcomes.

6. There are numerous patterns of substance abuse in the population. Self-change is a determinant of these patterns of interrupted initiation as well as the patterns of early or late discontinuation of substance use more typically defined as natural recovery.

7. It is important to promote self-change at every opportunity. Individuals who are misusing substances need encouragement, advice, consequences, and feedback whenever they come in contact with health care, social, and legal systems in order to foster the self-change process.

8. Treatment interacts with the process of self-change and seems to be a time-limited event in the course of the larger self-change process. All recovery from substance abuse can be envisioned as natural recovery, with treatment as a facilitator of that process.

9. The perspective that takes natural change seriously and as the foundation of the recovery process shifts the focus from an overemphasis on interventions and treatments and gives increased emphasis to the individual substance abuser, his or her developmental status, his or her values and experiences, the nature of the substance abuse and its connection with associated problems, and his or her stage of change.

Acknowledgments

I would like to thank Miranda Garay for her assistance in researching articles for this chapter and acknowledge funding from the Robert Woods Johnson Foundation Innovators Grant that help to support this project. Data and research that support the observations discussed here have come from grant funding from the National Cancer Institute; the National Institute on Alcohol Abuse and Alcoholism; the National Heart, Lung, and Blood Institute; and the National Institute on Drug Abuse.

Suggested Readings

Bischof, G., Rumpf, H.-J., Hapke, U., Meyer, C., & John, U. (2001). Factors influencing remission from alcohol dependence without formal help in a representative population sample. *Addiction, 96,* 1327–1336.

Chassin, L., Presson, C. C., Pitts, S. C., & Sherman, S. J. (2000). The natural history of cigarette smoking from adolescence to adulthood: Multiple trajectories and their psychosocial correlates. *Health Psychology, 19*(3), 223–231.

DiClemente, C. C. (2003). *Addiction and change: How addictions develop and addicted people recover.* New York: Guilford Press.

DiClemente, C. C., & Prochaska, J. O. (1998). Toward a comprehensive, transtheoretical model of change: Stages of change and addictive behaviors. In W. R. Miller & N. Heather (Eds.), *Treating addictive behaviors* (2nd ed., pp. 3–24). New York: Plenum Press.

Flory, K., Lynam, D., Milich, R., Leukefeld, C., & Clayton, R. (2004). Early adolescent through young adult alcohol and marijuana use trajectories: Early predictors, young adult outcomes, and predictive utility. *Development and Psychopathology, 16,* 193–213.

Kaplow, J. B., Curran, P. J., Dodge, K. A., & The Conduct Problems Prevention Research Group. (2000). Child, parent, and peer predictors of early-onset substance abuse: A multi-site longitudinal study. *Journal of Abnormal Child Psychology, 30*(3), 199–216.

King, M. P., & Tucker, J. A. (2000). Behavior change patterns and strategies distinguishing moderation drinking and abstinence during the natural resolution of alcohol problems without treatment. *Psychology of Addictive Behaviors, 14*(1), 48–55.

Prochaska, J. O., DiClemente, C. C., Velicer, W. F., Ginpil, S., & Norcross, J. C. (1985). Predicting change in smoking status for self-changers. *Addictive Behaviors, 10,* 395–406.

Randall, C., Roberts, J. S., DelBoca, F. K., Carroll, K. M., Connors, G. J., & Mattson, M. E. (1999). Telescoping of landmark events associated with drinking: A gender comparison. *Journal of Studies on Alcohol, 60,* 252–260.

Sobell, L. C., Klingemann, H. K.-H., Toneatto, T., Sobell, M. B., Agrawal, M. S., & Leo, G. I. (2001). Alcohol and drug abusers' perceived reasons for self-change in Canada and Switzerland: Computer-assisted content analysis. *Substance Use and Misuse, 36*(11), 1467–1500.

Spooner, C. (1999). Causes and correlates of adolescent drug abuse and implications for treatment. *Drug and Alcohol Review, 18,* 453–475.

Tarter, R. E., Kirisci, L., Mezzich, A., Cornelius, J. R., Pajer, K., Vanyukov, M., et al., (2003). Neurobehavioral disinhibition in childhood predicts early age at onset of substance use disorder. *American Journal of Psychiatry, 160*(6), 1078–1085.

Tucker, J. A., Vuchinich, R. E., & Rippens, P. D. (2004). Different variables are associated with help-seeking patterns and long-term outcomes among problem drinkers. *Addictive Behaviors, 29,* 433–439.

Vailiant, G. E. (2003). A 60-year follow-up of alcoholic men. *Addiction, 98,* 1043–1051.

Zapert, K., Snow, D. L., & Tebes, J. K. (2002). Patterns of substance use in early through late adolescence. *American Journal of Community Psychology, 30*(6), 835–852.

CHAPTER 7

Developmental Perspectives on the Risk for Developing Substance Abuse Problems

VICTOR M. HESSELBROCK
MICHIE N. HESSELBROCK

The vulnerability for developing alcohol and other drug use disorders results from two broad classes of factors. The first class of factors includes genetic mechanisms that contribute to the predisposition for developing alcohol/drug problems. There is no doubt that a parental history of alcohol or drug dependence, particularly paternal substance dependence, is related to a substantially increased risk for developing substance abuse problems in both male and female offspring. The familial nature of substance abuse problems and the transmission of the risk for substance abuse problems from parents to offspring are well documented. Family pedigree studies, twin studies, and adoption studies have provided significant evidence of an increased risk for developing substance use problems when a biological parent is affected. More recently, the nature of the risk due to a family history of alcoholism has been decomposed into genetic and environmental factors. Although the proportion of the risk for developing substance dependence determined by either environmental or genetic factors has not been conclusively determined, it appears that genetic factors account for about 50% of the variance. Consequently, familial factors (including parenting behavior), peer relations, cognitive factors (including alcohol expectancies), and other nongenetic variables may represent important direct and indirect effects on substance use behaviors, including pathological drug use involvement.

The second class of factors that may contribute to the variable risk for and expression of alcohol and drug use problems includes personal and environmental factors. Examples of personal factors include personality traits, psychopathology, and cognitive functioning; examples of environmental factors include such things as family environment and peer relations. These factors may influence the initiation of drug use, the maintenance of drug use behavior, the development of drug-related problems, treatment-seeking behavior, treatment outcomes, and the life course of alcohol/drug use dependence by moderating or mediating its genetic expression.

Personal Factors That May Influence Alcohol/Drug Abuse Risk

Temperament Traits

Temperament has been identified as an important factor in several theoretical formulations related to the development of substance use behaviors, including pathological use. While prior research has shown that the predisposition toward the development of substance abuse problems is partially due to the individual's genetic makeup, several studies suggest that this genetic predisposition may be expressed, in part, through the individual's temperament. *Temperament* is a set of behavioral and emotional reactions that varies among individuals, is moderately stable over time and situation, and appears early in life. Some temperament characteristics and deviations in temperament characteristics have been found to be highly heritable and to manifest early in a child's development. Several theoretical models of pathological alcohol involvement involve temperament as a key element. Tarter and colleagues proposed a temperament model of alcoholism based upon five temperament traits that increase an individual's liability for developing alcoholism. These traits include behavioral activity level, sociability, attention span/persistence, emotionality, and soothability. Each of the five traits is thought to be genetically influenced. The individual's liability is increased or decreased by the deviation of each trait from the population norm. Thus individuals whose personality traits are closer to the population norm are thought to have more control over their own behavior, including substance use. Those persons with behavioral and emotional dysregulation may be more prone to develop alcohol problems in relation to environmental influences and stressors, including seeking environments conducive to alcohol and drug use. Studies of adolescent problem drinkers, for example, have identified tolerance of deviance and related personality traits (e.g., distrust, aggressive sociality, cynicism) as being associated with acute alcohol problems in adolescence. Indeed, each of these traits and clusters of these traits constituting a "difficult temperament" constellation have been related to an increased risk for developing a substance use problem, including abuse.

Several temperament traits are likely to occur together under the rubric of behavioral undercontrol. For instance, the construct of *behavioral undercontrol* may include a wide range of traits including antisociality, novelty seeking, extraversion, impulsivity, and psychoticism. Conduct problems can be viewed as a measure of antisociality, a hypothesized outcome of behavioral undercontrol. A tendency to be disinhibited or easily bored may encourage the expression of externalizing behaviors (e.g., conduct problems, alcohol and drug use). A recent report found a negative association between age of first drink and disinhibitory behavior (oppositionality, impulsiveness, and inattention) assessed at age 11 that predicted alcohol use at age 14. It is likely that the temperament traits of behavioral undercontrol and behavioral disinhibition will initially lead to conduct problems and subsequently lead to early substance (tobacco, alcohol) use. Early-onset substance use has been associated with the early development of a variety of alcohol and drug use problems.

A separate but related dimension of temperament is *negative affectivity*. A tendency toward depression, neuroticism, and negative affect has been found to be overrepresented in some samples of offspring of substance abusers and individuals who later develop several alcohol problems. Negative affectivity may also contribute to the development of conduct problems and alcohol and drug involvement. For instance, some individuals may cope with a negative affect by using drugs and alcohol to relieve their unpleasant symptoms, while others may exhibit aggressive behaviors as attempts to distance themselves from painful feelings that they find extremely difficult to tolerate. Both behavioral undercontrol and negative affect may mediate the relationship of a family history of alcohol dependence to alcohol use and problems, either directly or through conduct problems. For instance, negative affectivity and behavioral undercontrol could, in the same person, lead to increased likelihood of alcohol (and drug) use because they play into the different processes suggested by different etiological models (e.g., affect regulation and deviance proneness).

More recently, personality research has focused on what has been termed the *five-factor model of personality*. With origins in the work of Allport and Cattell, the model focuses on five robust factors that characterize normal traits rather than deviations. These traits include (1) neuroticism—tendency to experience negative affect; (2) extroversion—gregariousness, activity; (3) openness to experience—intellectual curiosity, awareness of inner feelings, need for variety in actions; (4) agreeableness—altruism, emotional support, helpfulness; and (5) conscientiousness—will to achieve, dependability, responsibility. Reports suggest that a family history of substance abuse is positively associated with openness but negatively associated with agreeableness and conscientiousness.

In general, temperament traits can be maintained or moderated by environmental influences such as interactions with parents, friends, teachers, or other influential people. Thus temperament traits can have both direct and indirect effects on substance use patterns.

Childhood Psychopathology

Both cross-sectional and longitudinal studies over the past 40 years indicate that childhood problem behaviors predict both behavior problems and problems with alcohol and substance abuse in adolescence and young adulthood. An association between behavioral problems occurring in childhood and adolescence and consequent poor adult outcomes, including substance use problems, has been repeatedly found in longitudinal studies of child guidance clinic subjects, in community samples, and in studies of adoptees at risk for alcoholism. Many, but not all, of these individuals who develop substance use problems at an early age will go on to develop a severe form of the disorder. Even though problem behaviors typically begin in childhood for boys and in adolescence for girls, the relationship to later alcohol and drug problems holds for both boys and girls and across at least some ethnic minority groups. Importantly, recent studies indicate that the drug use problems among adolescents with conduct problems are not benign and do not resolve over time. For many, these substance use problems persist into young adult life and possibly beyond.

Conduct problems in childhood and adolescence are often accompanied by other externalizing behaviors such as attention deficit disorder, hyperactivity, and oppositional behavior. Childhood hyperactivity and attention deficit disorder have also been linked to an increased risk for developing alcoholism, particularly among children of an alcoholic parent. However, many of these studies often fail to take into account the effect of co-occurring conduct problems or sample children with only hyperactivity or attention deficit disorder. There is little evidence for the independent contribution of either hyperactivity or attention deficit disorder alone to the susceptibility for alcoholism.

Alcohol Expectancies

Many laboratory studies of alcohol and drug use focus on their ability to influence certain behaviors—for example, to promote aggression, to increase sexual arousal, or to reduce tension. All such studies assume a cognitive influence surrounding alcohol/drug use. An underlying assumption of such studies is that subjects have certain positive expectations of the drug effects being studied. This is especially true regarding alcohol use. A number of different alcohol-related expectancies have been identified including social facilitation, enhanced sexual performance and pleasure, increased personal power and aggression, social assertiveness, relaxation and tension reduction, as well as a general positive outcome that may result from drinking. Expectancies about alcohol's effects probably reflect not only a person's own experience with alcohol, but also result from advertising and from observing the behavior of others when they are drinking. For example, a study of children in elementary school found that positive expectancies regarding the effects of alcohol increased with age, most notably among 8- to 10-year-olds. Importantly, a variety of studies have shown that positive expectancies of alcohol's effects predict initiation of drinking, intention to drink, and drinking rates among middle-school students. Although originally linked to attitudes and beliefs about the reinforcing properties of alcohol, expectancies are thought to be related to memory processes. Thus, positive expectancies of alcohol use may be encoded in close association with usual drinking practices and be easily retrieved from memory in future drinking situations. Negative expectancies arising from unpleasant drinking experiences, on the other hand, may be more closely tied to heavy drinking episodes rather than being associated with usual drinking practices. Consequently, among light to moderate drinkers, negative expectancies of alcohol's effects are less likely to play an inhibitory role in most drinking situations.

Positive expectancies of alcohol's effects predict initiation of drinking, intention to drink, and drinking rates among middle-school students.

Cognitive Functioning

A growing number of studies have implicated heritable cognitive factors, including electrophysiological features related to central nervous system functioning, as being related to the vulnerability for developing alcohol and other substance use problems. A number of studies have found poorer cognitive performance among substance-dependent individuals, particularly alcohol-dependent patients, compared to controls on neuropsychological tests of memory, attention span, abstract thinking, verbal reasoning, and visual–spatial skills. A key element of the vulnerability for developing pathological substance involvement is the role of cognitive factors as possible mediators of the vulnerability posed due to a family history of substance dependence. For example, among a sample of female substance abusers, the majority was either abusing or dependent on alcohol, and had reduced cognitive abilities on measures of language skills, sustained attention, and perceptual efficiency compared to normal controls. Even though the findings are in the small effect size range, they are theoretically relevant to understanding substance abuse etiology (impulsive, inability to use language to cognitively regulate behavior, poor foresight). These particular cognitive deficiencies could compromise educational attainment and impair psychosocial development among individuals at high risk for alcoholism.

To date, specific cognitive deficits in persons at risk for developing substance abuse problems have not been consistently reported. However, tests of frontal and temporal lobe functioning among young adult males with susceptibility for developing alcoholism were predictive of the age of taking their first drink and their frequency of drinking to get intoxicated. Furthermore, there does appear to be a positive association of measures of executive cognitive functioning, aggressive behavior, and externalizing behavioral traits. Offspring of substance abusers (including persons with a family history of alcoholism) who are at increased risk for developing substance problems display poor behavioral inhibition and perform poorly on tests of executive cognitive functioning.

Differences in cognitive functioning as measured by electroencephalographic and event-related potential (EEG/ERP) methods have been found between adult alcoholics and controls. Similar findings have been reported among children and adolescents at risk for developing alcoholism and other substances prior to the onset of heavy use. Typically, differences in EEG and ERP brainwave patterns are found in the frontal brain region, an area thought to be responsible for the cognitive skills of attention, planning, and foresight. Importantly, a reduced P300 ERP amplitude may be predictive of an early onset of substance use apart from the family density for substance abuse. Possibly, the reduced P300 amplitude ERP and disinhibitory behavior as manifested through conduct problems reflects, at least in part, a common underlying vulnerability. Although these electrophysiological measures of brain activity do provide a "marker" of risk for a poor adult outcome, including an increased risk for developing substance abuse problems, the exact relationship between electrophysiological measures and behavioral/neuropsychological measures of cognitive functioning are not well established.

Environmental Influences on the Development of Alcohol/Drug Use Problems

Several possible environmental risk factors are presented here. However, two cautions are urged. First, even though certain environmental conditions/risk factors may characterize alcoholic homes, such conditions are not necessarily related to the later development of alcohol use disorders in the offspring unless variations in the environmental conditions are related to specific outcomes. Second, even when the environmental factor of interest is associated with a particular outcome, "cause" cannot be assumed. A third variable, such as a comorbid psychiatric condition in either the parent or the child, may falsely lead to the appearance of causation when the effect is almost entirely due to this unexamined third variable. It should also be recognized that children in a family can, and do, influence the amount and type of interactions with their parents and other family members. For example, one study has found that frequency of interactions with oppositional children may increase alcohol consumption among adults who provide such children care.

Family Violence

Alcohol use by the perpetrator is present in a substantial proportion of domestic violence incidents reported in the general population. An estimated 67% of persons who victimize an intimate partner (e.g., spouse or boy-/girlfriend) use alcohol compared to 38% who victimized an acquaintance or 31% who victimized a stranger. Thus it is often assumed by clinicians and other social service workers that there is a strong relationship between parental alcoholism and family violence. However, a careful reading of the research literature does not provide a clear and consistent answer because many published studies are based upon small samples, do not adequately separate or assess the different types of abuse, often sample from populations or agencies that are likely to have high rates of both parental alcoholism and violence, and frequently do not use an adequate comparison group. While alcohol use and violence are clearly associated, the causal relationship between parental alcoholism, family violence, and later alcohol problems among the offspring has not been firmly established.

Family Interaction

Implicit in the discussion to this point is that alcohol and other drug use disorders are multiply determined by a complex association of genetic, environmental, personality, and other factors. Frequently more than one member of the nuclear or extended family is substance-dependent. This complicates the identification of specific influences that family environment, childrearing practices, or interparental interaction may play on the development of alcoholism. Three general contemporary models can be identified: a family disease model, a family systems model, and a behavioral family approach.

The family disease model is based upon the assumption that all family members suffer from either alcoholism or codependency. Furthermore, alcoholism and codependency are interrelated such as to enable (perpetuate) the alcohol problem. Although the specific etiology is biological in origin, the family disease in this model maintains alcoholism.

In the family systems model, the etiology of alcoholism and substance abuse is focused on family members' behavior around drinking, with particular attention paid to the family of origin and the role of the spouse/partner. The model assumes that alcohol use stabilizes families and that the family organizes their interactions and structure around alcohol use to achieve "homeostasis," that is, to maintain the alcohol problem despite the problems associated with such a family system. However, "family rituals" such as dinnertime or the celebration of holidays may serve to protect offspring against the development of alcohol and other forms of drug abuse. The continuing interaction between adult offspring and their alcoholic parents is associated with increased rates of alcoholism, at least among the male offspring.

A third model is the behavioral family approach that focuses on the family's behaviors (especially those of the spouse/partner) as antecedents to and reinforcers of the consequences of alcohol or substance use. These behaviors are thought to help promote and maintain the drinking problem. Similarly, it is the behaviors of the family members that also influence the alcoholic individual to consider change, to act to change, to maintain the change, or to relapse to drinking.

Peer Influences

Peer influences have been consistently cited as risk factors for the initiation of alcohol, tobacco, and other drug use among children and adolescents. Peers influence adolescents' values, behaviors, attitudes, and choice of other friends. However, the closeness of the relationship is an important determinant of the strength of peer influence on drinking and drug use behavior. Alcohol use by an adolescent's best friend is more predictive of his or her alcohol use and maintenance than reports of use by other friends. Reports of use by same-age peers do not appear to be related to either initiation or maintenance of drinking in adolescence.

Associating with deviant friends tends to promote the acceptance of deviant behaviors, including the use of alcohol and other drugs.

However, it is not clear whether the association with deviant peers is a risk factor for, or the result of, maladaptive behaviors because deviant peer group involvement interacts with several other risk factors such as family problems, other mental health problems, low self-esteem, and stress, as well as with alcohol availability. Deviant peer group involvement is typically higher among adolescent boys than girls.

Still, adolescents often cite as reasons for alcohol and substance use an increased ability to socialize with friends; to reduce tension and anxiety, especially in mixed-gender situations; to reduce boredom; and to get high. As indicated above, expectations of alcohol's effects in these areas are associated with both initiation of alcohol use and drinking rates, particularly among adolescents. Drinking behavior in adulthood, however, is less influenced by peer and friend relations than it is during adolescence.

Social Support

An additional aspect of peer influence is social support. The people to whom one can turn in times of trouble and from whom one can confidently expect caring, valuing, and love can be defined as a *social network*. A strong social network has been reported to decrease vulnerability to both mental and physical health problems, help moderate the need for medication, and aid an individual to recover more quickly following an illness. Conversely, an increase in health problems has been reported in the context of high life stresses in the absence of social support. Implicit in these studies is the notion that the perception of potentially available social supports from family and friends may be as important as their actual existence. Social support is distinguished from sociability, a personality trait, which may not be directly related to alcohol use, even among persons at risk for developing alcoholism.

The role of social support both from family and from friends has been examined in relation to the development and maintenance of alcohol and substance use and to substance-related problem behaviors among affected individuals and persons at risk for developing substance use problems. However, these influences are probably not direct, but are mediated/moderated by other factors such as temperament. One study found that perceived social support from friends and from family did not vary according to a positive or negative paternal history of substance abuse. However, adolescent females perceived greater social support from their friends than the adolescent male subjects did from their friends. Furthermore, no association was found between perceived social support from family and friends and the age of onset of experimental drug use for any drug tried, including marijuana, amphetamines, sedatives, cocaine, hallucinogens, opiates, PCP, or inhalants. Social support from families has been associated with a later onset of tobacco and marijuana use. While social support from friends was not associated with initiation of substance use, friend social support did predict frequency of use. Adolescents with high levels of perceived social support from friends got drunk more frequently than those with low levels of perceived social support from friends. Among adult persons living together in a stable relationship, however, social support from close family members is more predictive of drinking behavior than social support from friends.

In general, a variety of social and environmental factors that may affect a person's risk for developing alcohol and other substance use problems have been proposed in the literature. As described in both social learning and social control theories of the development of alcoholism, social environments are thought to provide a wider context for the interaction of biological, psychological, and personality factors to determine a person's susceptibility for developing alcohol abuse problems. Peer influences to initiate or maintain use, stressful and negative life events, and family environment (including poor parenting styles) appear to further enhance the likelihood of developing alcohol- or drug-related problems among adolescents and young adults at high risk due to a family history of alcoholism. However, an adolescent's exposure to alcohol and other drugs tends to be more limited in the presence of good relations with nonusing peers (particularly best friends), family rituals that actively seek to prevent alcohol use, and consistent parental supervision and discipline. Reduced exposure to alcohol and drug use, in turn, limits the opportunity for expression of genetic, psychological, and personality susceptibility risk factors for developing alcoholism.

A General Model of Risk for Developing Alcohol/Drug Use Problems

An extensive literature indicates that the biological offspring of an alcohol- or drug-dependent parent are at higher risk for developing substance-related problems than offspring of non-substance-dependent parents. Importantly, several general classes of personal and environmental factors, including cognitive difficulties, temperament, and environmental influences, have been shown to influence the

Cognitive difficulties, temperament, and environment influence the developmental pathway between family history and the individual's susceptibility for developing substance use problems.

developmental pathway between a family history of substance abuse problems and the individual's susceptibility for developing substance use problems. There is a conceptual model, the deviance proneness model (see Figure 7.1), that integrates these potential different sources of influence to the development of pathological alcohol/drug involvement. Indicators of pathological alcohol/drug involvement may include the age of onset of first use, the age of onset of substance use problems, the frequency of use, and the severity of substance use problems. As shown in Figure 7.1, the deviance proneness model begins with a family history of alcohol/drug dependence as a background variable and predicts direct effects on several personal factors such as conduct disorder, temperament traits, and cognitive functioning. These personal factors, in turn, have direct effects on other aspects of the child/adolescent's life such as peer relations, affectivity, and expectancies concerning alcohol/drug effects, which may influence the vulnerable person's family environment. As can be seen from this conceptual model, the developmental pathway from a family history of substance abuse to pathological alcohol/substance involvement is quite complex, with many different factors contributing either vulnerability or protective effects.

Secular Trends/Birth Cohort Effects

Most people first experiment with tobacco and alcohol in their early teens and experience alcohol intoxication by their late teens. Furthermore, the primary age of risk for developing alcohol and other substance dependencies is from late adolescence to the late 20s. The large

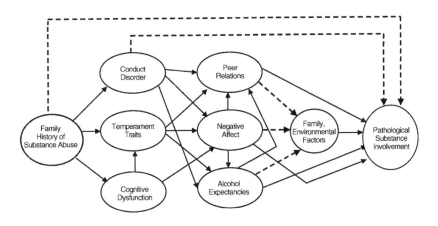

FIGURE 7.1. Deviance proneness model of risk.

majority (90%+) of those who develop alcoholism do so by their early 30s. However, alcoholism and other forms of substance abuse typically have a variable developmental course that is frequently interspersed with periods of remission and relapse. Once alcohol use resumes after a period of remission, it is probable that drinking will escalate and that serious problems will develop again. Because an age effect is present for most medical disorders, age-specific rates and age-of-onset distributions are typically presented for most disorders. This conceptualization is problematic for traits such as alcohol dependence, substance abuse, or other psychiatric conditions such as depression where epidemiological studies find lifetime rates in younger individuals already exceeding those in older individuals. This is illustrated by the finding of a 1.8% lifetime rate of DSM-III-R alcohol dependence in women born before 1940 as contrasted to a 13% rate in women born after 1960 in the Collaborative Study on the Genetics of Alcoholism (COGA) data set. A 15% rate was observed in males born before 1940 as contrasted to a 28% rate in males born after 1960. A similar effect is noted in the relatives of alcohol-dependent probands. As expected, the lifetime rates in relatives were elevated when compared to controls. Using survival analyses to examine the time to onset of alcohol dependence, highly significant risk ratios (RRs) were observed for gender (RR = 2.3), cohort of birth (RR = 1.5 over a decade), daily smoking (RR = 2.0), and comorbid diagnoses of antisocial personality (RR = 2.3) and depression (RR = 1.6).

Gender Differences

Gender differences have been noted in patterns of substance use, particularly in drinking behavior, the metabolism of alcohol, the course of developing alcohol problems, the point and lifetime prevalence of alcohol problems (including alcohol abuse and dependence), comorbid psychiatric conditions, the physical consequences of chronic alcohol use, and treatment utilization. Typically women are less likely to consume alcohol than men are, but when they do, women typically drink smaller amounts per occasion. Mortality rates are higher from a variety of causes such as accidents, violence, suicide, and medical illnesses among women than men who drink heavily.

Still, there are many similarities among male and female alcoholics. There is a high level of correspondence in the temporal sequencing of the occurrence of major alcohol-related life problems among male and female alcoholics, as well as between drinking but nonalcoholic men and women. Although the age of first appearance of symptoms examined may vary by gender, the order of appearance was very similar between males and females. Furthermore, once alcohol depend-

ence develops, the clinical manifestations of the disorder show few gender differences at either the low or the high end of severity. At an
intermediate level of severity of alcohol dependence, women often
manifest more anxiety and depressive symptoms but lower levels of antisocial behaviors compared to males. An antisocial type of alcoholism
predominates at the more severe end of the alcohol-dependence spectrum and few male–female differences are noted. However, women
tend to do as well as men following treatment for alcoholism, and in
some settings they may have a better outcome.

Ethnicity

Ethnic differences in the onset of substance use and in the developmental course of substance abuse problems have been consistently reported in the literature. Among persons in the United States, Caucasians typically begin using tobacco and alcohol at an earlier age than
African Americans, with African American women typically beginning
use last. Among Caucasian males, the proportion of heavy drinkers
peaks between ages 18 and 25 and then declines with increasing age.
Among Hispanic and black men, the proportion of heavy drinkers
peaks between the ages of 26 and 30 and then declines with age; however, the proportion of heavy-drinking black men is consistently lower
at each age compared to heavy-drinking Hispanic men. In a sample of
treated alcohol-dependent individuals, it was found that the developmental course of alcohol dependence did not appear to vary according
to the ethnicity of the proband. However, even after controlling for
socioeconomic status, ethnic minorities in treatment for alcohol dependence tended to be younger and more economically disadvantaged.
Alaska Natives reported the highest levels of alcohol-related depression. The rate of antisocial personality disorder was highest among
Hispanics and Alaska Natives. Female Hispanics and Alaska Natives reported violent behaviors as frequently as the male Hispanics and
Alaska Natives. Alaska Native men and women reported the earliest
age of onset of alcoholism and the highest frequency of serious alcohol
symptoms, including morning drinking, seizures, DTs, and liver disease. An earlier age of onset of alcohol dependence appeared to increase the risk for developing polydrug use among all groups, except
among African Americans who typically develop cocaine and opiate
dependence much later than alcohol dependence.

The familial transmission of alcohol dependence differs between
European American and African American families. Caucasian families were found to have a greater clustering of alcohol dependence and
habitual smoking, while African American families had the highest lev-

els of cocaine dependence. Other findings suggest that a higher rate and on earlier onset of tobacco use is found among alcohol-dependent African Americans versus nonalcoholic African Americans.

Does Biology Matter?

As indicated above, many aspects of the initiation of use, the maintenance of use and the development of alcohol and drug use problems are "familial" in nature. For example, similar styles of alcohol use and the presence of alcoholism can be found in the same family, running from parent to child and across multiple generations of biologically related individuals. However, many other traits or behaviors, such as religious or political affiliation, that have no biological basis and therefore cannot be under genetic control, also run in families. Still, the contribution of genetic factors contributing to the susceptibility to develop alcohol and other substance abuse problems cannot be discounted (see Hasin, Hatzenbuehler, & Waxman, Chapter 5, this volume). There are multiple sources of evidence pointing to a genetic basis for alcohol and substance dependence. While no single source of information definitely confirms the genetic hypothesis, the confluence of findings from extended pedigree studies, studies of monozygotic (identical) and dizygotic (fraternal) twins, and studies of adoptees raised apart from their alcoholic parent persuasively argues for a genetic component to the vulnerability for developing alcoholism.

The findings from the three types of studies hold for both males and females, although the evidence for the importance of genetic factors in alcoholism risk currently appears to be stronger for males than for females. These gender differences may reflect a real difference in male/female genetic risk, although to date no sex-linked genes have been identified for alcoholism. It is more likely that the gender differences found are due to the moderating role of cultural and social factors that may limit females' exposure to heavy drinking. More recent epidemiological studies suggest that gender differences in the incidence and prevalence of alcoholism are declining, particularly among more recent birth cohorts.

It is also important to remember that all studies to date report only an increase in the statistical probability, or the "risk," for developing alcohol and substance abuse problems among biological family members. While the statistical probability or risk of developing alcohol problems is higher among biological relatives of an alcoholic, in fact most offspring of an alcoholic parent *do not* develop alcohol use problems or disorders in their lifetime. Still, important progress is being made in terms of identifying genes that confer increased susceptibility for developing alcohol and other substance abuse/dependence problems. COGA, a large-scale multisite family study, has identified several chromosomal regions that likely contain genes that increase a person's susceptibility for developing alcohol and drug dependence. A careful examination of a region of chromosome 4 has identified a gene, GABRA2, that codes for the type A receptor of the inhibitory neurotransmitter gamma-aminobutyric acid (GABA) that has been associated with alcohol dependence by COGA and in three other independent studies. Although this gene is not a vulnerability gene that is specific for alcohol or other drug dependence, it is likely to be one of many genes responsible for increasing an individual's susceptibility for developing alcohol- and other substance-related problems. However, the question of what is biologically inherited from an affected parent that increases an offspring's risk for developing an alcohol or substance use problem remains unanswered.

Gene–Environment Interaction

Understanding the genetic contribution to alcohol and other substance dependence is only one piece of understanding the etiology and developmental course of substance use disorders. Some individuals carry predisposing genes but never manifest the disorder, whereas others may not harbor predisposing genes but do develop the disorder. These complexities are thought to be due, in part, to the interplay between genes and environmental factors, whereby the environment moderates the expression of predisposing genes. Twin studies have documented that both genes and the environment play a role in drinking patterns—for example, data from the Australian twin register indicate that marital status moderates the relative importance of genetic effects on alcohol consumption in females. Having a marriage-like relationship reduced the impact of genetic influences on drinking. More recently, religiosity has been found to have a moderating effect on alcohol use among females. In subjects without a strong religious upbringing, genetic effects played a large role, dwarfing the influence of shared environment; however, in individuals with a religious upbringing, there was no evidence of genetic influence, while the environment played a large role. In Finnish adolescent twin data, regional residency exhibited strong moderating effects on influences on alcohol use, with genetic factors exerting a larger role in urban settings than rural settings from ages 16–18.5, while common environmental factors assumed greater importance in rural settings. Further examination of socioregional variables, such as neighborhood stability and neighborhood alcohol sales, provided further evidence for gene–environment interaction, with more than fivefold differences in the magnitude of genetic effects between environmental extremes.

Clearly, environmental factors must also play an important role in substance abuse susceptibility. Most current gene–environment models assume a synergy between genetic and environment factors that may contribute either to an increased susceptibility for developing a substance use disorder or produce a level of protection for vulnerable individuals (i.e., attenuate possible genetic risk). However, specific environmental factors such as those found in a family environment, social relationships, parenting styles, and so on that contribute in general to the development of alcohol use disorders have not been definitively identified.

Social Policy Considerations for the Development of Substance Problems

Social policy factors, even though often ignored in etiological formulations, can have a wide influence on the risk for developing alcohol and substance abuse problems. Social policy influences the availability of beverage alcohol to the general population and provides punitive measures for violation of purchase and consumption laws and regulations. To some extent, lack of exposure and limited access to alcohol would serve to protect against the development of alcohol problems and abuse or dependence.

Over the years, local, state, and federal governments have used a variety of measures to restrict the availability of both illicit and licit substances such as beverage alcohol. Prohibition, local option for alcoholic beverage sales, and minimum legal age for alcoholic beverage purchase have had both short- and long-term effects in restricting the availability of alcohol. In the 1970s, lowering the legal age for purchase lead to increased alcohol consumption and increased auto injuries and fatalities among adolescents. These trends were reversed when the minimum legal drinking age was again raised. The direct effect of changes in legal drinking age on other alcohol-related behaviors (e.g., assaults, teen pregnancies, sexually transmitted diseases, and drowning) is more difficult to assess because the minimum drinking age varied considerably from state to state for several years.

Taxation has also been viewed as a method for controlling the availability of alcohol since higher local and federal taxes on alcohol typically lead to higher prices. In general, raising taxes on beverage alcohol has been associated with decreased drinking. However, light and heavier drinkers appear to be less responsive to increased prices than moderate drinkers, but this effect may be due to a lack of information about the health consequences of heavy drinking among these groups. It has been noted

Raising taxes on beverage alcohol has been associated with decreased drinking.

that better informed drinkers, including heavy drinkers, showed greater reductions in drinking due to price increases than less informed drinkers. The use of taxes to increase the cost of obtaining alcohol-containing beverages is not straightforward. Even though many taxes are applied uniformly to all units of beverage alcohol produced, different manufacturers and retailers operating in different locales and competitive markets may choose to differentially pass along the cost to the purchaser. Furthermore, cost of a unit of beverage alcohol can vary considerably by beverage type, by geographic region, and by the type of establishment where the beverage is purchased.

Robust Principles

1. Genetic factors are important in determining the vulnerability to substance abuse, but they are not deterministic. Personal and environmental factors play an equally important role.
2. Based upon existing studies of risk for troublesome substance use, prevention must begin at an early age.
3. Prevention efforts must be multifaceted, targeting the individual, family, peer group, and the community.
4. Prevention efforts must be focused not only on substance use but on a broader range of outcomes.
5. The risk factors mentioned above pertain to all substances in important ways.
6. Each of the risk factors identified has important clinical considerations. However, their importance varies depending upon whether the client is in the development of the condition, in active treatment, or in recovery. The effectiveness of different intervention strategies in assisting change may vary according to the developmental phase of the problem.

Acknowledgment

This work was supported, in part, by Grant Nos. P50 AA-03510 and U10-AA08403 from the National Institutes of Health.

Suggested Readings

Bierut, L. J., Dinwiddie, S. H., Begleiter, H., Crowe, R. R., Hesselbrock, V., Nurnberger, J. I., Jr., et al. (1998). Familial transmission of substance dependence: Alcohol, marijuana, cocaine, and habitual smoking. *Archives of General Psychiatry, 55,* 982–988.

Hesselbrock, M., & Hesselbrock, V. (1999). Etiology of addictive disorders. In B. McCrady & E. E. Epstein (Eds.), *Comprehensive text of addictions* (pp. 50–74). New York: Oxford University Press.

Hesselbrock, M., & Hesselbrock, V. (1999). Substance abuse in adulthood. In R. Tarter, R. Ammerman, & P. Ott (Eds.), *Sourcebook on substance abuse: Etiology, methodology, and intervention* (pp. 98–112). Needham, MA: Allyn & Bacon.

Hesselbrock, V. M. (1995). The genetic epidemiology of alcoholism. In H. Begleiter & B. Kissin (Eds.), *Alcohol and alcoholism* (Vol. 1, pp. 17–39). New York: Oxford University Press.

Sher, K. J. (1991). *Children of alcoholics: A critical appraisal of theory and research.* Chicago: University of Chicago Press.

Tarter, R. E., & Vanyukov, M. (1994). Stepwise developmental model of alcoholism etiology. In R. A. Zucker, G. Boyd, & J. Howard (Eds.), *The development of alcohol problems: Exploring the biopsychosocial matrix of risk* (NIAAA Research Monograph 26, pp. 303–329). Washington, DC: U.S. Department of Health and Human Services.

CHAPTER 8

Comorbid Substance Use Disorders and Psychiatric Disorders

KIM T. MUESER
ROBERT E. DRAKE
WIN TURNER
MARK MCGOVERN

Problems with substance use and mental illness are inextricably linked. Comorbidity worsens the course of each problem area, complicates personal adjustment, and profoundly affects treatment needs. The possible reasons for the overlap between the problems are many, as are the potential implications for treatment. Understanding the roots of comorbidity, and effectively treating them, must be informed by an appreciation of their vast heterogeneity.

Prevalence and Consequences of Comorbid Disorders

Abundant evidence demonstrates that psychiatric and substance use disorders co-occur more often than would be expected by chance alone, and that comordibity worsens the course of each disorder.

Prevalence of Comorbid Psychiatric and Substance Use Disorders

Two types of research studies document high comorbidity rates: epidemiological surveys and studies of clinical populations. Several large-scale, population-based epidemiological surveys have shown that people with a mental illness are more likely to have a substance use disorder (and by definition, vice versa). In addition, the more incapacitating psychiatric disorders are related to higher rates of substance use problems than the less severe disorders. For example, the lifetime prevalence of substance use disorders in persons with the more severe illnesses of schizophrenia or bipolar disorder is about 50%, compared to about 25–30% in persons with depression or anxiety disorders, and 10–15% for persons with no mental illness. Furthermore, comorbidity is associated with increased service use, indicating that as problems mount due to multiple disorders, so does the need for treatment. For practical purposes this means that people who seek treatment for either a mental illness or a substance use problem are more likely to have a comorbid disorder than people with a disorder who do not seek treatment, a phenomenon observed for any comorbid medical condition over 50 years ago called "Berkson's fallacy."

People who seek treatment for either a mental illness or substance use problem are more likely to have a comorbid disorder than people with a disorder who do not seek treatment.

The high rate of comorbidity found in epidemiological studies is supported by many more studies of clinical samples. For example, studies of persons in alcohol or drug treatment typically report rates of comorbid mental illness in the 60–80% range, and studies of people in psychiatric treatment settings find rates of comorbid substance abuse in the 40–60% range. Thus comorbidity is a dominant clinical reality in most treatment settings.

Consequences of Comorbidity

As suggested by epidemiological studies showing that comorbidity increases the need for treatment, people with comorbid disorders tend to have a more severe course of illness than those with only a single disorder. For example, among persons with a severe mental illness, substance use problems contribute to worse symptoms, more frequent relapses, and more problems with family, housing, money, health, victimization, and the law than similar persons without a substance use disorder. Similarly, in addiction treatment settings, the severity of psychiatric disturbance predicts worse outcomes across a range of areas, including substance use and the social, health, and legal consequences of such use.

The impact of antisocial personality disorder (ASPD) on the course of substance abuse warrants special mention. The behavioral traits that characterize ASPD have long been associated with a more severe course of addiction, including an earlier age of onset, abuse of a greater variety of substances, more rapid progression to dependence, and experience of more negative consequences. The importance of ASPD as a correlate of substance abuse severity is reflected by the inclusion of some variant of it in all the major subtypes of alcoholism proposed over the past 50 years. Furthermore, the relationship between ASPD and substance abuse outcomes has also been extended to persons with severe mental disorders, such as schizophrenia and bipolar disorder. Thus, while any comorbid psychiatric disorder is related to more severe substance abuse problems, ASPD has an especially pernicious effect on the course and outcome of addictive disorders.

Understanding High Comorbidity

The high rate of comorbid psychiatric and substance use disorders leads to the question What accounts for their increased comorbidity? Understanding the reasons underlying increased comorbidity could lead to more effective prevention and treatment.

Numerous theories have been proposed to explain the high comorbidity between substance use and mental health disorders. Individual theories can be summarized in terms of four sets of overarching meta-models: *secondary psychopathology models*, *secondary substance abuse models*, *common factor models*, and *bidirectional models*.

Secondary Psychopathology Models

According to these models, increased comorbidity is due to substance use causing some cases of mental disorders, perhaps in vulnerable individuals. These theories can only be considered in relation to the effects of specific substances on specific disorders, with most evidence pertaining to schizophrenia, depression, and personality disorders.

For many years, it has been speculated that psychotomimetic substances (e.g., stimulants, LSD [lysergic acid diethylamide], phencyclidine, cannabis), which can cause transient psychotic episodes, might also precipitate long-term psychotic disorders in vulnerable individuals. Evidence shows that various drugs can trigger an earlier age of onset of schizophrenia, and that individuals who develop long-term psychosis following drug use are more likely to have a family history of psychosis. It remains unclear whether these individuals would have developed mental illness in the absence of drug use. Several recent studies indicate that cannabis use prospectively predicts the development of schizophrenia, and it has been hypothesized that cannabis can precipitate the illness. However, this theory is discordant with the stable or declining rate of schizophrenia in countries that have experienced an increase in cannabis use in the general population over the past several decades. Other explanations for the association include the possibility that cannabis use masks or overlaps with prodromal signs of the schizophrenia.

In regard to depression, many possibilities have been raised. Just as some drugs are psychotomimetic, alcohol, barbiturates, and some other drugs are inherently depressant. Their prolonged use is associated with high rates of depressive symptoms, most of which resolve with prolonged abstinence. For a significant minority of individuals, however, depression persists after weeks of abstinence. As in the situation of cases of schizophrenia that emerge in the context of drug abuse, the association between depressant drugs and depressive disorders could be due to a causal relationship. There is also speculation that stimulants, such as amphetamines and cocaine, which briefly enhance but subsequently deplete neurochemicals related to mood, might cause prolonged as well as transient episodes of depression in vulnerable individuals (see Koob, Chapter 3, this volume). In addition, the negative consequences of substance use disorders, such as the loss of work and housing, and problems with close relationships, health, victimization, and the criminal justice system, can deprive people of important reinforcers in their lives. Moreover, depression may occur in some individuals when they attain sobriety and begin to take stock of their disordered lives and the losses they have suffered.

Substance use disorder has a profoundly disorganizing effect on behavior as individuals constrict their lives to the pursuit and use of substances, often through illegal means and criminal behaviors. Different substances also disinhibit, reduce, or transform behaviors in extreme ways that are deviant from socially prescribed and normally patterned interpersonal behaviors. Thus people with extreme substance use problems often appear to exhibit personality disorders, but their dysfunctional patterns often disappear with stable remission. Even long-term antisocial behavior sometimes disappears with sobriety. Another issue is whether long-term substance use disorder, with its attendant neurological damage, interpersonal and cerebral trauma, and dysfunctional patterning of behavior, can produce personality disorders that persist beyond periods of use. There is little evidence on this issue, though long-term follow-up studies tend to show a normal range of personalities among those who are in recovery.

Secondary Substance Abuse Models

According to these models, increased comorbidity could be due to mental disorders causing some cases of substance use disorders, again perhaps in vulnerable individuals. These causal relationships could be driven by self-medication, general dysphoria, supersensitivity, or secondary psychosocial effects.

The *self-medication hypothesis* states that people with psychiatric illnesses use substances (and develop substance use disorders) in pharmacologically specific ways to ameliorate the symptoms of their mental disorders. In general, the evidence supporting the self-medication hypothesis is weak for most psychiatric disorders. That is, people with particular disorders or particular symptoms do not in general select specific substances for their specific pharmacological impact on those disorders or symptoms. In fact, many individuals seem to select drugs that exacerbate their symptoms and illnesses (e.g., schizophrenia patients who use cocaine). Somewhat stronger evidence exists for the anxiety disorders. For example, among individuals who develop both posttraumatic stress disorder and an alcohol use disorder, the posttraumatic stress disorder tends to precede the alcohol disorder and alcohol use appears to be motivated in part by its anxiolytic effects. There is also some evidence that nicotine use has an ameliorative effect on the attentional deficits that characterize many cases of schizophrenia, although nicotine use appears to be high for persons with all severe mental illnesses, not just those with schizophrenia.

The *general dysphoria theory* postulates a less specific motivation for substance use based on the historical observation that substance use tends to relieve many kinds of suffering, at least temporarily, and therefore people who suffer from unhappiness or pain of any kind, including loneliness, boredom, insomnia, physical trauma, medical illnesses, and psychiatric disorders, are generally predisposed to use psychoactive substances repeatedly, and therefore to develop addictions. In these situations, the short-term effects of many substances, such as anxiolytic, sedating, and anesthetic effects, can be reinforcing, even though the long-term effects actually worsen problems. This general mechanism of negative reinforcement probably obtains for many cases of substance use disorder and is probably what the general public refers to as "self-medication." People who have unhappy or painful lives are also prone to use substances to pursue the euphoric effects of the drugs—another mechanism that applies to many cases of substance use disorder. The notion that general dysphoria predisposes to substance use has little specific application to psychiatric disorders and hardly rises to the level of a theory. It may, however, account for the high predisposition to substance use disorders of all kinds among children and adolescents who develop early cases of chronic illnesses, including depression, anxiety, attention-deficit/hyperactivity disorder, and other psychiatric disorders.

The *supersensitivity model*, which has been applied mainly to psychotic disorders, posits that specific psychiatric disorders predispose individuals to be more sensitive to the effects of psychoactive substances on functioning, leading to their increased vulnerability to substance use problems that define the disorder. This model is unique in that it suggests that some of the increased comorbidity is not due to *greater amounts* of substance use in people with a psychiatric illness, but to *greater sensitivity* to the effects of relatively moderate or culturally normative substance use. The basis for the supersensitivity could be neurobiological, that is, related to the brain abnormalities that define mental disorders, but it could also be due to the marginal social, work, and self-care functioning of individuals with severe mental disorders that renders even modest deterioration in these areas problematic. Evidence supporting this hypothesis is mainly limited to schizophrenia. People with schizophrenia are less able to sustain moderate substance use over time without problems; "challenge tests" show high sensitivity to the effects of specific substances (e.g., small doses of stimulants or cannabis often precipitate episodes of severe symptoms); and individuals often develop substance use problems when using relatively low amounts of substances.

The *secondary psychosocial effects model* suggests that the cognitive, social, educational, vocational, housing, and economic consequences of mental illness may predispose people to substance misuse. Cognitive impairment, including difficulty planning ahead, may prevent people from anticipating the long-term consequences of substance use. Poor judgment related to cognitive difficulties leads to victimization of many kinds. The stigma of and poor functioning associated with mental illness may deprive individuals of many social opportunities, forcing them to develop social connections with other groups on the margins of society, including homeless, addicted, and antisocial persons. Low economic standing due to mental illness often results in people living in poor housing in neighborhoods where heavy and illicit substance use is the norm and drugs are readily obtainable. While it is established that social adversity contributes to increased substance use problems, limited research has attempted to disentangle the role of such adversity to the increased rate of substance use disorders in people with mental illness.

Common Factor Models

According to these models, another underlying variable independently increases risk for both mental illness and addiction, thereby increasing comorbidity. Underlying common variables could be genetic, neuro-cognitive, familial, social, or environmental. Genetic factors have been explored as a possible common factor, but the preponderance of evidence suggests that genetic vulnerability is disorder-specific, without increasing risk for other disorders except through associated comorbidity. ASPD (and its precursor conduct disorder) represents a neurocognitive dysfunction that has been proposed as a common factor that independently increases risk of developing schizophrenia and substance use disorder, and some data support this hypothesis. Severely abusive family or cultural environments, including torture and ethnic war, may be examples of stressful environments that predispose to psychiatric and substance use disorders. A variety of other potential common factors have been identified to explain the high comorbidity between substance use and severe mental disorders, including cognitive impairment (antedating onset of either disorder) and poverty, but few systematic attempts have been made to formally test these hypotheses.

Bidirectional Models

According to these models, different factors related to mental illness and substance abuse can contribute to the onset and maintenance of comorbid disorders. For example, a substance use disorder may trigger the onset of a psychotic disorder, with ongoing substance use maintained by the social facilitation afforded by use in social situations. Although research has documented the effects of substance abuse on psychiatric illness and vice versa, little research has examined these effects longitudinally, which is a prerequisite for a true test of a bidirectional model. One exception is research indicating that posttraumatic stress disorder is associated with the subsequent development of substance use disorders, which can in turn worsen the severity of posttraumatic stress disorder symptoms. Intuitively, bidirectional models are attractive because they take into account both the mutual effects that psychiatric and substance use disorders have on each other and the notion that these influences may change over time. These models are also the most difficult to test, which explains the relative paucity of relevant research.

Synopsis

A variety of models have been proposed to explain the high comorbidity of psychiatric and substance use disorders. Within each of the four meta-models described above, a number of specific models have been evaluated. No model has received strong support for explaining substance abuse comorbidity across the range of different psychiatric disorders. Researchers have therefore focused on specific relationships (e.g., secondary substance use disorders among people with posttraumatic stress disorders, schizophrenia that is possibly induced by cannabis use disorder).

The lack of strong support for any one specific model or a meta-model of comorbidity, either within a specific combination of comorbid disorders or across different types, points to the clinical challenges of preventing comorbid disorders and treating established comorbidity. No prevention or treatment program based on a single theory of comorbidity can be expected to be effective for the broad range of persons affected, even within a specific pair of comorbid disorders. Interventions based on etiological factors that underlie comorbid conditions may need to be individually tailored in order to address the possible range of different factors contributing to the onset and maintenance of comorbid disorders. The basic monolithic fact is that we understand relatively little about the etiologies of individual psychiatric and substance use disorders. Therefore accounting for comorbidity is a complex conundrum. Explaining the etiology of individual disorders more specifically through future research may have a profound effect on prevention and treatment.

Systemic Approaches

Despite universal agreement that treatment systems need to change in order to accommodate individuals with comorbid disorders, the exact form of a new system remains unclear. Two overarching systemic approaches have been proposed to guide the organization of interventions for persons with co-occurring disorders. Both of these models, the *integrated treatment model* and the *quadrant model*, address the organization of mental health and substance abuse services for the treatment of people with dual disorders.

Integrated Treatment Model

The integrated treatment model addresses the treatment of substance use disorders among people with severe mental disorders in public mental health settings, where the great majority of these individuals receive care due to federal and state funding. Research throughout the 1980s showed that despite the

Parallel (or sequential) treatment approaches proved ineffective.

high rate of substance use disorders in this population, detection was minimal and clinical management was ineffective in mental health treatment settings. The most common treatment approach was to refer individuals with comorbid substance use disorders to addiction treatment programs. However, such parallel (or sequential) treatment approaches proved ineffective, as many people did not follow through on treatment referrals (lacking sufficient motivation), and those who did frequently encountered either barriers to access (e.g., due to eligibility requirements) or stressful, confrontational treatment methods that precipitated dropouts from treatment. In contrast to parallel treatment, integrated treatment involves the same team of clinicians combining mental health and substance abuse treatments in the same setting to ensure access to coordinated care for both disorders. Various forms of integrated treatment have evolved steadily since the mid-1980s to address the problem of poor detection and management of substance use disorders among people with severe mental disorders in mental health treatment settings.

Variants of the integrated treatment model share a fundamental commitment to concurrent provision of mental health and substance abuse services by the same team of clinicians in the same setting. In addition, they usually include assertive outreach to engage reluctant persons in treatment, stage-wise motivation-based treatment, comprehensive services, long-term commitment, and an emphasis on minimizing the harmful effects of substance use. A variety of interventions are typically offered in integrated treatment programs including individual, group, family, residential, and pharmacological modalities.

Research on the integrated treatment model has focused almost exclusively on adults with severe mental illnesses, with more than 30 controlled studies. Many of these studies have significant methodological limitations, but several randomized controlled trials plus some quasi-experimental studies permit some tentative conclusions. First, people receiving integrated treatment for their dual disorders tend to have better substance abuse outcomes than individuals receiving traditional parallel or sequential treatment. Second, different service models for integrating treatment (such as different case management models) tend to produce similar positive results. Third, brief interventions based on motivational interviewing are associated with better substance abuse outcomes for some individuals, although results are mixed. Fourth, group interventions have been the most widely studied psychotherapeutic modality, with the preponderance of results favoring cognitive-behavioral approaches. Fifth, a significant proportion of individuals with dual disorders seem to require long-term residential interventions. Sixth, despite general support for the overall concept of integrating treatment, the critical components of effective integrated treatment programs remain uncertain.

Note that the integrated treatment model is silent about services for individuals with co-occurring disorders in non-mental health settings, such as in primary care, substance abuse, and criminal justice settings, where co-occurring disorders encompass the less severe psychiatric disorders, typically a combination of mood, anxiety, and personality disorders. Though some studies have indicated that adding mental health counseling within these settings can improve outcomes, there has been minimal consensus on how to address co-occurrence in these settings and even less research on specific care models. Several approaches to concurrent mental health and substance abuse services have been proposed, including not only team-based approaches but also various forms of collaboration and referral, but thus far there is little research on their effectiveness or clinical consensus on how to transform care in these non-mental health settings. Administrators and clinicians in substance abuse treatment settings have suggested that programs might be categorized as addiction only, dual diagnosis capable, or dual diagnosis enhanced, based on training, resources, and capabilities. This approach assumes that not all programs need to be able to provide mental health treatments on site and that efficiency might occur with some specialization. Though these categories do capture the capabilities of current addictions programs, there is as yet no research to support the effectiveness of such a division of labor.

The fundamental issue for non-mental health programs is the absence of validated models of clinical effectiveness. It may be premature to prescribe a system model until effective clinical models are available. Nonetheless, encouraging programs and clinicians to attend to co-occurrence seems likely to spawn clinical approaches and outcomes research, and hence lead to research and valid clinical models.

Quadrant Model

The quadrant model presents a heuristic framework for conceptualizing different subgroups of persons with co-occurring disorders in terms of the severity of each disorder. Four different subgroups are proposed, corresponding to combinations of high and low severity of mental illness and substance abuse. The working hypothesis of the quadrant model is that individuals who differ in the severity of their addictions and mental illnesses have different treatment needs, and consequently should receive treatment in different settings. The quadrant model proposes organizing treatment services to meet the different needs of persons in each quadrant. For example, one approach based on the framework suggests that different levels of service (consultation, collaboration, or integration) should be provided depending on the extent of the treatment need:

Quadrant I (low severity of both substance abuse and mental illness) services are found in primary health care settings and typically involve a *consultation model* (i.e., substance abuse or mental health experts are consulted as needed).

Quadrant II (low severity of substance abuse; high severity of mental illness) services are found primarily in mental health settings, and may involve either a *collaboration model*, where related but autonomous substance abuse and mental health service providers work in tandem, or an *integrated model*, where services are blended within a single team of providers. Collaborative versus integrated models of care are determined by severity (i.e., the more severe, the more integrated treatment is indicated).

Quadrant III (high severity of substance abuse; low severity of mental illness) services are found primarily in addiction treatment settings, and may again involve either a collaboration model (an addiction treatment agency working in tandem with a mental health provider) or an integrated model (services for the comorbid disorders are blended within a single team or agency).

Quadrant IV (high severity of both substance abuse and mental illness) services are typically provided in state hospitals, jails/prisons, and emergency rooms and may utilize providers in either the mental health or addiction treatment delivery system. It is for persons in Quadrant IV for whom the integrated service model is hypothesized to be most indicated.

The quadrant model has been proposed to conceptualize the service needs of the broad population of persons with co-occurring disorders, but it has not been empirically validated. As a simple heuristic, it does draw attention to the wide diversity of individuals with comorbid disorders, their diverse needs, and the diverse treatment settings in which they receive care. This goal appeals to policy planners because they are appropriately concerned about improving services for all individuals with comorbid disorders, not just those with severe mental disorders. Beyond its intuitive appeal, however, the quadrant model breaks down immediately when it is applied to routine clients or treatment settings. The four categories of service recipients do not correspond to valid treatment approaches; a majority of individuals shift categories over time; the clinical groups do not appear consistently in the proposed service settings; there is no research (other than the research on integrated treatment for individuals with severe mental disorders cited above) to indicate that they should receive services in the proposed settings; and clinicians in these settings are faced with diverse populations. In other words, although the quadrant model does focus administrators' attention on the diverse service needs of individuals with co-occurring disorders, it suffers a lack of empirical support.

Synopsis

Both the integrated treatment model and the quadrant model identify the need for closer integration of services for individuals with the highest levels of severity. This convergence reflects a clinical truism that individuals whose lives have been severely disorganized by two or more severe and persistent illnesses are more likely to need help in accessing, combining, and maintaining connections to services. The argument and related empirical supports extend to services beyond mental health and substance abuse treatments (e.g., to housing, general medical care, vocational training). Beyond this point the two models diverge because of the lack of empirical support for the quadrant model.

Rather than starting with hypothetical clinical groups with unrealistic stability and treatment settings with imaginary homogeneity, a more useful approach to system reform might begin with the clinical realities of current treatment settings, which are firmly entrenched by current financial, administrative, professional, and training structures, and build a series of systemic models based on the evidentiary base as it develops. Following this approach, existing clinical programs might be modified steadily to reflect clinical needs and our understandings of effective treatments. For example, since surveys show that addiction treatment programs are filled with individuals who suffer from non-severe comorbid mental disorders, especially anxiety, mood, and personality disorders, researchers, policymakers, and administrators should consider how these programs would need to be modified to provide adequate assessment and treatment for the clients they are actually serving. If the empirical models that emerge involve close integration of mental health treatments for some types of comorbidity, efforts should be made to provide such expertise. If, on the other hand, research shows that other types of linkage, such as a visiting mental health specialist or referral to a mental health specialist, are warranted for certain types of co-occurrence, these arrangements could be established as systemic goals. On parallel tracks, systemic goals could be developed for other treatment settings, such as jails/prisons and primary care settings.

Comorbid Disorders in Adolescents

Recent increased attention on adolescent mental health and substance use disorders has led to new findings that illuminate similarities with and differences from adults with comorbid disorders. Unlike adults, the majority of youth are referred for substance abuse services from juvenile justice agencies, schools, or families. The overall prevalence of adolescents with comorbid disorders and their negative impact is similar to that for adults, but youth present with very different developmental, cognitive, and social needs; risks; strengths; and symptom profiles.

Youth referred for substance abuse treatment report high levels of delinquency and acute victimization/past trauma that often go unidentified and untreated. Principles emerging for the treatment of youth with co-occurring disorders suggest the necessity to build a quick therapeutic alliance; administer and repeat age-appropriate comprehensive assessment; include family and/or legal guardians; utilize motivational, behavioral, and family-based interventions; and continue assertive engagement to address the chronic nature of symptoms and long-term recovery periods.

Comprehensive Repeated Assessment

For youth, a fluid conceptualization of comorbidity is especially necessary due to the strong influence of developmental and environmental factors. Table 8.1 summarizes a few fundamental differences between youth and adults with comorbid disorders.

Critical to our understanding comorbidity in youth is an evaluation of resiliency (connections to support, competencies, positive view of self and future, expectations), the strengths and risk factors, symptoms, and impairment across family, culture, school, community, peer relations, criminal justice, and work environments. The evaluation and treatment of youth needs to be multidimensional and include collateral information from external supports (e.g., parents, teachers, coaches), with frequent reassessment to refine treatment as needed. In general, parents/guardians are more accurate reporters of youth emotional and behavioral symptoms, while youth are more accurate reporters of their own substance use. Youth, compared to adults, are said to be opportunistic in their use of substances, and hence seem to change between substance dependence and abuse for particular substances according

TABLE 8.1. Differences between Adults and Youth with Comorbid Disorders

Category	Youth	Adults
• Family	• More family involvement	• Less family involvement
• Developmental	• Invincible and concrete	• Vulnerable and abstract
• Typical substance abuse and mental health presentation	• Substance abuse/ dependence and behavioral health	• Substance dependence and serious mental health
• Groups	• Potential harmful influence	• Foundational support
• Abstinence perspective	• Sobriety is for adults	• Sobriety: an option
• Consequences	• About "getting caught"	• Bottoming-out process
• Life perspective	• Lack of past knowledge and possible future	• Experience informs choice
• Resiliency and recovery	• Increase resiliency: monitor, model, and motivate to build assets and decrease risk	• Support recovery: empower existing and new coping skills
• Mandated requirements	• Family, school, and juvenile justice system	• Criminal justice system
• Motivation	• Externally motivated	• Internally motivated
• Pattern of use	• Opportunistic use	• Drug of choice

to what and how much is available. Child and family psychologists use the term "ecologically contextual" to describe the strong interaction between youth expression of symptoms with their environmental setting and context.

Prevalence

Prevalence of comorbid disorders in youth referred to mental health, substance abuse, or juvenile justice institutions vary depending on system-level factors (e.g., referral/access to the setting, level of care, and assessment techniques) and client-level factors (e.g., gender, race). Community samples of substance-abusing adolescents report high rates of co-occurrence (60%), with the most common psychiatric conditions being disruptive behavior disorders, especially conduct disorder; depression; anxiety; and attention-deficit/hyperactivity disorder. Studies have also found that conduct disorder is associated with earlier onset of substance use and abuse, in line with other research showing that ASPD (of which conduct disorder is a required precursor) is associated with an earlier onset of addiction.

Comorbidity *within* psychiatric disorders, as well as *between* mental and substance use disorders, for youth is high, with about 45% of youth having both internalizing and externalizing disorders. The complexity of problems is illustrated by the fact that youth with comorbid disorders report high levels of vicitimization as well as high levels of criminal behaviors. Rates of comorbidity tend to be higher among girls referred for substance abuse treatment or in juvenile justice settings, which may be related to the lower rate of substance misuse in girls as well as the lower rate of referral for treatment of girls with substance use problems compared to boys with similar problems. Youth with comorbid disorders who are referred to outpatient treatment reported the most problems with (1) substance use, (2) criminal activities, (3) trauma experience, and (4) family environment.

Negative Impact of Comorbidity

Similar to adults, youth who present with comorbid disorders have poorer treatment outcomes than those who present with a single disorder. It has been hypothesized that untreated mental illness makes it more difficult to engage an adolescent in treatment, resulting in poor retention in substance abuse treatment. In addition, externalizing disorders such as conduct disorder and attention-deficit/hyperactivity disorder are characterized by a lack of control over impulses, which naturally make substance abuse treatment more challenging, even when the disorder is recognized. Depression is less likely to remit with sobriety in adolescents than in depressed adults with chronic alcohol or drug dependence. In addition, research indicates that treatment of psychiatric disorders alone does not tend to improve substance abuse in adolescents with comorbid disorders.

Victimization is consistently correlated with increased comorbid psychiatric and substance use disorders, as well as with negative peer and family influence, HIV risk behaviors, health problems, and mental problems. The findings are in line with those for adults, involving a cycle of trauma and posttraumatic reactions leading to substance misuse, which then increases subsequent victimization and worsening of psychiatric, social, and health adjustment. This apparent cycle also suggests that early intervention designed to address the psychological effects of victimization (or even to prevent it?) could prevent substance use problems that culminate in complex comorbid disorders.

Prevention Opportunities

The early onset of mental health disorders predicts school failure, teen childbearing, early marriage and divorce, adult relationship violence, and adult economic instability. The failure to treat these problems represents an important lost opportunity for the prevention of subsequent substance use disorders. Research findings now clearly support more investigation into the efficacy of early mental and behavioral interventions as prevention for thwarting the onset of adolescent substance disorders. Data from multiple studies document that the age of onset of mental disorders in adolescents is several years younger than the age of onset of substance use disorders.

Early treatment of mental and behavioral health childhood disorders supports the secondary substance abuse meta-model (e.g., the secondary psychosocial effects and self-medication models). Studies of the early use of stimulant therapy for children diagnosed and medicated for attention-deficit/hyperactivity disorder and the early treatment of anxiety suggest preventative effects. The youth treated at a young age reported fewer days of substance use and fewer consequences of use. To capture the preventative effect, mental health counselors and/or researchers will need to extend follow-up periods beyond the typical 1- to 3-year outcome periods and add substance use measures.

Treatment for Comorbid Disorders in Youth

Several recent published articles based on separate evaluations of substance abuse and mental health interventions now illustrate "best practice" principles for the effective treatment of youth with comorbid disorders. Unlike treatment models for adults with severe mental illness and substance use problems, no specific treatment models for youth with comorbid disorders have been rigorously evaluated, but data do indicate what is not successful and suggest what could be most effective. Similar to adults, there is little evidence to support the use of *sequential treatment models* for adolescents, and in fact it is likely contraindicated.

The *parallel or simultaneous model* of treatment for youth is the most commonly used approach for comorbid disorders. Community and residential programs often deliver mental health and substance abuse services by separate staff with different licensure. By their very nature, the success of parallel programs depends on communication, collaboration, coordination, and timing of interventions across settings and staff, regardless of the location or colocation of services. The most typical example is when one provider recognizes a need in substance or mental health and refers for that treatment in another location. The effectiveness of this approach, as compared to more fully integrated treatment, remains to be determined.

Integrated treatment for youth, like that for adults, assumes that communication, collaboration, and coordination of interventions is purest when one agency and a single cross-trained staff deliver the majority of services. No large-sample comparison studies of an integrated treatment for youth with comorbid disorders exist, but recent studies of comprehensive adolescent interventions have helped to shape this practice model, which includes intensive services (weekly or two to three meetings per week, for 12–24 weeks); small therapist-to-client ratios (1:6); community- and home-based delivery of services; family involvement (parent behavior training); the use of one accountable care manager and/or therapist; 24-hour availability to each family; psychiatrist for medication evaluation/management; and stage-wise interventions using combinations of cognitive-behavioral, motivational, and family therapy.

Two integrated evidenced-based practices, multisystemic therapy (MST) and multidimensional family therapy (MDFT), have potential application to this population of youth, and each is designed for specific targeted populations. MST is designed to treat youth involved in the juvenile justice system, and MDFT is designed to treat youth with substance abuse disorders. Both of these models use a home-based service delivery model and have a family focus for treatment. Both models have reported positive outcomes in long-term reductions of substance use, family problems, and delinquent behavior. Similarly, positive outcomes have also been reported in several studies for youth with co-occurring disorders when cognitive-behavioral interventions are used in adolescents with depression and substance abuse.

Synopsis

Youth who enter the substance abuse treatment system typically present with a complex symptom picture that most often includes a combination of internalizing and externalizing disorders. Intervention models are needed that monitor and teach skills for coping and changing the interactive nature of multiple emotional and behavioral symptoms, including substance use. There are few controlled studies evaluating standardized models of care or providing guidance for treatment matching of youth with comorbid disorders. Perhaps most importantly, the failure to treat emotional and behavioral disorders soon after they appear in youth represents a potential missed opportunity for the prevention of subsequent substance use problems that follow in the wake of mental illness.

Failure to treat emotional and behavioral disorders soon after they appear in youth represents a missed opportunity for the prevention of subsequent substance use problems.

Robust Principles

1. Comorbidity of mental health and substance use disorders is high in the general population, and even higher in persons receiving treatment for either disorder, with rates upwards of 50%.
2. The co-occurrence of mental health and substance use disorders worsens the course of both illnesses and compromises treatment response compared to either disorder alone.
3. There is no single explanation that sufficiently accounts for why comorbid disorders occur more often than would be expected by chance alone, either across all disorders or within a subgroup, including the "self-medication hypothesis."
4. High substance abuse comorbidity in people with schizophrenia is partly explained by their increased sensitivity to the effects of substances, while increased alcohol abuse in people with anxiety problems is partly related to the anxiolytic effects of alcohol.
5. Traditional treatment approaches for comorbid disorders that involve providing separate mental health and substance abuse treatments have met with limited success.
6. Integrated treatment models that combine mental health and substance abuse interventions have empirical support for persons with severe mental illness, but have not been adequately tested for persons with mood, anxiety, or personality disorders.
7. Youth with emotional or substance use problems have very high rates of comorbid disorders, which are often combined with multiple other life challenges, including trauma, family instability, school problems, and involvement in the juvenile justice system.
8. Standardized programs for treating comorbid disorders in youth have not yet been empirically validated.
9. Early intervention in the course of mental illness or substance use problems, both in youth and adults, has the potential for preventing the development of comorbid disorders and their untoward effects on people's lives.

Suggested Readings

Babor, T. F., Hesselbrock, V., Meyer, R. E., & Shoemaker, W. (Eds.). (1994). Types of alcoholics: Evidence from clinical, experimental, and genetic research. *Annals of the New York Academy of Sciences, 708,* 1–258.

Blanchard, J. J. (Ed.). (2000). Special issue: The co-occurrence of substance use in other mental disorders. *Clinical Psychology Review, 20*(2), 145–287.

Center for Substance Abuse Treatment. (2002). *Assessment and treatment of patients with co-existing mental illness and alcohol and other drug abuse.* Rockville, MD: Author.

Centre for Addiction and Mental Health. (2001). *Best practices: Concurrent mental health and substance use disorders.* Ottawa: Health Canada.

Donald, M., Dower, J., & Kavanagh, D. J. (2005). Integrated versus nonintegrated management and care for clients with co-occurring mental health and substance use disorders: A qualitative systematic review of randomised controlled trials. *Social Science and Medicine, 60,* 1371–1383.

Drake, R. E., Mueser, K. T., Brunette, M. F., & McHugo, G. J. (2004). A review of treatments for clients with severe mental illness and co-occurring substance use disorder. *Psychiatric Rehabilitation Journal, 27,* 360–374.

Kaminer, Y. (2004). Dually diagnosed teens: Challenges for assessment and treatment. *Counselor: The Magazine for Addiction Professionals, 5*(2), 62–68.

Kessler, R. C., Crum, R. M., Warner, L. A., Nelson, C. B., Schulenberg, J., & Anthony, J. C. (1997). Lifetime co-occurrence of DSM-III-R alcohol abuse and dependence with other psychiatric disorders in the National Comorbidity Survey. *Archives of General Psychiatry, 54,* 313–321.

Mueser, K., Drake, R., & Wallach, M. (1998). Dual diagnosis: A review of etiological theories. *Addictive Behaviors, 23,* 717–734.

Mueser, K. T., Noordsy, D. L., Drake, R. E., & Fox, L. (2003). *Integrated treatment for dual disorders: A guide to effective practice.* New York: Guilford Press.

Nunes, E. V., & Levin, F. R. (2004). Treatment of depression in patients with alcohol or other drug dependence: A meta-analysis. *Journal of the American Medical Association, 291,* 1887–1896.

Regier, D. A., Farmer, M. E., Rae, D. S., Locke, B. Z., Keith, S. J., Judd, L. L., et al. (1990). Comorbidity of mental disorders with alcohol and other drug abuse: Results from the Epidemiologic Catchment Area (ECA) study. *Journal of the American Medical Association, 264,* 2511–2518.

Riggs, P. (2003). Treating adolescents for substance abuse and comorbid psychiatric disorders. *Science and Practice Perspectives, 2,* 18–32.

Sacks, S., & Ries, R. K. (Eds.). (2005). *Substance abuse treatment for persons with co-occurring disorders: A treatment improvement protocol (TIP)* (DHHS Pub. No. [SMA] 05-3992). Rockville, MD: U.S. Department of Health and Human Services, Substance Abuse and Mental Health Services Administration, Center for Substance Abuse Treatment.

CHAPTER 9

Motivational Factors in Addictive Behaviors

WILLIAM R. MILLER

Addiction is fundamentally a problem of motivation. That is my central thesis, and I hasten to clarify what I do *not* mean in stating it. I do not mean to say that addictive behavior is merely the result of people being unmotivated and therefore morally blameworthy, nor do I mean that it's all a matter of effort and willpower. Neither do I mean to dismiss the substantial biological aspects of addiction so capably addressed in other chapters in this volume. Quite to the contrary, the neuroscience of addiction points precisely to central systems of reinforcement and motivation.

What I do mean to say is that the troubles we summarize within the rubric of "addiction" are well understood as a function of potent motivations, and often of competing motivations that are mirrored in subjective experiences such as craving, broken resolutions, restraint, resisting temptation, compulsion, and impaired control. I believe that a motivational understanding of addiction also helps us to make sense of puzzling behavioral phenomena as diverse as cyclic relapse, reactance, response to brief intervention, jury verdicts, psychotherapy processes, and transformational change of the variety observed in Alcoholics Anonymous (AA).

Motivation as Intrapersonal

Perhaps the most common way to think about motivation is as an intrapersonal trait or force, something that resides within the individual. Clients may be judged as "highly motivated" or "unmotivated" for change. Indeed, as discussed later, measures of personal motivation are often good predictors of subsequent behavior change, or lack thereof.

Psychometric Constructs

The addiction field has no shortage of ways for measuring intrapersonal motivation. A common approach for measuring motivation is through paper-and-pencil questionnaires, some of which have well-established psychometric properties. Clinicians also assess motivation via structured or unstructured interviews. Motivational constructs for which there are reliable measures include (1) craving, urges, and temptation; (2) decisional balance, pros and cons; (3) desire or willingness; (4) expectancies for the positive and negative effects of a drug; (5) intention or readiness to change; (6) perceived need or importance of change; (7) problem recognition; (8) perceived ability or self-efficacy for change; and (9) stages of change. These are far from interchangeable dimensions that load on a single latent factor of motivation. Knowing an individual's position on one of these scales reveals relatively little about his or her position on the others. Motivation does not seem to be a single trait or even a fluid internal state that can be measured for depth. Instead what we mean by "motivation" seems to be comprised of multiple, loosely interrelated subjective phenomena that are primarily measured via self-report.

Inference from Natural Language

If motivation is a term of speech that refers loosely to multiple dimensions, and if verbal self-report is the typical means for ascertaining it, then one option is to study the natural language that is used to request, negotiate, and agree to change. From what forms of speech do people judge each other's level of motivation for and probability of action? In other words, how do we predict (or at least develop expectations about) what other people will do? Psycholinguistic studies indicate that people communicate and judge the probability of action from *committing language*, specific speech acts that signal various levels of intention. Strength of commitment or intention predicts behavior, albeit imperfectly. In turn, commitment strength is predictable from expressions of desire, ability, reasons, and need for change. These are probably the same verbal cues that clinicians use in judging client motivation for change.

Inference from Behavior

Motivation is also inferred from observed behavior. In animal research, this is necessarily so: behavioral scientists measure motivation by attending to variables such as activity level, frequency of bar presses, and persistence despite aversive consequences. People similarly infer level of human motivation from observed levels of effort (e.g., trying), performance of requested actions (e.g., adherence, compliance), and persistence (e.g., retention). Confidence in motivation is increased when speech acts and behavior converge ("walking the talk"). These are all proxies for change, motivational markers that signal the probability of subsequent behavior. Finally, motivation is sometimes judged retrospectively from behavior change itself: if the person stopped drinking, he or she must have been motivated. Here the inference becomes completely circular.

Motivation for What?

No one is unmotivated. The question is what a person is motivated *for*, what he or she values, what reinforcers are effective for him or her. In human discourse, discussions of motivation often emerge in the context of competing goals: the desire of one person (e.g., a counselor) for a particular change or outcome is not shared by another person (e.g., a client).

Motivation is therefore necessarily judged with regard to a *particular* action or outcome. The transtheoretical stages of change, for example, are measured in relation to a specific behavior or goal. A person's level of motivation (e.g., desire, self-efficacy, readiness, problem recognition) is action-specific. A person might be quite motivated for change but not for treatment, or for one form of treatment but not another. Polydrug users commonly show levels of motivation (e.g., stages of change) that differ depending upon the drug. A client might be highly motivated (in the action stage) to quit cocaine, considering cutting down drinking (in the contemplation stage), and uninterested in quitting tobacco (in the precontemplation stage).

Finally, it is worth noting the absence of scientific support for popular beliefs that people with substance use disorders have a distinct "addictive" personality, or manifest abnormally high trait levels of immature defense mechanisms such as denial and projection. Such attributions of low motivation to intrapersonal pathology are unfounded and countertherapeutic stereotypes. People with alcohol/

drug problems and dependence are widely distributed on nearly all personality characteristics, and are as richly variable as the rest of humanity.

Summary

Intrapersonal motivation appears to be a fluid state, specific to particular goals and methods for achieving them. It is multidimensional rather than unitary in structure, with modest intercorrelations among measured dimensions. Subjective motivational states are inferred from psychometric instruments, natural language, and behavior, again with modest correlations across these sources of data.

Motivation as Interpersonal

If denial and low motivation for change are not intrapersonal traits of people with substance use disorders, then what does influence their motivation? There is substantial evidence that a person's strength of motivation for change in substance use is strongly influenced by interpersonal factors. In this way, motivation can be thought of as both an interpersonal and an intrapersonal process.

Therapist Effects

One indication of interpersonal influence on motivation is the frequent presence of therapist effects in substance abuse intervention research. When clients are randomly assigned to counselors in the same program or using the same treatment, often one of the strongest predictors of client motivation (retention, adherence, behavior change) is the counselor to whom they were assigned. Treatment dropout, often regarded as an indication of poor client motivation, tends to be differentially distributed among treatment staff. In randomized trials, a single follow-up phone call or handwritten note after an intake interview doubled the percentage of clients returning for a second session.

What accounts for these differences among counselors in patient retention and outcome? One robust predictor is the therapeutic skill of accurate empathy, as defined by Carl Rogers in person-centered counseling. The more a counselor listens to clients and can accurately reflect their meaning, the better that counselor's clients fare in treatment outcome. This is so even when the treatment approach is behavioral in focus. It matters how a counselor interacts with clients. Another study found that doctors' rates of dropout were predictable from the doctor's tone of voice when talking about alcoholic patients: the more anger in the doctor's voice, the higher the patient dropout rate. In still other studies, a relatively brief period of empathic counseling dramatically increased the rate of return for substance abuse treatment among emergency room patients presenting with alcohol-related injuries and problems. Something important happens between counselor and client that can substantially increase or decrease motivation for change.

Commitment

By definition, much that happens in "talk therapy" involves language. It is through verbal transactions that people normally request and agree to change. Psycholinguistic analyses of such transactions have identified at least five themes that occur in behavior change conversations, reflecting (1) desire, (2) ability, (3) reasons, (4) need, and (5) commitment to change. Of these, only committing language seems to predict subsequent behavior change. To say that one wants to, could, has reasons for, or needs to change is not to make a commitment to do so. A cognitive psychology literature on implementation intentions similarly indicates that behavior change is facilitated when an individual verbalizes a clear intention and a specific plan.

> *To say that one wants to, could, has reasons for, or needs to change is not to make a commitment to do so.*

Such commitment is usually negotiated in the context of interpersonal conversation. Successful negotiation emerges from a match between (1) the requester's level of demand and magnitude of change, and (2) the level of willingness of the one from whom change is requested. When the requester's level of demand and change exceeds the other's range of willingness, both parties usually leave the transaction dissatisfied and change negotiation fails.

Motivational Interviewing

Consistent with these findings is the outcome literature for motivational interviewing, a person-centered goal-oriented approach for facilitating change through exploring and resolving ambivalence. Clinical trials with a wide range of populations and problems have supported the efficacy of this interviewing method, which was originally designed to facilitate change in problem drinking. Typically offered in one to four sessions, motivational interviewing focuses on evoking the client's own statements of intrinsic desire, ability, reasons, need, and ultimately commitment to change. Ambivalence is conceptualized as a principal obstacle, and the method focuses on helping the client to decide about and commit to change. It appears that once the person has made this commitment, change often proceeds apace without additional intervention. When used as a prelude to other interventions, motivational interviewing has shown synergistic effectiveness.

Intervening through Family Members

The family is an important natural source of interpersonal influence. It is now abundantly clear from research that an individual's motivation for changing substance abuse can be enhanced by unilateral intervention through concerned significant others, usually close family members such as a spouse or parent. An early form of unilateral family intervention with "unmotivated" problem drinkers was pioneered by the Johnson Institute. Family members were prepared for a group meeting to confront the individual with the negative consequences of his or her substance use, and to trigger entry into treatment. A consistent problem with this approach is that up to 80% of families find the confrontational meeting unacceptable and refuse to go through with it. Among those families who complete an intervention, however, a high percentage of their loved ones do enter treatment.

Several other approaches have been developed for helping family members whose loved ones refuse to change or seek help for substance abuse. One of these, the 12-step Al-Anon program, provides mutual peer support for family members, advising self-care and "loving detachment" that avoids efforts to change the loved one. Studies indicate that family members themselves benefit from involvement in Al-Anon groups, with decreased distress, depression, negative emotions, and health problems. Family involvement in Al-Anon does not, however, significantly increase treatment engagement for the loved one. This is unsurprising, because efforts to change the loved one are specifically discouraged in Al-Anon.

In contrast, unilateral family counseling approaches have been successful both in relieving family distress and in engaging a high percentage (usually two-thirds to three-fourths) of substance-abusing loved ones in treatment. Here a professional counselor helps family members to learn strategies for decreasing their loved one's substance use and for initiating treatment. In an approach conceptually opposite to Al-Anon, family members are counseled that they can have substantial influence on their loved one, and are taught how to use principles of behavior change. Even when the loved one does not enter treatment, family members have reported substantial reduction in substance use and problems after such unilateral counseling.

Summary

To a significant extent, motivation for change is transactional, reflected in and affected by interpersonal interaction. In natural discourse, change is negotiated in dynamic processes for requesting and committing to action. Motivation for change appears to be enhanced by an empathic, accepting facilitator, rather than by high demand and confrontation. Significant others can also reinforce or deter change through the interpersonal influence inherent in close relationships. Reaching a decision and making a commitment may be a final common pathway to change, having both intrapersonal and interpersonal components.

> *Motivation for change appears to be enhanced by an empathic, accepting facilitator, rather than by high demand and confrontation.*

Motivation as Contextual

Motivation also occurs in context. Sitting one-to-one with a client in a consulting room, the therapist naturally searches for intrapersonal determinants of motivation, or perhaps looks to the client's closest relationships for motivational keys or obstacles. But there is a much larger social–environmental context within which the person lives, the impact of which is easily underestimated by therapist and client alike.

Norms

Perhaps the most common motivational obstacle to early behavior change or help seeking is the perception that one does not "have a problem" serious enough to warrant change. In the language of the transtheoretical model, this is characteristic of individuals in the precontemplation or contemplation stage, which is where roughly 80% of those with substance use disorders can be found at any given time. People compare their own substance use to that of people around them, or to perceived norms. If they find no discrepancy—for example, if heavy drinking is normative rather than sanctioned in the person's reference group—change is unlikely to occur. In a common phenomenon known as the *false consensus effect*, people tend to perceive their own behavior as falling within and often below social norms. Judgments about how much drinking is "normal" are strongly related to the person's own volume of alcohol consumption: the more a person drinks, the more he or she is likely to overestimate normal levels of drinking in the general population or reference group (and vice versa). This can be understood as self-serving defensive perception: people justify their own behavior by inflating the norms against which they compare themselves. This may be true, but causality clearly works in the other direction as well: permissive norms favor increased use.

Several factors are likely to promote norm inflation. First, salient behavior attracts differential attention. Modeling studies have demonstrated that it is the heaviest drinker at a table who tends to set the pace. Adding one heavy drinker (confederate) tends to increase the average alcohol consumption of others at the same table, whereas adding a moderate drinker exerts little or no effect on others' drinking. A minority of visible smokers in a school attract differential attention, inflating norm perceptions. As substance use progresses, people also tend to gravitate toward peers who use at a similar or higher rate. Smokers associate with smokers, heavy drinkers with heavier drinkers, promoting a consensus of higher use norms. Insulation from corrective feedback and from negative consequences (sometimes called "enabling") can further deter problem recognition.

Self-regulation theory emphasizes the comparison of status against standards, of behavior against norms. When no discrepancy is perceived, no need for change is apparent. A detected discrepancy of current status (or behavior) with norms or goals, however, triggers a search for change options. If an acceptable and accessible option is found, behavior change may be initiated. (There is a direct parallel here with the precontemplation, contemplation, preparation, and action stages of the transtheoretical model of change.) This is the conceptual basis for norm correction interventions. Feedback regarding actual use norms has been found to reduce use among heavier drinkers (who also tend to have inflated norm perceptions), and also shows promising effects in primary prevention applications.

Obstacles

Relatively straightforward practical matters can be substantial obstacles to change. In one study, for example, the best predictor of clients' attendance at aftercare sessions was the distance they had to travel in order to reach the meetings.

Anticipating and surmounting such barriers can enhance steps toward change. In another study, placing a referral call and scheduling an appointment while the client was still in the office doubled the likelihood of completing the referral, as compared with giving the client the telephone number to call him- or herself. In a randomized trial, clients were either encouraged to attend AA or linked with an AA member who offered to transport and accompany them to a meeting. The corresponding percentages of clients attending a first AA meeting were zero and 100%.

Contingencies

Another potent contextual factor is found in social contingencies for nonuse, use, and heavier use of substances. Certain drugs of abuse, particularly stimulants, provide primary reinforcement through direct stimulation of reinforcement channels in the brain. Mammals will self-administer such drugs when given free access to them. Beyond the reinforcement inherent in drug use, social contingencies can also reinforce or diminish use. Even severely alcohol-dependent or cocaine-dependent individuals can and do moderate or refrain from use of available alcohol or cocaine in response to such contingencies. At a societal level, drug use is curtailed by social norms and policies that sanction and increase the cost of use. Easy access and low response cost (e.g., an "open bar" at a reception) tend to increase use.

Summary

Instigation to change is triggered by a perceived discrepancy between present and desired states. Social norms and influences affect an individual's judgment regarding the range of states that are ideal, desirable, and acceptable. Deviation from this range may trigger intrapersonal motivation for change as well as social sanctions and pressure for change. In seeking change, people also encounter practical situations and social contingencies that may facilitate or hinder the change process.

Predicting Change

Increasing motivation for change is seldom an end in itself. Motivational factors are of interest presumably because they predict and influence future behavior. An intervention that increases scores on a measure of motivation without impacting behavior would usually be of little interest to clinicians or makers of social policy.

Indeed, one way to operationalize motivation is as behavior probability. A "motivational" intervention is one that actually alters the probability of subsequent behavior. This is the pragmatic operant definition of reinforcement or punishment. Something is not a reinforcer *unless* when applied in contingent fashion is does increase behavior probability. This means that what constitutes a reinforcer (or motivator) will vary across individuals, time, and dependent measures (behaviors to be modified).

What is the target behavior for motivational interventions? An obvious target is substance use itself, but motivational principles can also be used to encourage proximal behaviors likely to lead to reductions in substance use. One strategy for changing a target behavior is to modify such intervening steps. Self-control is sometimes described as engaging in specific behaviors *in order to* modify others. Motivational strategies have been used successfully to increase treatment initiation, attendance, and retention, and to support adherence to change strategies. Social support can also be mobilized to increase adherence with intermediate steps toward reaching a goal, as in "buddy" systems where partners commit to exercise together at a particular time and place.

Relatedly, one of the more consistent predictors of successful change in substance abuse is adherence to change efforts. The more treatment sessions or 12-step meetings a person attends, the better the outcome. The more faithfully a person takes a prescribed medication to reduce substance use, the greater the reduction (even, in one study, when the medication was a placebo). The more a person is taking active steps toward making change, whether prescribed or not, the more likely change is to occur and be maintained.

Another reasonably reliable predictor of change is self-efficacy. More successful changers are those who believe that there are effective ways to accomplish change (general efficacy) and that they themselves are able to make use of them (self-efficacy). Responses to the question "How likely are you to remain abstinent for the next month?" are fairly good markers of the actual probability.

Self-reported motivation for change also predicts behavioral outcomes. Paper-and-pencil measures of readiness, stage of change, commitment, goals, and taking steps have all been found to predict the probability of behavior change. Often motivational measures compare favorably with other prognostic factors in predicting outcome.

The quality of a counseling relationship is also linked to treatment outcome. A client's rating (more so than the therapist's rating) of the quality of the working alliance after two sessions of counseling is often related to outcome. As noted above, observer ratings of the quality of therapist empathy have also predicted substance use outcomes.

Finally, as described earlier, behavior change may be predictable from certain aspects of client speech during an interview or treatment session. The strength of commitment language in particular has been found to predict drug use outcomes, more than statements reflecting desire, ability, reasons, or need for change.

Summary

Expressed motivation for, and particularly commitment to, change predicts movement into action. The taking of specific steps (e.g., attendance, adherence, self-regulation efforts) is a still more proximal predictor of change.

Influencing Motivation for Change

To enhance motivation for action is to increase the probability that a specific behavior change (e.g., smoking cessation) will occur. Thought about in this way, motivation seems less mysterious and more manageable. There is an enormous psychological literature on factors that influence the probability of behavior in general, and of substance use in particular.

What Doesn't Work?

Examining approaches that fail to motivate change may be instructive not only in planning interventions, but also in understanding the nature of addiction itself. There are many interventions that have been tested and found wanting in a trial or two, but there are three broad approaches in particular for which there is strong evidence of ineffectiveness.

Enlightenment

The first of these ineffective strategies is based on the assumption that substance abuse occurs because people lack sufficient information, knowledge, or insight. It follows that the needed intervention would be some form of education or persuasion to enlighten the person as to the true nature and dangers of substance abuse. In U.S. treatment programs, this often takes the form of educational lectures or films. Knowledge-focused education and insight-oriented persuasion have been spectacularly unsuccessful in changing substance abuse once established or in deterring its establishment.

> *Knowledge-focused education and insight-oriented persuasion have been spectacularly unsuccessful in changing substance abuse.*

Education does produce measurable increases in knowledge about substance use and problems, but its effects on attitudes are marginal and on behavior negligible. Insight-oriented (e.g., psychoanalytic) psychotherapies similarly yield little or no change in addictions.

Confrontation

A second ineffective strategy is confrontation, which has a particularly strong history of use in U.S. addiction treatment. In a sense, confrontation is education and persuasion "with the volume turned up," delivered with a forcefulness intended to evoke fear, shame, or humiliation. Support for this approach is usually offered in the form of anecdotes, but controlled trials consistently reflect either no benefit or a paradoxical detrimental effect. Illustrative are studies of victim impact panels (VIPs) widely promoted by Mothers Against Drunk Driving. In a typical VIP, an audience of offenders hear heartrending firsthand descriptions of how victims' lives have been devastated by a drunk driver. Offenders who attend such events are often quite moved emotionally, and leave the auditorium feeling remorseful, embarrassed, and ashamed. Yet the outcome consistently observed in well-designed studies of VIPs is no beneficial effect on recidivism. In one randomized trial, reoffenders showed a significant increase in the probability of repeating their offense when mandated to attend a VIP, as compared with those given the same court sanctions without a VIP. Other confrontational approaches simply lack persuasive evidence of efficacy for want of properly designed research.

Punishment

One of the paradoxes of substance abuse is its persistence in spite of substantial negative consequences. If aversive consequences cured alcoholism and drug addiction, their prevalence would be quite low. Criminal sanctions for substance use may deter initial experimentation, but they are at best ineffective in decreasing established abuse and dependence. Moreover, the secondary effects of imprisonment contribute to more general deterioration of prosocial functioning and cycles of recidivism. From a learning perspective, punishment suppresses behavior while aversive contingencies are in effect, but does nothing to shape and reinforce alternative behavior.

Beyond these three broad themes, there is also evidence that substance use disorders do not respond to attention alone. Here is a seeming paradox. As discussed above, retention is a reasonably consistent predictor of substance abuse treatment outcome. The longer people voluntarily remain in treatment, the better they do. Equally consistent is the finding that when clients are randomly assigned to longer versus shorter or to more intensive versus less intensive (e.g., inpatient vs. outpatient) treatment, the groups show similar outcomes. Most such studies have evaluated undifferentiated treatment as usual, and it is possible that dose effects would emerge with a more efficacious treatment. In any event, larger doses of attention in the form of generic treatment do not seem to enhance outcome in randomized trials.

What Does Work?

If enlightenment, confrontation, punishment, and attention fail to motivate change in substance abuse, what strategies are more successful? These too may shed light on the nature of addictive disorders and how best to address them.

One surprising finding is the relatively strong and consistent support in dozens of clinical trials for the efficacy of brief interventions for alcohol problems. One might not intuitively expect that one or two sessions of counseling would yield a significant reduction in such long-practiced and persistent behavior. Yet there is solid scientific evidence for precisely that, at least with clients having lower levels of alcohol problems and dependence, both in help-seeking samples and among people screened in health care settings who are not seeking consultation with regard to their drinking. If brevity is not the active ingredient, then what accounts for the impact of such brief interventions? Our analysis revealed six components that were often present in effective brief counseling with problem drinkers, summarized in the acronym FRAMES:

- Feedback regarding personal status, relative to norms, of drinking and its consequences.
- Responsibility for change is left with the client, honoring the person's autonomy.
- Advice and encouragement to reduce or stop drinking.
- Menu of options for how to change one's drinking.
- Empathic counseling style that listens to the client.
- Support for self-efficacy, and optimism about the possibility for change.

The counseling style of motivational interviewing shares many of these attributes, and its adaptation in motivational enhancement therapy specifically includes personal feedback of clients' own assessment results. Noticeably absent in effective brief interventions are general education, confrontation, or efforts to teach specific change skills. Fewer studies have tested brief interventions for illicit drug abuse, although some positive findings have been reported with motivational interviewing for marijuana use. Brief physician advice has also been found to exert modest effects in smoking cessation.

A second effective strategy to increase motivation for change in substance use is positive reinforcement for nonuse and alternative behaviors. Financial incentives (e.g., vouchers) for abstinence clearly have been effective in reducing alcohol, cocaine, and opiate use. In controlled laboratory settings abstinence- or moderation-contingent access to social reinforcers substantially suppressed drinking by alcohol-dependent individuals of freely available alcohol. More generally, interventions based on positive reinforcement principles (rather than extinction or punishment) have a strong track record in treatment outcome research, including an approach that emphasizes helping clients to access alternative drug-free sources of positive reinforcement.

Emphasis here has been on interventions designed to enhance motivation for change in substance use. A broader summary of treatment outcome research is found in Part V of this book.

Summary

Substance abuse does not appear to be the result of insufficient knowledge, insight, shame, or suffering. Interventions designed to evoke these conditions have been consistently ineffective in motivating change in individuals with substance use disorders. More effective are methods that provide individuals with positive incentives for nonuse and facilitate reliable drug-free sources of natural positive reinforcement.

Putting the Pieces Together

The research considered here focuses on the instigation of change, that which sets the process in motion. Instigation appears to be a highly significant process, and one that is often ignored or assumed in substance abuse interventions. Several lines of evidence indicate that the instigation process is a necessary and often sufficient condition for change. Brief interventions and motivational interviewing trigger behavior change that is often similar in magnitude and duration to that resulting from longer interventions. In longitudinal treatment studies that document week-to-week substance use, the majority of change occurs within (and sometimes before) the first few weeks of intervention. Motivation and adherence measures are good predictors of subsequent behavior change, or the lack thereof.

Ambivalence is the resting state, the status quo from which instigation to change begins. For abused substances, drug use is reinforcing. The incentives for continuing involve a combination of the primary reinforcing properties of the drug itself and secondary reinforcement from the social environment. Over time drug use results in at least periodic aversive consequences, escape from which offers incentive (negative reinforcement) for nonuse. The subjective result is "I want it, and I don't want it," understandably leading to cycles of use and nonuse. Less often there is also positive reinforcement for nonuse. In the absence of positive incentives for abstinence, the person is left with a choice between (1) substance use and its attendant positive reinforcement and punishment, or (2) the absence of negative consequences in exchange for the absence of a behavior. This is the motivational dilemma of substance abuse and dependence.

If instigation is a key in changing substance abuse, then what factors influence it? (See Figure 9.1.) Through schedules of reinforcement and discounting slopes, it is possible to identify points at which the pros and cons of substance use balance. Instigation also occurs during brief interventions that involve no change in real-life contingencies, although perceived contingencies may shift. Research on brief intervention and on therapist effects points to certain characteristics of an interpersonal alliance (e.g., empathy) that facilitate instigation, mirroring the early writings of Carl Rogers on the necessary and sufficient conditions for change. The balance of positive incentives and obstacles for change (pros and cons) involves intrapersonal, interpersonal, and contextual considerations, and can tip in the direction of change (literally a "decisional balance"). Intrapersonal factors such as desire, ability, reasons, and need can favor change or the status quo. Interpersonal contingencies can likewise provide incentives or disincentives for change. Contextual aspects of the social environment influence judgments about what is normative and acceptable.

Within this confluence of continuous factors, instigation nevertheless has the appearance of a reasonably discrete process. Something "clicks" or "snaps." Studies of natural change (see DiClemente, Chapter 6, this volume) and of transformational change point to discrete events that are turning points, often reflected in statements like "I just decided." Ambivalence diminishes, and the person gets unstuck. In subjective experience, instigation comes down to a decision, a choice point.

We come full circle here to the risk of simply blaming people for not doing the right thing. Yet the evidence is overwhelming that substance use is a matter of choice, even under conditions of severe dependence. Courts and juries regularly hold offenders accountable for their actions under the influence of drugs, implicitly regarding substance use (and nonuse) as volitional—that the person could have chosen to do otherwise. Through the long binary debate over free will versus determinism, what we have failed to develop is a coherent psychology of volition. Choice is not unconstrained. It occurs in the presence of and taking into account the rich context of social environment,

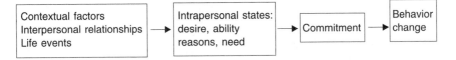

FIGURE 9.1. Instigation to change.

interpersonal relationships, and intrapersonal motives. The choices that people make can be influenced, and yet they remain choices. Instigation to change still necessarily passes through a variably conscious decisional process.

In natural speech, this is reflected in the phenomenon of commitment, the volitional act of saying "I will." There is in natural language a continuum of strength of commitment. To say "I swear" or "I promise" or "I do" is to make a stronger commitment than one does in saying "I'll try" or "I'll think about it." These speech events literally signal behavior probabilities in natural discourse, and normally emerge in the context of interpersonal communication. To be sure, people can and do knowingly overstate their actual level of commitment, or for other reasons fail to live up to their promises. Yet the language process itself tells us something about the underlying phenomenology of reaching a decision, making a commitment as a final common pathway to change.

Robust Principles

1. Once substance abuse/dependence has been established, education, persuasion, confrontation, punishment, and attention typically yield little or no beneficial effect, and sometimes exert a paradoxical effect.
2. Substance use is highly responsive to contingent positive reinforcement. Even severely dependent substance users can and do abstain from or modify their drinking or drug use in response to positive incentives to do so.
3. The most common motivational obstacle to early help seeking is ambivalence and the perception that one does not "have a problem" serious enough to warrant change or treatment.
4. Instigation to change occurs when a person perceives significant discrepancy between his or her present state and his or her desired goals or values.
5. Motivation and instigation to change often emerge in the context of interpersonal communication.

6. Relatively brief interventions including motivational interviewing can instigate behavior change in people with substance use disorders.
7. Outcomes vary widely across therapists. A positive therapist–client alliance is associated with better outcomes in substance abuse treatment, and therapist empathic skill in particular predicts greater reduction in drinking.
8. Motivation for change is not unitary, but is comprised of multiple dimensions that are at best modestly intercorrelated.
9. Decision or commitment is a final common pathway to change.
10. Once instigation occurs, change may proceed without much additional support.

Related Readings

Amrhein, P. C., Miller, W. R., Yahne, C. E., Palmer, M., & Fulcher, L. (2003). Client commitment language during motivational interviewing predicts drug use outcomes. *Journal of Consulting and Clinical Psychology, 71*, 862–878.

Heather, N., Miller, W. R., & Greeley, J. (Eds.). (1991). *Self-control and the addictive behaviours*. New York: Maxwell Macmillan.

Hettema, J., Steele, J., & Miller, W. R. (2005). Motivational interviewing. *Annual Review of Clinical Psychology, 1*, 91–111.

Miller, W. R., & Rollnick, S. (2002). *Motivational interviewing: Preparing people for change* (2nd ed.). New York: Guilford Press.

Miller, W. R., Wilbourne, P. L., & Hettema, J. (2003). What works?: A summary of alcohol treatment outcome research. In R. K. Hester & W. R. Miller (Eds.), *Handbook of alcoholism treatment approaches: Effective alternatives* (3rd ed., pp. 13–63). Boston: Allyn & Bacon.

Moyer, A., Finney, J. W., Swearingen, D. W., & Vergun, P. (2002). Brief interventions for alcohol problems: A meta-analytic review of controlled investigations in treatment-seeking and non-treatment-seeking populations. *Addiction, 97*, 279–292.

Orford, J. (2001). *Excessive appetites: A psychological view of addictions* (2nd ed.). New York: Wiley.

Project MATCH Research Group. (1998). Therapist effects in three treatments for alcohol problems. *Psychotherapy Research, 8*, 455–474.

Smith, J. E., & Meyers, R. J. (2004). *Motivating substance abusers to enter treatment: Working with family members*. New York: Guilford Press.

Vuchinich, R. E., & Heather, N. (Eds.). (2003). *Choice, behavioural economics and addiction*. New York: Pergamon Press.

Part IV

Social Factors

CHAPTER 10

Racial and Gender Differences in Substance Abuse

What Should Communities Do about Them?

HAROLD D. HOLDER

Epidemiological studies of alcohol and other drug consumption have shown important differences in drinking and other drug use according to racial and ethnic group membership, as well as according to gender. These studies provide us with a picture of substance use that is rich in texture and context. This richness can provide greater understanding of the epidemiology of alcohol consumption and associated social, personal, legal, health, and safety problems resulting not only from the use of alcohol but also from the use of other drugs.

Differences in substance use can have potential implications for treatment and prevention. Looking across research papers, we can identify at least four areas of concern expressed: (1) lack of racial-/ethnic- or gender-appropriate measurement for treatment and prevention, (2) need for racial-/ethnic- or gender-specific services, (3) varying impact of policy changes that do not reflect such differences, and (4) typical exclusion of racial/ethnic subgroups and women from health research.

How practically important are differences according to racial heritage/ethnicity and gender and what are the implications for communities that are faced with finding real approaches to these issues? Is our necessary response obvious? This chapter has three major goals. First, I want to summarize the quite diverse and sometimes contradictory differences in substance use and associated problems according to racial and ethnic groups as well as by gender. Second, I summarize some of what is known about differences in effects on different racial and ethnic groups as well as gender from substance abuse treatment and from prevention. Third, I consider the implications of these findings for future efforts to reduce substance abuse problems in designing community systems to reduce substance use and abuse and associated problems that might be considered. The last objective suggests a break from traditional parallel approaches, that is, treatment and prevention, and suggests a new perspective (a "community integrated systems model") for reducing substance abuse problems in a community. The epidemiological data presented are neither exhaustive nor complete. I have chosen this data specifically to illustrate various patterns reported in the research literature.

Epidemiological Data about Differences in Consumption of Substances and Associated Problems

Alcohol and other drugs have significant and unique patterns of use and problems associated with this use. In addition, each substance may also have quite different use and misuse patterns that are associated with subgroups of users. In this chapter I focus specifically on racial/ethnic subgroup differences and gender differences. I only occasionally consider age-specific differences.

General Consumption Patterns

National studies of the health and well-being of children typically report that male youth are more likely to drink than female youth; and as adolescents grow older, this gender difference becomes more pronounced. Heavy drinking is more likely among white and Hispanic youth than black youth. In general, self-reported underage drinking during the past 30 days is highest among whites (12 years and older) followed by Native Americans/Native Alaskans, Hispanics, blacks, and Asians. Asian and black youth report less binge drinking than Hispanics, Native Americans, Native Alaskans, or whites.

Male youth are more likely to drink than female youth; as adolescents grow older, this gender difference becomes more pronounced.

Regarding drinking patterns, men and women in general had similar ages for peak drinking, even though men typically drink more than women. On average whites' total alcohol consumption exceeds that of blacks and Hispanics over the entire life course, blacks' and Hispanics' average drinks per occasion exceed that of whites in later adulthood— even though white frequency of drinking is typically higher in the same age range. In general, transition to marriage affects drinking patterns, but while whites decrease their frequency of heavy drinking and alcohol dependence over the early marital years, blacks remain relatively stable in terms of frequency and dependence. Both groups appear to have similar alcohol problem patterns, but white men report a decline in alcohol problems after marriage and black men report an increase in alcohol problems.

White women report the highest risk of alcohol-related problems as heavy drinking increased. These effects were more pronounced among the genders for whites than for blacks. Overall, there appears to be less problem vulnerability among black women than among black men, possibly due to psychological differences and differences in the normative climate concerning women's drinking.

When epidemiological analyses of drinking by racial/ethnic groups include ethnic origin, pronounced differences are observed within racial groups as well as across racial groups. People of Hispanic and Native American origin are less likely to drink than whites of European heritage but consume more per drinking occasion. Whites whose ancestry is southern and eastern European drink proportionately more wine and exhibit more moderate drinking patterns than those whose ancestry is northern and central European. Blacks from the English-speaking Caribbean report more moderate drinking than other blacks. Asian drinkers, in particular those of non-Japanese origin, have the most moderate drinking patterns of all racial/ethnic groups.

Considering ethnic group membership by itself is not sufficient to understand patterns because there are important racial/ethnic and gender differences in patterns of alcohol use among ethnically diverse black and Hispanic urban youth. Hispanic youth typically report greater experience with alcohol than black youth. Dominican adolescents drink more frequently and drink more per occasion than Puerto Rican adolescents. Similarly Caribbean/West Indian youth report drinking more frequently, becoming drunk more often, drinking more per occasion, and planning to drink more in the future relative to African American youth. Epidemiological studies have documented substantial differences among Hispanic subgroups relating to drinking patterns and alcohol-involved problems; no single variable can explain the observed differences. A number of factors also seem to contribute to subgroup patterns of drinking among blacks, including individual and environmental characteristics. In addition, subgroups of Asian Americans also vary in drinking rates and heavy drinking. The widely varying drinking patterns among different tribal groups of Native Americans are also likely shaped by a variety of influences.

In general, the national household surveys of drug use find higher rates of current illicit drug use by blacks than by whites or Hispanics. While combined use of alcohol with marijuana has increased for all groups over the past decade, this increase is greater among blacks and Hispanics than among whites. Among college undergraduates, men and women are equally likely to use ecstasy. Moreover, there is a significant relationship between ecstasy use and other substance use such as binge drinking in the past 2 weeks, marijuana use in the past month, and daily smoking.

Among whites, marijuana use is most often associated with less prestigious occupations and lower family income. Among blacks, marijuana use seems unrelated to occupation. Also among blacks, cigarette smoking is negatively associated with drinking. In general, substance use, particularly smoking, is associated with reduced occupational attainment in blacks as compared to whites.

Problems Associated with Alcohol and Other Drugs

White and Hispanic men rank the highest in self-reported drinking and driving. Not surprisingly, they also have the highest lifetime arrest rates for DUI (driving under the influence). Alcohol-involved pedestrian fatalities are higher for black adults ages 25 and older, and for Hispanic males and Native American males ages 15 and older. While white male heavy drinking has declined, according to recent studies, there was no equivalent decline among black and Hispanic males. Problem prevalence remains very high for black and Hispanic men. Heavy drinking remains stable and relatively low among women of all three ethnic groups. Over the past decade, rates of self-reported drinking problems have declined among whites, but have increased among Hispanics; there was no change for blacks. The overall drinking problem incidence is higher for Hispanics than for whites and blacks, but problem remission (repeated self-reported problems) appears to be higher among whites. Women report a lower problem incidence but a higher problem remission than men, independent of ethnicity, but this could be a type of telescoping effect resulting from so few cases for women.

The rate of violent victimization among Native Americans is well above that for other U.S. racial/eth-

Among all racial/ethnic groups Native Americans seem to be the most likely victims when the perpetrator has been drinking.

nic subgroups. Among all racial/ethnic groups Native Americans seem to be the most likely to be victims when the perpetrator has been drinking. The perpetrator's use of alcohol and other drugs is less likely in violent crimes committed against whites or blacks. The arrest rate for alcohol-related offenses (e.g., DUI, liquor law violations, public drunkenness) for Native Americans is more than double that of all other races. There exist racial and gender differences in adolescent risk behavior associated with alcohol. For example, female students are more likely to ride with a drinking driver than male students, and whites and Hispanics are more likely to do so than blacks. Disposition to risk taking is a better predictor of injury than either drinking or drug use for white patients, while none of these variables were significant for blacks or Hispanics. Based upon emergency room interviews, white patients are more likely than black or Hispanic patients to report drug use.

Alcohol-related problems are associated with intimate partner violence among blacks and whites but not among Hispanics. Black and Hispanic couples are approximately three times at greater risk of male-to-female partner violence than of female-to-male partner violence. Their risk is twice as high as that for white couples.

Evidence of Treatment Effect Differences

Given the obvious differences in substance use according to subgroups and the associated substance problems, how might these differences show up in dependency risk, seeking care, and treatment outcomes? No claim is made here that this review is complete or exhaustive. However, the review below does illustrate the possibilities in subgroup differences associated with substance use treatment.

Risk- and Treatment-Seeking Behavior among Subgroups

The age of initial self-reported drug use has been shown to be associated with drug abuse over the life course in general. Early onset is often associated with development of lifetime alcohol dependence. The general implicit principle is that early exposure to substance use increases the future risk of heavier and often dependent use. This has been found to be true among males, females, and non-blacks. However, this association is not consistently found among blacks whose identification at an initial interview as alcohol abusers may not be followed by a subsequent depend-

> *Early exposure to substance use increases the future risk of heavier and often dependent use.*

ence diagnosis. In other words, there are likely biases in abuse diagnoses such that females, blacks, and high-school dropouts may be less likely to receive such a diagnosis at a baseline survey.

Hispanics in some studies have an increased likelihood to seek help for their drinking (when there exist three or more alcohol-related problems) compared to whites or blacks (who seek help comparably to whites). However, there are studies that find opposite patterns in treatment-seeking behavior among racial/ethnic subgroups. While alcohol use disorders are more prevalent in men compared to women, psychiatric comorbidities (especially depression and eating disorders) are more common in women.

Applying DSM-IV criteria in a treatment sample of whites, blacks, and Mexican Americans, studies have found that drug use is higher among blacks and Mexican Americans than among whites. Among alcohol-dependent individuals, almost 50% of the whites, about 75% of the blacks, and almost 50% of the Mexican Americans report using at least one drug other than alcohol once a week or more in the 12 months prior to interview for the study. The drug most frequently used by whites is marijuana, followed by cocaine and amphetamines. The drug most frequently used by blacks and Mexican Americans is cocaine, followed by marijuana. In short, there appear to be distinctive patterns of multidrug use among racial/ethnic subgroups and the recording of abuser or dependency appears to have racial/ethnic and gender biases in practice. This means that developing a universal principle or practical strategy for working with abuse among racial/ethnic subgroups is difficult if not impossible.

Effectiveness of Treatment According to Racial/Ethnic and Gender Differences

Neither gender nor race differences are found to be significant in predicting retention in treatment. There are no significant outcome differences between blacks and whites in treatment—for example, no ethnic main effect appears to exist on drinking intensity after 1-year follow-up. Across studies of substance abuse treatment for women, such factors as provision of childcare, prenatal care, women-only programs, supplemental services and workshops that address women-focused topics, mental health programs, and comprehensive programming increased positive outcomes for women in treatment. There is some evidence that women in treatment improve their drinking patterns even if their mental health risks are higher than those of women in the general population. Women with depression had poorer drinking outcomes, as did subjects with schizoid personality disorder.

There appear to be few consistent gender differences for treatment outcomes even allowing for differences in family history of alcoholism, later onset of drinking, marital disruption, and comorbidity.

Evidence of Prevention Effect Differences

There are limited data concerning relative effectiveness of prevention programs according to racial/ethnic group membership or gender. At this point, one can make the distinction between culturally specific interventions and culturally tailored prevention interventions. *Culturally tailored interventions* are those that are designed for a general population that are subsequently adapted to a specific ethnic minority, generally by translating program curricula and by hiring bilingual-bicultural program staff. *Culturally specific interventions* are those designed for a specific ethnic minority population, generally incorporating ethnically specific and sociocultural norms and values into the theories of change that underlie program curricula and intervention activities. Such norms and values may include ethnically specific family structures, notions of health and wellness, and practices related to substance use, as well as educational and therapeutic methods.

Prevention strategies can be simplistically grouped according to whether they target specifically identified individuals and subgroups or whether the prevention effort seeks to change the larger social system including neighborhoods and communities. Targeted programs, for example, are most often directed at a subgroup with a goal to alter risk behavior. One area of prevention that has given some attention to ethnic/racial group effects is school-based education, but in fact there are few well-designed school-based education strategies that have shown demonstrated effects for minority groups. One example is a substance abuse prevention school curriculum for elementary-age children that is based on the classroom alcohol and other drug use prevention curriculum life skills training (LST), which suggests that LST reduced reports of cigarette use in the past month and number of new smokers relative to control conditions with white, suburban, middle-class and with urban, multiethnic, and predominantly black samples.

A recent review of published and unpublished evaluations of prevention programs concluded that cultural tailoring of general population strategies is more effective for environmental prevention approaches (prevention interventions that seek to change the overall community system rather than target specific subgroups) and culturally specific interventions may be more effective for programs directed at individuals and families. At this point there have been no substantive outcome evaluations of culturally specific interventions.

Implications of Epidemiological Differences

Overall, the epidemiological evidence demonstrates that there are substantial differences in use of alcohol and other drugs and associated problems according to racial/ethnic group membership as well as gender, and some evidence of differential effects of treatment and prevention. Many studies end with an admonition that treatment and prevention must be adjusted to account for these subgroup differences. From my point of view, it is difficult to derive unequivocal and consistent statements about unique patterns of drinking and other drug use (as the effects of treatment and prevention) according to ethnic/racial subgroup and gender that can be consistently utilized to increase effectiveness. Very little has been presented here about age-group differences. The possible interactions of age with race/ethnic heritage and gender are so complex that they defy even broad conclusions. Frankly, all of these possible combinations overwhelm me and most likely most health service planners.

Therefore, in thinking about the future and how to reduce reoccurring alcohol and other drug problems in communities, we are faced with two alternative perspectives. The first view is that because of the gender and ethnic/racial differences (and possible age-group differences) in level of use, age of initial substance use, and associated problems with substance use, we must alter existing approaches to substance abuse problems to account for these differences. This might suggest, at the extreme, gender- and racial-/ethnic-specific addiction programs only, that is, treatment programs for each racial/ethnic group that reflects the cultural differences and support systems associated with each group as well as its cultural symbols and norms. A similar argument has and could be made that prevention programs should similarly be customized for all of the unique subgroup differences linked with high-risk substance use and associated problems.

An alternative view, given the stated purpose of this book, is to question if, in fact, these differences suggest that all forms of treatment and prevention should be customized for the subgroups that are targets for treatment and/or prevention. The point of view of this chapter (written by a heretic) is "no." A number of factors support my position.

Substance use and associated problems are public health and safety concerns. The public response should be a cost-effective approach to these problems. Thus a public health and safety response to alcohol and other drug use and associated problems should be supported, even mandated.

Resources for substance abuse treatment and prevention (as we currently know them) will most likely be insufficient to produce population-level reductions of substance use and abuse, even if we adjust for racial/ethnic and gender differences. Now this perspective is not to be taken as supporting a "one size fits all" approach to treatment and prevention or that gender-specific or racial-/ethnicity-specific programs are not necessary. Rather, I wish to turn the issue upside-down.

Community responses to reoccurring substance abuse problems demand effectiveness and accountability. Current responses exist like silos such that even within the recovery/treatment community, there may be many alternative approaches, approaches that often compete for funding and public support. Similarly, local prevention efforts operate separately from one another, compete for funding among themselves and with treatment programs, and are isolated from the treatment programs in the same community. This silo approach creates no accountability for overall reduction in substance use and associated problems.

I propose that we need to create a *community system for reducing substance use and abuse problems* such that effectiveness is measured by population-level reductions in use and associated problems and that is challenged to select the mix of strategies for prevention and treatment that maximizes this effect. This community system's effectiveness would be measured initially in terms of population-level effects. A second level of accountability would be reductions in problems in subgroups whose members have clearly identified individual problems. Thus treatment and prevention would lose their individual identities and would be employed according to local needs and the potential to achieve desired effects.

There are many reasons why custom-designed system services and programs may be necessary. Thus a type of "backup" would be created in which the failures of more general or universal strategies (people who fall out, drop out, resist, or have unique individual needs) could be served via more customized strategies. In this case, existing barriers to recovery or seeking recovery services would be essential. For example, if a community had large number of female Hispanic drug users for whom existing services were not effective, then a specific service intervention that addressed these gender and ethnic attributes would be required.

This chapter challenges the assumption that all differences must be addressed. Frankly, there are insufficient research resources to design, field test, implement, and evaluate a full range of approaches that can address all possible combinations of individual characteristics and special groups. Customized strategies for reducing problems come into play primarily as a result of demonstrated failures in more general strategies, rather than assuming that all strategies must be customized for differences at the start. In such a system, we would be required to expect failures, dropouts, and individual resistance. This is not because each personal problem is not important but because of limited resources.

With a public health and safety approach, our primary challenge is to determine the overall effectiveness of the mix of strategies utilized in reducing specific population-level problems. For example, how effective are programs/policies to reduce alcohol-involved traffic crashes in general and/or crashes with women, especially young women? How effective are community programs to increase the age of initial drinking and other drug use for young African Americans, Native Americans, or Hispanics/Latinos?

Historically, local approaches to reduce substance abuse addressed individuals who shared geographical proximity. For example, if the reduction of rates of breast cancer is the prevention goal, then increased breast examinations could be the goal for prevention interventions targeted at all women who live within a geographical area or catchment area. Women who live within this area may share a number of social and economic factors and are likely exposed to common environmental risk factors. The incidence of the disease is not necessarily related to any social interaction among them or others. In this case, the use of a catchment area is a cost-efficient way to define a target group that is to receive the interaction—in this case, a program to encourage breast examination. This does not deny the contribution of the social or physical environment to the development of the disease condition. But no particular changes in the social and economic structure of the community are usually proposed other than those that make treatment and rehabilitation more available.

For the most part, planners using the catchment area approach most often select strategies that seek to alter individual decisions and behavior or that provide direct services to individuals. One-on-one and group treatment and counseling may often be used. Many community prevention trials for heart disease and cancer have employed some form of a catchment area approach—for example, educational and clinical strategies where individual decisions and behavior are emphasized. Thus the mass media, focus groups, targeted communication, health promotion, social marketing, and health awareness efforts are all excellent and potentially effective strategies, as are specifically tested clinical strategies.

However, it is simply not possible to permanently "inoculate" a community population against substance-related problems by only employing individual target group strategies. The community is itself a dynamic system. The system changes and adapts as new people enter and others leave; as alcoholic beverage or cigarette marketing and promotion evolve; as there are changes in the availability of alcohol and other drugs; and as social and economic conditions, including employment and disposable income, change. No single program, no matter how good, can sustain its impact, particularly if system-level changes are not accomplished. Existing approaches to substance use and abuse have stimulated a mixed set of individual programs in each community, normally labeled as "treatment and prevention."

A basic premise of the community systems approach advocated here is that the collective risk of substance use and abuse will be reduced by intervening to change the processes that contribute to alcohol problems, smoking, and illicit drug use. Prevention strategies focused on the community at large can potentially be more effective than those focused on specific individuals at risk.

A systems perspective to substance problem reduction, rather than addressing a single problem behavior or condition, considers simultaneously a potentially wide-ranging set of problem behaviors. By identifying "individuals at risk," the entire population within the community is engaged in concert. Rather than basing strategies on fixed interventions, the community (system) can constantly mix interventions that can shift the population away from problem-causing contexts.

Such a system for reducing substance abuse problems actually exists: general strategies backed up by subgroup-specific strategies in the case of reducing drinking and driving. Population-level countermeasures for drinking and driving are designed to reduce overall incidents of driving during and after drinking. Such countermeasures, including the use of random breath testing, lower limits for legal blood alcohol concentration (BAC), suspension of driving licenses, and routine enforcement, have been shown to have effects in reducing traffic crashes at the population level. Individual drivers do come to the attention of the police as a result of routine drinking and driving surveillance (enforcement) but also as a result of breath testing in conjunction with a traffic crash. Most arrested drinking drivers are "first-time offenders" who have not previously been arrested for drinking and driving or who have not had a traffic accident related to drinking. They rarely repeat their offense or are rearrested because arrest and sanctions are sufficient to reduce future problems—that is, a general intervention program including possible clinical assessment appears to be sufficient in reducing recidivism.

A unique but highly significant group within the DWI population are multiple offenders who are arrested several times, continue to drink and drive, come to the attention of the police (largely because of their overall exposure to detection and the many driving trips they make while impaired), and individually cause a well-above-average number of traffic accidents. This subgroup clearly requires a specific mix of incarceration and other sanctions and rehabilitation because they are often less affected by more general population strategies to prevent drinking and driving. In terms of racial and ethnic differences, it has been shown that there is a need for specific designs for racial and ethnic subgroups within the multiple-offender population to decrease recidivism.

Thus, this specific alcohol-involved problem, alcohol-involved traffic crashes, in any community provides a simple example of the concept of how general universal prevention can be used to affect most of the population at risk (general driving population) backed up by programs/strategies to reduce future risk of alcohol-involved traffic crashes.

Robust Principles

1. There are many significant but complex differences in substance use and associated problems related to racial/ethnic groups and gender.
2. While there are some demonstrated differences in racial/ethnic group responses to current treatment and prevention modalities, these complex differences in themselves do not guide the creation of long-term cost-effective community responses to alcohol and other drug problems.
3. Current separation of treatment and prevention is unlikely to be capable of achieving a long-term reduction in current use patterns and problems.
4. What is needed is a unified system (one that combines prevention and treatment into a total system) at the community level for response to alcohol and other drug problems that is accountable for finding the best mix of evidence-based treatment and prevention strategies for reducing population-level problems.
5. In such a system, the challenge is to find the most cost-effective mix of strategies, whether for individual- or community-level interventions that can reduce problems.
6. Treatment and prevention responses to subgroups can come into play when there are demonstrated failures of more general strategies.
7. The system should respond to the general needs of the community *and* to the special needs/requirements of important subgroups as necessary to achieve an overall reduction of alcohol and other drug problems.

Suggested Readings

Brienza, R. S., & Stein, M. D. (2002). Alcohol use disorders in primary care: Do gender-specific differences exist? *Journal of General Internal Medicine, 17*(5), 387–397.

Caetano, R., & Clark, C. L. (1998). Trends in alcohol-related problems among whites, blacks, and Hispanics: 1984–1995. *Alcoholism: Clinical and Experimental Research, 22*(2), 534–538.

Caetano, R., & Clark, C. L. (2000). Hispanics, blacks and whites driving under the influence of alcohol: Results from the 1995 National Alcohol Survey. *Accident Analysis and Prevention, 32*(1), 57–64.

Caetano, R., Clark, C. L., & Tam, T. (1999). Alcohol consumption among racial/ethnic minorities: Theory and research. *Alcohol Health and Research World, 22*(4), 233–241.

Caetano, R., & Kaskutas, L. A. (1996). Changes in drinking problems among whites, blacks, and Hispanics: 1984–1992. *Substance Use and Misuse, 31*(11–12), 1547–1571.

Caetano, R., & Schafer, J. (1996). DSM-IV alcohol dependence and drug abuse/dependence in a treatment sample of whites, blacks, and Mexican-Americans. *Drug and Alcohol Dependence, 43*(1–2), 93–101.

Caetano, R., Schafer, J., & Cunadi, C. B. (2001). Alcohol-related intimate partner violence among white, black, and Hispanic couples in the United States. *Alcohol Research and Health, 25*(1), 58–65.

Cherpitel, C. J., & Borges, G. (2002). Substance use among emergency room patients: An exploratory analysis by ethnicity and acculturation. *Journal of Drug and Alcohol Abuse, 28*(2), 287–305.

Dawson, D.A. (1998). Beyond black, white, and Hispanic: Race, ethnic origin and drinking patterns in the United States. *Journal of Substance Abuse, 10*(4), 321–339.

Greenfeld, L. A., & Smith, S. K. (1999). *American Indians and crime.* Washington, DC: U.S. Bureau of Justice Statistics.

Henderson, G., Ma, G. X., & Shive, S. E. (2002). African American substance users and abusers. In G. X. Ma & G. Henderson (Eds.), *Ethnicity and substance abuse: Prevention and intervention* (pp. 59–86). Springfield, IL: Thomas.

Holder, H. D. (1988). *Alcohol and the community: A systems approach to prevention.* Cambridge, UK: Cambridge University Press.

Holder, H. D. (2001). Prevention of alcohol problems in the 21st century: Challenges and opportunities. *American Journal on Addictions, 10*, 1–15.

Jones-Webb, R. (1999). Drinking patterns and problems among African-Americans. *Alcohol Health and Research World, 22*(4), 260–264.

Lisansky-Gomberg, E. S. (2003). Treatment for alcohol-related problems: Special populations. Research opportunities. In M. Galanter (Ed.), *Recent developments in alcoholism* (Vol. 16, pp. 313–333). New York: Kluwer Academic/Plenum Press.

Prevention Research Center. (2004). *Preventing minority drinking problems.* Unpublished report for the National Institute on Alcohol Abuse and Alcoholism, National Institutes of Health. Berkeley, CA: Author.

Tonigan, J. S. (2003). Project Match treatment participation and outcomes by self-reported ethnicity. *Alcoholism: Clinical and Experimental Research, 27*(8), 1340–1344.

CHAPTER 11

Family and Other Close Relationships

BARBARA S. MCCRADY

Some Framing Comments

Defining Close Relationships

Any discussion of families and other close relationships must begin with some consideration of what constitutes a "family" or a "close relationship." We have many images of the family: the family in the agrarian economy, with parents and children working together; the family during the Industrial Revolution, with a father who left the home to work in the factories and a mother who stayed home to care for the home and family; the family from the early days of the women's movement, when men and women both worked outside of the home and collaborated in childrearing. Today, although all of these family forms still exist, the definitions and images of the "family" in contemporary society have broadened and changed. Contemporary families may be a traditional nuclear family living together in one household, with one or, more commonly, both parents working; a nuclear family that includes extended kin living together; a household headed by a single parent; a grandparent raising her grandchildren; a blended family as a result of divorce and remarriage; a cohabiting couple with or without children in a committed or more transitory relationship; a same-sex couple with or without children; or roommates who are long-term friends who do not share a sexual bond but consider themselves a family. Research on family functioning and clinical trials of family-based interventions have not always been designed and executed with these broader definitions in mind.

Nuclear families exist within broader social networks of extended family, friends, coworkers, neighbors, and acquaintances. These various social networks may function harmoniously in providing needed emotional, tangible, and guidance support to an individual, but more often an individual's experience of family and the extended social network is mixed, with some individuals being sources of support, others primarily adding stress to the individual's life, and still others serving as sources both of support and stress.

The role and importance of family and extended kin networks varies across ethnic groups. For example, for many blacks/African Americans, the church, pastor, and network of members of the church are central to their social network. Native Americans live within an extended kin network that is part of everyday activities, discussions, and ceremonies. For Asian Americans, family also may be a major focus for both social and cultural activities, and behavior may be strongly motivated by the desire to avoid bringing shame to the family. For individuals from a Latino/Hispanic background, family gender roles are distinct, and respect for others and attentiveness to the thoughts and needs of other family members is an important motivator of behavior.

In addition to the social networks that occur naturally through family and community ties, individuals with substance use disorders may become involved in a constructed social network, such as a self-help group, that creates new opportunities for support and friendships, and that interacts with existing relationships. These networks are the primary focus of Chapter 16 in this volume, and are not addressed further here.

Some Broad Issues

Families and other social systems are not static entities. Rather, families are systems that evolve over time. Individuals enter and leave the family or the individual's extended social network. Individuals in the family and extended social network develop new ties and connections of their own through dating, marriage, residence, and work, and some of these new individuals become part of the social network and exert their own effects on the family. Individuals in the family grow and age, and their roles and influence in the family may change accordingly. The child becomes an adult; the parent becomes a grandparent; the grandparent ages and needs care. Any understanding of the influence of the family and social network on an individual's substance use must take account of the changing and evolving nature of each family. Family-based interventions require tailoring to the current circumstance of an individual's family constellation, roles, and functioning, and must also attempt to anticipate the relative stability or instability of the current family constellation.

Although family members and members of the extended social network have strong influences on each other, individuals also bring their own personal characteristics, personality, temperament, intelligence, and genetic strengths and vulnerabilities to their relationships. Each relationship represents interactions between individuals who have distinct characteristics that influence how they behave and how others respond to them. Thus, no individual is a passive recipient of "social support" or "encouragement to use alcohol or drugs," but rather may, because of his or her own characteristics, elicit or discourage certain kinds of support. Similarly, individuals may be relatively more or less inclined to provide support for or to undermine others based on their own background and personal qualities. Thus family and other social interactions are a product of what each person brings to the relationship. Although research suggests certain broad principles about family functioning and the nature of social networks in relation to the etiology, maintenance, course, and resolution of substance use disorders, there is considerable variability in research findings. In particular, the interrelationships between substance use and social networks seem to differ depending on individual characteristics such as gender, sexual orientation, culture/ethnicity, and comorbid conditions. Policies and principles of intervention must take account of individual differences that may require different approaches.

What Do We Know about Families, Social Networks, and Substance Use Disorders?

Persons with Alcohol and Other Drug Use Disorders Live in and Have Relationships with a Network of Family and Friends

Despite stereotypic images of substance users as estranged from family and friends, in fact most have a complex network of relationships. The network includes individuals who use and abuse alcohol or drugs, as well as individuals who do not. The social network includes individuals who support and encourage the individual to continue to use alcohol or drugs, and others who support and encourage change and help seeking.

Nonetheless, the size of alcohol and drug users' social networks may be somewhat constricted for several reasons. First, some family members and friends will distance themselves from the user or effectively terminate their relationship with him or her. Second, husbands, wives, or other intimate partners may eventually dissolve the marriage or intimate relationship if the consequences of the alcohol or drug use are too severe and the husband, wife, or intimate other becomes convinced that the user will not change. In general, wives are more likely than husbands to remain with their alcoholic or drug-abusing partner. A third reason for the constricted network is that, over time, drug users may gravitate toward other drug users, and heavy drinkers may associate more and more with other heavy drinkers. Members of the social network who neither drink heavily nor use drugs may become estranged from the user.

The composition of these social networks is important to understand. Drinkers tend to have drinking and heavy-drinking social networks; drug users tend to be part of drug-using social networks. Women often are introduced to drugs by a male partner, and the husbands of women with alcohol dependence have a high rate of alcohol dependence themselves. Any attempt to change drinking or drug use occurs in the context of a network of drinking or drug-using friends and family members, and some of these friends or family members may undermine change attempts. Individuals whose family supports change generally are more likely to be successful.

The significance of the size of the social network also is important to understand. Although it would be simple to think that larger social networks are better, the connections between network size and network support are complicated. For example, there are good data suggesting that individuals with good coping skills and lower stress have larger social networks, but it is hard to know whether the larger social network fosters better coping skills, whether individuals with larger social networks simply have better coping skills that attract people to them, or, most likely, that there are interactions among the individual's skills, level of stress, and the size of his or her network. People may be attracted to competent and relaxed individuals, who in turn may draw support from these others. Seeking support from the social network is common, and people who have more problems ask for more support. However, individuals who ask for a great deal of support are less satisfied with the support they receive, perhaps because their problems seem so extensive to them and to those around them.

The reciprocal nature of close relationships also influences the degree to which individuals engage with a social network. People tend to avoid support if they know they cannot reciprocate, and their avoidance may foster greater isolation, which then decreases their access to potential resources. This social isolation because of a self-perceived inability to reciprocate support is observed most with lower income samples, especially of women. Social isolation may protect them from having to deal with other people's problems when they have a lot to deal with themselves, but also may isolate them from needed support.

The composition of an individual's social network varies with gender, race, ethnicity, and other individual factors. In general, women tend to have larger social networks than men. African Americans and Native Americans are part of larger extended kin and community networks, and single black mothers in particular are more likely to be involved with an extended family/kinship network than with nonkin friends. Living with extended kin is associated with less stress for these women.

Family Relationships May Protect against the Development of Alcohol or Drug Problems

Parental behavior and family functioning have a clear relationship to the development of drug and alcohol problems in adolescents. Several parental influences are important. For example, adolescents are strongly affected by their parents' disapproval of, indifference to, or acceptance of drug use. Even seniors in high school care about their parents' opinions and are less likely to use drugs if they know unambiguously that their parents disapprove of drug use. The ways that parents interact with their children also influence drug use. If parents provide consistent supervision, maintain consistent discipline, and have clear family values that they communicate to their children, the children are less likely to use drugs.

As youth reach adulthood, marriage becomes a salient protective factor. For example, marriage generally leads to decreases in drinking. However, men's drinking prior to marriage predicts their wives' drinking after a year of marriage and men who use drugs may influence their wife or girlfriend to use drugs. As development continues, becoming a parent also is protective in terms of developing drinking problems, but only for women. The importance of the intimate partner as protective against heavy drinking also is suggested by findings that the loss of the spousal role often leads to increased drinking, particularly among women.

Families and Others Close to the Drinker or Drug User May Contribute to the Development and Maintenance of Substance Use/Substance Use Disorders

Hesselbrock and Hesselbrock (Chapter 7, this volume) provide a more detailed review of etiological factors in the development of substance use disorders, so my comments here focus on familial factors that contribute to the development and maintenance of substance use disorders in adults. The interplay between alcohol or drug use and family responses is dynamic and evolves over time. At first, family members may not recognize use as problematic. However, over time, families do react. Persons with substance use disorders are likely to have received comments about their use and recommendations to cut down from multiple family members. Mothers are most likely to comment, even on adult behavior. For men, their wives are a major source of feedback; for women, their mothers and children are more likely to comment than are their husbands.

As families continue to develop an awareness of the drinking or drug use as problematic, they develop ways to cope with and respond to heavy drinking and drug use. Some of these ways of coping may help maintain use, while other responses may motivate the individual to change. Families may become overly engaged with the drinker or drug user, and inadvertently perpetuate the use through their attempts to get the person to change. Use of coercive communication strategies, such as nagging or verbal attempts to control the user, may backfire and lead the user to want to continue to use. Families also may protect the user from experiencing naturally occurring negative consequences of drinking or drug use. Although protecting a family member from physical or emotional distress may be understood as a natural and positively motivated response, such protection may help to perpetuate use because the drinker or drug user is unaware of the extent or severity of the potential consequences from his or her use. In general, three types of coping responses have been described: *tolerant* coping that accepts the use, *engaged* coping that attempts to change the user's behaviors, and *withdrawal* coping in which the family member withdraws from the user and spends time in separate activities and interactions with others. These broad categories of coping have been observed among families in Great Britain, among families in Mexico, and among aboriginal peoples of Australia, suggesting some universality to these experiences. Some types of coping may be more effective than others in facilitating change in the user; however, other types of coping may be more adaptive for the individual family member.

Three types of coping responses have been described: tolerant, engaged, and withdrawal coping.

Once a substance use disorder is established, its negative financial, emotional, and physical effects on the family are clear. However, research also points to identifiable positive or adaptive consequences of alcohol or drug use in terms of family roles and communication. These adaptive consequences also may help to maintain the drinking or drug use. Drinking or drug use may allow the user to become more assertive or to express emotions otherwise unexpressed. Family members may learn, over time, to treat the user kindly when he or she is high as a way to avoid arguments or physical violence. However, that same kindness may also serve to perpetuate the use.

Individual differences may be associated with different relationships between drinking or drug use and family functioning. For example, different drinking styles may have different impacts on relationship functioning. Drinkers who drink at home in a daily, steady pattern may be less disruptive to the family than drinkers who drink episodically and outside of the home. This latter pattern is associated with a more antisocial personality style. Compared to families of steady drinkers, families with antisocial types of drinkers interact with more hostility and experience more relationship disruption, and spouses experience more distress. There also are sex differences in the relationship between drinking or drug use and family functioning. Women tend to be influenced by their male partner's drinking or drug use pattern, often begin drinking heavily after rather than prior to marriage, and may be introduced to drug use by their partner. In female alcoholic couples, drinking may decrease conflict and help regulate negative affect.

Families and Others Close to Drinkers and Drug Users Play a Role in Helping a User Recognize a Problem and Seek Help

How do individuals realize that their drinking or drug use is problematic? What factors lead to motivation to change their behavior? Miller (Chapter 9, this volume) provides a nuanced contemporary view of motivation, so the discussion here focuses on family aspects of motivation. When asked, individuals with alcohol use disorders typically do not view family problems as the major marker of their drinking being a problem, instead stating that realizing how much they were drinking was a major factor in recognizing that their drinking had become problematic. However, recognizing a behavior as problematic and making a decision to change are two related but different facets of motivation. Drinkers often cite family or interpersonal problems as an important factor contributing to a decision to seek help.

Families engage in a number of actions that may provide motivation for an individual to change independently of treatment or to seek help to change. Generally, families discourage and comment on drinking more than they encourage it. For men, family members, especially spouses, encourage help seeking. Women experience opposition to help seeking, particularly from their husbands, but may experience support and encouragement from their mothers and children. Although the family may use their own resources and ingenuity to motivate a user to seek help, specific treatment models also have been developed and tested that focus on helping the family to foster help seeking and change. These are described in detail later in this chapter.

Families and Others Close to Drinkers and Drug Users Have a Significant Impact on the Change Process and Treatment Success

There is a robust research literature on the role of the family in the change process. Family and social network factors predict a positive response to treatment. Family predictors of positive outcome include the presence of an intimate relationship, having a cohesive family that does not argue much, having a family that values a drinker, having a partner who is clear and direct about drinking, having a larger social network, having nondrinking friends, and receiving support for abstinence from family, friends, and coworkers. Conversely, negative characteristics of the family and social network predict a poorer response to treatment. Negative influences on outcome include marital dissatisfaction; high levels of expressed emotion; having a partner who withdraws, tolerates use, or is passive about use; having more drinking friends and keeping them; and having even one friend that uses the same drug that the substance abuser uses.

Research on family-involved treatment suggests that specific interventions do make a difference. For adolescents, family therapy is strongly associated with better retention in treatment as well as better treatment outcomes. For adults, most research has focused on couple therapy. Here too the results are positive. Behavioral couple therapy leads to greater improvements in drinking or drug use than individually oriented therapy. Couple therapy also results in more stable and happier intimate relationships, better functioning of children, and greater decreases in domestic violence than therapy that does not involve the partner.

> *Behavioral couple therapy leads to greater improvements in drinking or drug use than individually oriented therapy.*

What happens in the couple or family therapy is important. Specific aspects of family-involved treatment are effective, including contingency contracting, relationship enhancement interventions, and communication training. Other types of interventions are less effective, particularly interventions that provide separate treatment for the user and family members. For example, separate treatment for parents and adolescents is substantially less successful than family treatment that includes all family members in the same therapy session.

Although research here is more limited, tailoring family-involved treatment to specific characteristics of the user seems to be important, particularly in fostering engagement in the treatment. One important dimension for adjusting family-involved treatment appears to be the degree to which the couple has a pattern of interaction char acterized by demands from one partner being met with withdrawal by the other partner. In couples that have a strong "demand–withdraw" pattern, structured approaches to couple therapy, such as cognitive-behavioral approaches, appear to result in more attrition from treatment than treatments based on systemic models of therapy. A second dimension that has been researched is the tailoring of treatment to the needs of specific racial or cultural groups. For example, including relevant themes in family sessions, such as those related to alienation, respect, and rage, appears to be important to engaging and developing a therapeutic alliance with African American adolescent males.

Families and Others Close to Drinkers or Drug Users Play an Important Role in the Maintenance of Change

As a drinker or drug user decreases or stops using, the composition of his or her social network may change. Family and close friends are affected by changes in the user, who in turn is affected by the actions of those in his or her social network. Naturalistically, social networks tend to evolve to include fewer drinkers and more nondrinkers. Nondrinkers become more important to the former drinker. Caucasian (but not African American) cocaine users have better outcomes if they have no contact with drug-using former friends. In general, having support for abstinence reduces the odds of drug use by 50%. Individuals in recovery cite their spouses as the most important factor in maintaining their successful self-change.

Conversely, maintaining substantial contact with drinking friends increases the risk of relapsing. Individuals who enter treatment with strong support from their friends for continued drinking appear to do well only if they are able to extract themselves from their heavy-drinking social network and establish a new network of nondrinking friends. Similarly, living with a drug or alcohol abuser after treatment is particularly difficult, increasing the odds of relapse by a factor of 2.5–3. Even if the user is not in close contact with family or friends who are actively using and abusing alcohol and drugs, family and social network factors may contribute to relapses. Marital, family, and other interpersonal stressors are common precipitants of relapse, suggesting that a possible mechanism by which family-involved treatment is effective may be the reduction in marital and family stressors.

Violence Is Prevalent in Families with a Member with a Substance Use Disorder and Should Be a Major Concern in Treatment and Prevention

Intimate partner violence is prevalent in couples, with or without substance use disorders, but rates are higher in couples in which one partner has an alcohol or other substance use disorder. Violence typically does not develop as a direct consequence of alcohol or drug use, but instead tends to develop early in relationships. The relationship between alcohol or drug use and increased violence is true whether the user is male or female, whether a woman is Caucasian or Latina, and whether the couple is a heterosexual or a gay male couple. Violence is not an isolated event in alcoholic relationships, is associated with greater unhappiness among women, and is a marker of greater marital dissatisfaction and instability.

Increasing aggression develops over time in intimate relationships. For example, verbal aggression early in a marriage predicts later physical aggression; physical aggression at one point in time predicts more physical aggression later on. Alcohol use makes these relations (between earlier and later aggression) even stronger.

Despite the high prevalence of domestic violence among individuals with substance use disorders, clinicians do not routinely assess for or deal with domestic violence as part of substance abuse treatment. Even when they do, they may apply inappropriate models of intervention for the domestic violence, such as providing separate referrals for the male and the female, or assuming that the female is never the initiator of violence.

What Works?

A substantial body of research supports the effectiveness of certain family-based treatment interventions both to prevent and to effectively treat substance use disorders.

Effective Preventive Family Interventions

Family-based approaches are effective in preventing alcohol and drug use and associated problems among high-risk youth. Several important principles are common to effective family-based prevention efforts. Multicomponent programs address multiple aspects of risk, family relationships, and family communication, and increase parents' skills and motivation to monitor their children's behavior. With very high-risk families, treatment needs to be fairly intensive. If the parents have extensive problems themselves, then interventions for the children should begin very early to be most effective. There are significant challenges to retaining very dysfunctional families in treatment, but salient incentives related to the family's need for childcare, food, housing, and transportation can help to retain these families. Treatment is effective when it is structured, goal-oriented, and includes practice during therapy sessions, homework between sessions, and other active learning experiences. Finally, preventive family interventions are most effective in keeping families in treatment if they are tailored to the developmental needs of the children and the cultural traditions of the family.

Effective Family/Social Network Approaches for Substance Abusers

Problem Recognition and Help Seeking

Family and friends often hear that they can do nothing to motivate a drinker or drug user to change. They may be counseled to detach from the drinker or drug user, hoping that he or she will become motivated to change through accumulated negative experiences. However, as Miller (Chapter 9, this volume) emphasizes, motivation is a state that is strongly influenced by experience. Family and friends can engage in very specific behaviors that will facilitate "motivation" through experiences that they create or foster through their own actions.

Specific treatments have been developed to help families motivate the user to change or seek help. Generally described as "unilateral family therapies," these treatments focus on changing three major aspects of family behavior: (1) communication, (2) consequences of use, and (3) self-care. Family members are taught assertive communication skills, how to give feedback about the consequences of use, and how to make specific requests for change. Families are taught to rearrange consequences so that users experience more negative consequences when using and more positive consequences when not using. And families are taught to take care of themselves and protect themselves from potential violence in the home. Research suggests that these unilateral models are effective, with about two-thirds of substance users seeking treatment after the family has received unilateral family therapy. Family members also report feeling better, which is an additional benefit of the approach. To date, unilateral approaches have not been tailored specifically to culturally defined

About two-thirds of substance users seek treatment after the family has received unilateral family therapy.

differences in family structure and family roles even though the populations studied have been ethnically diverse. It may be that certain types of unilateral interventions may be difficult to implement for persons of certain ethnic backgrounds. Thus, for example, making assertive requests for change might be particularly difficult for the adult child of an Asian American drug-using parent. Or firm limit setting about unacceptable behaviors might be particularly difficult for the Latina wife of a Latino drinker. Or trying to attend to one's own needs rather than taking care of an intoxicated and sick spouse might be culturally incompatible with the beliefs of a Native American woman.

Treatment/Active Change

Conventional lore encourages clinicians to provide treatment to the drinker or drug user, and to involve families only to address their own problems and coping responses. Typical clinical advice is to delay conjoint or family therapy for at least a year while the user focuses solely on his or her individual recovery. Findings from controlled research studies suggest a different approach. Family involvement from the outset of treatment and family therapy that includes important family members and the user together in the therapy session are important strategies to enhance treatment retention as well as to improve treatment outcomes.

A number of specific clinical interventions have strong empirical support for their effectiveness. These include contingency contracting for treatment-related behaviors (such as taking medication or attending support group meetings); a focus on improving daily interactions in the family, including shared recreational activities; increasing reciprocal positive exchanges; teaching constructive communication and problem solving; and enhancing family members' skills to support improvements and provide more effective responses to drinking or drug use.

Interventions also may focus on the drinker or drug user's larger social network. One focus of treatment should be on fostering the development of a social network that does not support drinking or drug use and that does support change. Such support may be enhanced within the client's existing social network, or may be accessed through some type of support group. Some clients are so lacking in resources or have such compromised social networks that active case management strategies may be necessary to foster their access to social resources.

Individual difference variables also must be considered in treatment planning that involves the family. An important variable is *social investment*, the degree to which the individual has and feels attachments to others, and how that social investment interacts with the degree of support that the individual receives from the social network. Social network-involved treatment tends to be more effective than individually focused treatment for drinkers with either a social network unsupportive of abstinence or with a low level of investment in their social network. Conversely, individually focused therapy seems to be more effective if drinkers have both a low level of support for abstinence from their social network *and* a low level of investment in their social network, or if drinkers have both high support for abstinence *and* high investment in their social network.

Couple therapy also should vary in its degree of structure, based on the nature of the couple's communication patterns, with less structured and task-focused therapy being appropriate for couples with a demand–withdraw pattern of interaction, who already are engaging in struggles around compliance.

When Should the Family Be Involved . . . or Not?

Although research supports the general value of involving families in treatment for individuals with substance use disorders, research has focused less on contraindications for family-involved treatment. Several factors seem to predict successful family-involved treatment, including (1) the absence of alcohol or drug problems in other family members; (2) a more severe alcohol or drug problem for the identified client; (3) some level of social and relationship stability such as having a job and being in a committed relationship; (4) coming to treatment after a crisis, particularly one that has threatened the stability or integrity of the family. There are, however, times when the family probably should not be involved in treatment, or at least in treatments that place the family together in the therapy room. If there has been significant domestic violence, resulting in injury or the need for medical attention, conjoint therapy is inappropriate. If the victim of domestic violence feels intimidated by the abuser or afraid of retribution after therapy sessions, then too it would be inappropriate to place the victim and the abuser in therapy together. Clearly, if there is a legal order that restrains the violent abuser from having contact with the victim, then treatment that involves them both would be inappropriate. Finally, there are some families in which interactions seem to be so "toxic" that placing them in the therapy room together may be inappropriate. Although research evidence is lacking, "toxic" families may (1) communicate in such cruel and destructive ways that involving them in therapy will increase the user's negative experience; (2) be unable to harness their hostility enough to be able to support the user's efforts at change; (3) be largely unresponsive to the therapist's interventions to teach constructive communication skills; or (4) have significant alcohol or drug problems themselves that they do not want to change. In such families, the focus of treatment may instead shift to assisting the user to focus on members of the social network outside the immediate family or development of additional sources of support that may provide more general emotional support as well as support for the user's attempts to change.

Robust Principles

1. Families are complex, dynamic, changing social systems. No single description can capture the range of family constellations.
2. Families exist within larger social networks of communities that have reciprocal patterns of influence with the functioning of the family.
3. Individual variables affect the ways that individuals seek, receive, and provide social support to others.
4. Persons with alcohol and other drug use disorders live in and have relationships with a network of family and friends, and that social network has a substantial influence on their use.
5. Family relationships may protect against the development of alcohol or drug problems.
6. Families and others close to the drinker or drug user may contribute to the development and maintenance of substance use/substance use disorders.
7. Families and others close to drinkers and drug users play a role in helping a user to recognize a problem and seek help.
8. Families and others close to drinkers and drug users have a significant impact on the change process and treatment success.
9. Families and others close to drinkers or drug users play an important role in the maintenance of change.
10. Violence is prevalent in families with a member with a substance use disorder and should be a major concern in treatment and prevention.
11. Specific elements of family-involved treatment are effective in preventing the development of alcohol and other drug problems. These include multicomponent programs to address multiple aspects of risk, a focus on family relationships and communication, enhancing parents' skills in monitoring their children's behavior, very early interventions with the highest risk families, and use of salient incentives to enhance treatment retention.
12. Generally, family-involved treatment may facilitate positive treat-

ment outcomes and families should be involved in the treatment process. However, under certain circumstances, family involvement may be counterproductive or even destructive. Specific approaches to family involvement that are effective in treating alcohol and other drug problems include sessions that include family members and the user together, use of contingency contracting procedures, a focus on relationship/family functioning as part of the treatment, tailoring treatment to individual characteristics of the user and his or her social network, fostering a social network that supports the user's goals, and use of case management strategies for individuals who lack functional social networks.

Suggested Readings

Castro, F., Proescholdbell, R. J., Abeita, L., & Rodriguez, D. (1999). Ethnic and cultural minority groups. In B. S. McCrady & E. E. Epstein (Eds.), *Addictions: A comprehensive guidebook* (pp. 499–526). New York: Oxford University Press.

Epstein, E. E., & McCrady, B. S. (2002). Marital therapy in the treatment of alcohol problems. In A. S. Gurman & N. S. Jacobson (Eds.), *Clinical handbook of couple therapy* (3rd ed., pp. 597–628). New York: Guilford Press.

Galanter, M. (1999). *Network therapy for alcohol and drug abuse.* New York: Guilford Press.

Havassy, B. E., Hall, S. M., & Wasserman, D. A. (1991). Social support and relapse: Commonalities among alcoholics, opiate users and cigarette smokers. *Addictive Behaviors, 16,* 235–246.

Jacob, T., & Johnson, S. L. (1999). Family influences on alcohol and substance abuse. In P. J. Ott, R. E. Tarter, & R. T. Ammerman (Eds.), *Sourcebook on substance abuse: Etiology, epidemiology, assessment, and treatment* (pp. 166–174). Needham Heights, MA: Allyn & Bacon.

Kumpfer, K. L., & Alvarado, R. (2003). Family-strengthening approaches for the prevention of youth problem behaviors. *American Psychologist, 58,* 457–465.

Leonard, K. E., & Mudar, P. (2003). Peer and partner drinking and the transition to marriage: A longitudinal examination of selection and influence processes. *Psychology of Addictive Behaviors, 17,* 115–125.

Longabaugh, R., Wirtz, P. W., Beattie, M. C., Noel, N., & Stout, R. L. (1995). Matching treatment focus to patient social investment and support: 18-month follow-up results. *Journal of Consulting and Clinical Psychology, 63,* 296–307.

Longabaugh, R., Wirtz, P. W., Zweben, A., & Stout, R. L. (1998). Network support for drinking: Alcoholics Anonymous and long-term matching effects. *Addiction, 93,* 1313–1333.

McCrady, B. S., Epstein, E. E., & Sell, R. D. (2003). Theoretical bases of family approaches to substance abuse treatment. In F. Rotgers, J. Morgenstern, & S. T.

Walters (Eds.), *Treating substance abusers: Theory and technique* (2nd ed., pp. 112–139). New York: Guilford Press.

Miller, W. R., Meyers, R. J., & Tonigan, J. S. (1999). Engaging the unmotivated in treatment for alcohol problems: A comparison of three strategies for intervention through family members. *Journal of Consulting and Clinical Psychology, 67,* 688–697.

O'Farrell, T. J., & Fals-Stewart, W. (1999). Treatment models and methods: Family models. In B. S. McCrady & E. E. Epstein (Eds.), *Addictions: A comprehensive guidebook* (pp. 287–305). New York: Oxford University Press.

O'Farrell, T. J., Van Hutton, V., & Murphy, C. M. (1999). Domestic violence before and after alcoholism treatment: A two-year longitudinal study. *Journal of Studies on Alcohol, 60,* 317–321.

Roberts, L. J., & McCrady, B. S. (2004). *Alcohol problems in intimate relationships: Identification and intervention: A guide for marriage and family therapists.* Bethesda, MD: National Institute on Alcohol Abuse and Alcoholism.

Stanton, M. D., & Shadish, W. R. (1997). Outcome, attrition, and family-couples treatment for drug abuse: A meta-analysis and review of the controlled, comparative studies. *Psychological Bulletin, 122,* 170–191.

CHAPTER 12

Social Contexts
and Substance Use

RUDOLF H. MOOS

How can we grasp the fundamental characteristics of social contexts
and the processes by which they affect and are affected by substance
use and misuse? Some contexts offer powerful inducements and modeling that enhance the likelihood of substance misuse, whereas others
provide social bonds that shield individuals from exposure to and use
of substances. To address these issues, I describe four theoretical perspectives that underlie most of the relevant research and use the research findings to formulate evidence-based propositions about social
contexts that may help shape effective interventions to reduce substance use and misuse.

Theoretical Perspectives

Four related theories have emphasized the role of social context in substance use and misuse. According to *social control theory*, strong bonds
with family, school, work, religion, and other aspects of traditional society motivate individuals to engage in responsible behavior and
refrain from substance use and other deviant pursuits. When such
social bonds are weak or absent, individuals are less likely to adhere to
conventional standards and tend to engage in rebellious behavior, such
as the misuse of alcohol and drugs. The main cause of weak attachments to existing social standards is social disorganization and inadequate monitoring of behavior, as exhibited by families that lack cohe-

182

sion and structure, school and work settings that lack supervision and vigilance, and disorganized neighborhoods.

Strong bonds with family, school, work, religion, and other aspects of traditional society motivate individuals to refrain from substance use.

Behavioral economics or behavioral choice theory, which is closely related to the social control perspective, focuses specifically on involvement in protective activities. In behavioral choice theory the key element of the social context is the alternative reinforcements provided by activities other than substance use. These alternative reinforcements can protect individuals from exposure to substances and opportunities to use them, as well as from escalating and maintaining substance use. The theory posits that the choice of one reinforcing behavior, such as substance use, depends in part on lack of effective access to alternative reinforcements, such as involvement in school and work pursuits, religious engagement, and participation in physical activity. For example, physical activity and substance use may both elevate mood and decrease anxiety, which may make them functionally similar and substitutable.

According to *social learning theory*, substance use originates in the substance-specific attitudes and behaviors of the adults and peers who serve as an individual's role models. Modeling effects begin with observation and imitation of substance-specific behaviors, continue with social reinforcement for substance use and expectations of positive consequences from substance use, and culminate in substance use and misuse. In essence, this model proposes that substance use is a function of the easy availability of substances, positive norms, and peer use.

Finally, *stress and coping theory* posits that the stressful life circumstances that often stem from social disorganization, including stressors emanating from family members and friends, school, work, and neighborhood, lead to distress and alienation and eventually to substance misuse. For example, the work stressors or alienation model suggests that employee substance use is a response to the problematic qualities of the workplace, such as interpersonal conflict with supervisors and coworkers, unfair treatment, meaningless and low-level work, high work demands, lack of participation in decision making, and physical hazards. Stressors are most likely to impel substance use among individuals with inadequate coping skills who try to avoid facing problematic situations and to escape from experiencing distress and alienation.

All four of these theories encompass the presence of both social causation and self-selection processes. Most of the relevant research reflects a social causation perspective in which the environment is seen as a causal factor that shapes individuals' substance use, such as when a youngster's peers model and reinforce smoking and drinking. From this perspective, social contexts tend to maintain or accentuate individual characteristics that are congruent with their dominant aspects. In a closely related self-selection process, individuals choose or alter social contexts, which, in turn, shape their subsequent behavior. Youngsters who smoke and drink may choose friends who smoke and drink and who then play a role in shaping and maintaining their substance use. Self-selection and social causation are ongoing interconnected processes that mold individual cognition and behavior.

The approach I take here is guided by these theories and a primary focus on social causation, that is, on how specific aspects of life domains shape attitudes and behaviors associated with substance use and misuse. I consider four domains in individuals' lives: families; friends and peer groups, including schools; the workplace; and neighborhoods. I also comment on the relevance of the four theories in understanding the role of intervention programs in altering substance use and misuse.

Families and Substance Use and Misuse

Families and Youth

The theories described earlier highlight the main processes that underlie the role of the family in the socialization of substance use. A general effect occurs when disruptions in parenting lead to a lack of nurturance (cohesion) and control (monitoring) and to social stressors that impair the bonding process and increase the likelihood of alienation and distress. A substance-specific effect involves social learning, the development of expectancies, and modeling family members' substance use. In general, these sets of influences have comparable effects on tobacco, alcohol, and marijuana and other drug use.

Bonding and Monitoring

Disruptions of basic family management processes, such as lack of support and abusive parental behavior, parent–child conflict, erratic and inconsistent discipline, and inadequate parental monitoring raise the likelihood of youngsters' substance use, are associated with earlier initiation of use, and predict accelerated growth trends in use. In contrast, high family involvement and support, age-appropriate parental supervision, and sanctions against nonnormative activities can foster youngsters' self-control and problem-solving orientation, and lessen the likelihood of their substance misuse. Parental support and monitoring enhance bonding with educational and social values and promote the likelihood of participation in activities that may protect youngsters from substance use.

Parental Modeling

On average, parents' modeling of substance use increases their children's future use. Parental alcohol use predicts youngsters' beliefs in the positive effects of alcohol, which is associated with earlier initiation of alcohol use and subsequent alcohol misuse. Youngsters who report that adults who are important to them smoke, parental approval of smoking, siblings who smoke, and offers of cigarettes are more likely to become daily smokers. In general, weak attachments with parents are a risk factor for substance use; however, when parents are substance users, strong child–parent attachments may enhance the likelihood of youngsters modeling their parents' substance use.

Stress and Coping

Youngsters who experience more negative life events are more likely to engage in substance use and show a sharper rise in use over time. Many of these events are associated with parent–child conflict, physical and sexual abuse, and parental separation and divorce, and thus are part of the syndrome of growing up in a high-risk family. Life stressors may shake youngsters' beliefs in the predictability of events and the relevance of conventional norms and lead to their alienation and loosening of social bonds. In contrast, high parental support and monitoring strengthen family bonds, reduce the likelihood of negative life events and help youngsters to interpret them when they occur, and enhance youngsters' self-esteem and coping skills, all of which protect against substance misuse.

Mutual Influence Processes

When a youngster engages in substance use or misuse, mutual influence processes occur. As parents try to manage a child's substance use, they may become less supportive and institute strict rules and discipline, thereby alienating the child and stimulating rebellious behavior. In a maladaptive spiral, parents sometimes strengthen family control and restrict independence in a vain attempt to keep the youngster's behavior within acceptable limits. In a continuation of this downward spiral, escalating substance use may lead to a decline in parental support and monitoring. Thus, parent–youth conflict is partly a response to

parents' attempts to influence and control the youngster's initial problem behavior. More generally, some families perpetuate a cycle in
which parental dysfunction and children's problems coexist in an ever-
worsening reciprocal relationship.

Long-Term Effects

Lack of bonding and supervision, modeling, and childhood stressors
associated with the family of origin can have a long-term influence on
substance use. Parental conflict and abuse, coercive and overcon-
trolling parenting, and family members who model substance use are
associated with more tobacco, alcohol, and drug use among young
adults. Childhood stressors, including parental neglect and family conflict, disruption of family routines and family separation, and physical
and sexual abuse, play an important role in young adults' and adults' alcohol misuse and in the intergenerational transmission of alcohol use
disorders. Overall, the factors that lead to and sustain alcohol use in
adolescence and early adulthood foreshadow problematic substance
use during the adult years.

Families, Young Adults, and Adults

Role Transitions and Social Bonding

Role transitions, such as completion of education, entering the workforce, and getting married typically involve social bonding in which
young adults change their substance use to make it more compatible
with the expectations associated with their new roles. In this respect,
individuals who marry and remain married tend to reduce their use of
tobacco, alcohol, and illicit drugs. Transitions to parenthood also are
associated with a decline in substance use. One mechanism through
which adult roles reduce the risk of alcohol problems is by social control or placement of new responsibilities and demands that are incompatible with heavy drinking or lifestyles that promote heavy alcohol
use. Individuals who do not get married or who divorce tend to consume more alcohol and are more likely to engage in heavy drinking
and marijuana use than are stably married individuals.

Selective Mating and Spouse Modeling

Similarity between spouses in substance use reflects both the selection
of mates who share certain attributes (self-selection or assortative mat-
ing) and the influence of one spouse on the other (social causation or
socialization). In this vein, young adults who have drinking problems

and/or are heavier lifetime users of marijuana are more likely to marry a spouse who drinks heavily and/or uses marijuana. In turn, spousal concordance in problem drinking and marijuana use increases over time. More generally, individuals who have a spouse or partner who misuses alcohol or drugs are more likely to use and misuse alcohol or drugs themselves.

Conjugal Family Bonding and Social Control

Conjugal family bonding and social control is involved in substance use among adults. In a compelling example, smokers who live in smoke-free homes modify their smoking behavior. Nonsmoking family members' preferences for a smoke-free home are associated with lighter smoking, intention to quit, recent quit attempts, and a longer time to relapse following a quit attempt among family members who smoke. Conversely, specific aspects of family climate that reflect poor bonding and control, such as high conflict and a lack of support, organization, and social integration, are associated with alcohol abuse among adults. Moreover, individuals with alcohol use disorders and their spouses tend to view their families as relatively low in support and structure.

Families and Entry into and the Outcome of Treatment

Family members can influence the onset, continuation, and outcome of treatment for substance misuse. Both bonding and modeling are involved in these effects. Family members tend to have a positive influence when they refrain from using substances themselves and support reduced substance use; they have a detrimental effect when they use substances or hinder an individual's attempts to abstain or reduce substance use. Consistent with the underlying theories, both abstinence-specific support and modeling and general support and bonding contribute to achieving and maintaining successful treatment outcome. In contrast, patients whose spouse or partner shows a lack of bonding by expressing criticism and hostility toward them are more likely to relapse.

Friends, Peer Groups, and Substance Use and Misuse

Friends, Peer Groups, and Youth

The key approach used to describe the initiation and progression of substance use among youth is the *gateway hypothesis*, which posits a developmental sequence of involvement with substance use such that initiation begins with substances like tobacco and alcohol, may continue with marijuana, and may eventually extend to other illicit drugs. The main models that have been used to explain this progression (or lack of it) are social learning theory, with its emphasis on modeling friends' and peer groups' behavior, and social control and behavioral choice theories, with their emphasis on the protective role of bonding to conventional norms and activities.

Peer Cluster Theory and Peer Modeling

Peer cluster theory posits that youngsters establish key aspects of their identity through relationships with peers and that, in most cases, these relationships exert positive influences that reduce the likelihood of exposure to substances and of substance use and misuse. Friends who model conventional norms and behavior and engage in activities that are incompatible with substance use may protect youngsters against association with deviant peers and subsequent problem drinking and drug use. Participation in traditional pursuits, such as academic achievement, sports, and religion, can strengthen social affiliation among youngsters who do not use substances and reinforce remaining substance-free.

On the other hand, peers may represent a haven from family problems and offer opportunities for escapism and deviant behavior through excessive substance use. Peers share ideas and beliefs about substances, shape attitudes toward them, and provide substances and the social contexts for their use. Three related forms of social influence affect youngsters' substance use: explicit offers of substance use, social modeling, and perceptions of friends' and other youngsters' substance use.

With respect to tobacco use, social learning and modeling, especially exposure to peers and friends who smoke; peer approval and offers of cigarettes; the availability of cigarettes; and the perceived prevalence of smoking among peers are all associated with an increased risk of smoking. When youngsters have close friends and/or a sibling who smokes, and when most of the peers in their friendship group smoke, they are more likely to begin smoking and to smoke more heavily. Comparable findings hold for alcohol and marijuana use.

School Norms, Modeling, and Social Control

One index of peer norms and behavior is the prevalence of substance use among students in a school. When a higher percentage of students in a school use cigarettes, alcohol, and marijuana, youngsters perceive that these substances are more acceptable and available. School norms for substance use, as measured by averaging the reported use of all the students in a school, may be independent predictors of substance use, over and above the prediction afforded by peer and best friends' use and being in a peer network of users. Importantly, peer influence or social causation effects may be especially strong when they occur in a social context in which tobacco and/or alcohol and drug use are highly prevalent. Friends' drug use is likely to be less influential in contexts in which most peers are not using substances.

Schools may also serve a social monitoring or social control function. Students in schools that emphasize student involvement (social bonding) and discipline are less likely to begin smoking or to transition into daily smoking; these schools also attenuate the link between poor emotional self-regulation and smoking. Specifically, students with poor emotional control who are in schools with more involvement and discipline are less likely to begin smoking than are similar students in schools with low involvement and lax discipline. A structured school milieu with well-articulated rules provides more monitoring and social control and thus can reduce students' substance use.

Moderators of Peer Influence

A present (vs. future) time perspective, avoidance (vs. approach) coping, low self-esteem, extroversion, and a preference for a submissive or follower role tend to foreshadow more susceptibility to social influence, which is associated with increased exposure to peer drinking and heightened alcohol use. In addition, youngsters who are social outsiders or isolates may be more susceptible to peer influence than are youngsters who are group or clique members. For example, youngsters who are social outsiders are more likely to begin smoking if their chosen best friend is a smoker than if he or she is a nonsmoker. To win favor and gain access to a friendship group, youngsters may be influenced by their future or desired friends as well as by their existing friends.

> *Present time perspective, avoidance coping, low self-esteem, extroversion, and preference for a follower role foreshadow more susceptibility to social influence.*

Mutual Influence Processes

Since mutual choice is involved in friendship formation, the association between a youngster's substance use and his or her friends' substance use depends on selecting and maintaining like-minded friendships (social selection), as well as on the influence of existing friends (social causation). Social selection contributes to peer group similarity in substance use; once formed, friendships tend to reinforce common behaviors and may operate as a stabilizing influence on substance use. In this regard, there is a positive, prospective, bidirectional association between adolescents' and peers' substance use. Adolescents who report more substance use subsequently tend to report more peer substance use, and vice versa.

Friends, Peer Groups, and Young Adults and Adults

Sources of Peer Group Influence

The main sources of peer influence on young adult substance use are the same as those for youth: direct modeling, offers to use substances, and perceived social norms. With respect to modeling, experimental studies have paired target individuals with confederates trained to consume particular amounts of alcohol. In general, individuals exposed to heavy-drinking models consume more alcohol than individuals exposed to light-drinking models or to no models at all. Active peer influence, which ranges from offering to get someone a drink to encouragement of drinking to commands to drink, is associated with more alcohol consumption. Perceived normative support for drinking (both perceptions of other people's approval of drinking and of how much they drink) also predicts more alcohol use and alcohol-related problems. Moreover, same-gender and opposite-gender friends' use of cigarettes and alcohol and their binge drinking predicts young adults' use of the same substances and the same behaviors.

Peer Modeling and College Students' Substance Use

Most generally, students in heavy-drinking college environments are more likely to have alcohol-related problems. College students exposed to "wet" environments, which include colleges with a pub on campus and social contexts in which drinking is prevalent and alcohol is inexpensive and easily accessible, are more likely to engage in binge drinking and marijuana use than are their peers without similar exposure. Students in relatively protected and isolated college settings may be especially prone to peer influences. However, probably because other social contexts become more important, the effects of college environments appear to be short lived: affiliation with a fraternity or sorority in college does not predict postcollege heavy drinking.

Peer Networks and Heavy Drinking among Adults

Friends' alcohol consumption, positive drinking norms, and approval of drinking are consistently associated with heavier alcohol consumption and drinking problems among adults. For example, among young married couples, a social network composed of friends who consume more alcohol tends to be associated with heavier drinking among both husbands and wives. Moreover, the alcohol consumption of the spouse's friends is associated with the partner's drinking; this connection holds for both husbands and wives, which suggests that mutual-influence processes shape a couple's drinking patterns and those of their social networks to be consistent with each other.

These findings hold among older adults and, in fact, friends' approval of drinking is one of the most consistent predictors of late-onset drinking problems among lifetime non-problem drinkers. Friends and peer groups who consume more alcohol and espouse heavy-drinking norms appear to promote heavier drinking among individuals in all stages of the lifespan, including old age.

Mutual Influence Processes

Both self-selection and social causation effects are involved in the association between friends' and own drinking. For example, compared with entering students who live in a dormitory or elsewhere, students who join Greek houses consumed more alcohol in high school (self-selection); in turn, residence in a Greek house is associated with an especially marked rise in alcohol consumption (social causation). In part, this is due to modeling the heavy drinking of student leaders and the strong peer pressure to drink. In general, selection effects seem to operate more strongly during the formation of social ties when individuals seek out and affiliate with others whose drinking habits are similar to their own, whereas social influence effects seem to operate more strongly in stable social networks.

Friends, Peer Groups, and the Process of Remission and Relapse

Friends and peer groups can affect the process of remission and relapse. More social network support for abstinence, fewer substance users in an individual's social network and an abstinence-oriented network, predict lower risk for relapse after attempts at self-change or treatment for substance use. In contrast, individuals whose friends or peers use substances are at heightened risk. These influences primarily involve social bonding and modeling.

Work and Substance Use and Misuse

Work and Youth

High-school students who work more intensively, especially 20 hours or more per week, are more likely to use substances and to experience increased levels of future use. Work intensity is an example of an "off-time" transition that is associated with a decrease in family bonding and conflict with parents, a decline in age-graded family controls, greater economic and social independence, lower academic aspirations, and more involvement with friends and dating. Work also is a locus of association with older adolescents and young adults, who may introduce a youngster to alcohol and drug use. Students' work intensity is associated with prior poor educational performance and adjustment problems and may be part of a "precocious development syndrome" and premature engagement in adult-like roles.

Work among Young Adults and Adults

In contrast to the link between intensive work and more substance use among adolescents, employed status generally is associated with less substance use among adults, especially with respect to alcohol use. In longitudinal studies, favorable job changes (such as moving from unemployed or underemployed to employed status) reduce the odds of binge drinking among prior binge drinkers. Working status is likely to keep substance use in check due to the monitoring, supervision, and social control imposed by a regular job, as well as the associated structure, stability, and curtailment of unmonitored leisure time. In contrast, unemployed status and financial stressors, which are associated with lower levels of bonding and monitoring, and alienation stemming from lack of material resources predict increased substance use.

Modeling, Norms, and Availability

Coworkers' alcohol use and a positive work-group climate for drinking, as reflected in availability of alcohol at work, permissive drinking norms, and attitudinal support for drinking, are associated with employees' frequent drinking, heavy drinking, and alcohol-related problems. For example, individuals in jobs in which there is more approval of alcohol use and social pressure to drink, more coworker drinking, and easy access to substances are more likely to misuse alcohol and drugs and to WUI (i.e., work under the influence of alcohol and drugs). When substances are available as an integral part of the workplace, such as alcohol among restaurant and entertainment workers and drugs among health care employees, coworker use and perceived pressure to use are especially strongly associated with a high risk of substance use and misuse.

Monitoring and Supervision

Lack of strong policies restricting or eliminating the use of alcohol at work, along with lax and inconsistent monitoring, are associated with the availability of alcohol and employee drinking at work. Changing schedules, such as shift and night work, and traveling and working away from home, which are associated with reduced monitoring and more unstructured free time, also enhance substance use. These aspects of the workplace tend to be reinforced by coworkers' approval of drinking and heavier drinking and are associated with negative workplace consequences of drinking, such as low morale and a higher likelihood of accidents.

Work Stressors and Coping

Work-related stressors, such as job role ambiguity and physical risk, powerlessness, and pressure; lack of social resources, especially supervisor and coworker support; and boredom and alienation from work are consistently associated with alcohol misuse. Two key variables involve heightened psychological and/or physical demands and a lack of job discretion or control. For example, compared to men in more benign work settings, men employed in work settings characterized by high demands and low job discretion or control, and low social support, are more likely to develop alcohol abuse or dependence.

Consistent with stress and coping theory, some of the influences of the workplace may be moderated or mediated by coping styles. In this vein, workplace stressors are more closely associated with heightened alcohol consumption and drinking problems among individuals who endorse escapist reasons for drinking than among those who do not. Moreover, employees' perceptions of high work pressure and lack of autonomy and supervisor support have been associated with escapist reasons for drinking and, in turn, heavy drinking and negative consequences of drinking.

Neighborhoods and Substance Use and Misuse

Substance Use Norms and Modeling

At a broad level, easier availability of alcohol in cities and neighborhoods, as reflected in the number of establishments that sell alcoholic beverages, is associated with more arrests for public drunkenness and more misdemeanor and felony drunk driving arrests. Neighborhoods characterized by more available drugs, street-corner drug sales, and drug paraphernalia have a higher concentration of adolescents who use alcohol and drugs and have drug problems. In a social causation or contagion process, persons who believe they are at risk for drug use, or who have used drugs, tend to cluster within neighborhoods in part because their neighbors expose and initiate them into drug use. In this vein, "exposure opportunity" to substances in disadvantaged neighborhoods may manifest itself among youngsters as early as in the sixth grade.

The number of establishments that sell alcoholic beverages is associated with more arrests for public drunkenness and more misdemeanor and felony drunk driving arrests.

Monitoring and Social Control

Lack of social cohesion and effective monitoring of residents' behavior are key mediators through which demographic and structural factors eventuate in heightened rates of neighborhood substance use. Indices of neighborhood poverty and the number of outlets for alcohol sales are associated with less social cohesion, which, in turn, is associated with more alcohol and drug use among neighborhood youth and higher rates of alcohol- and drug-related arrests. Aspects of neighborhood social disorganization, as reflected in poverty, residential mobility, unemployment, and higher population density, may render neighborhoods incapable of providing normative control over illicit behavior.

Neighborhood Deprivation and Stressors

Indices of neighborhood deprivation, such as dilapidated housing, a higher proportion of unemployed men, and more individuals living in overcrowded households, are associated with higher odds of being a smoker, even after controlling for individual-level socioeconomic status. In addition, some neighborhood risk factors, such as gang activity and violence, and the perceived need for toughness and emotional isolation, may reflect heightened individual-level stressors and engender hopelessness, alienation, and elevated substance use, especially among inner-city youngsters. Neighborhood risk is associated with a subsequent decline in protective factors, such as supportive family and peer relationships; in addition, lack of family bonding and monitoring may exacerbate the effect of neighborhood risk on drug use.

Cross-Domain Influences

A few studies have examined neighborhood factors in the context of family, peer, and school characteristics. For example, neighborhood deterioration may be associated with youngsters' drug involvement in conjunction with family conflict and lack of cohesion and peer models for drug use. Conversely, consensus about child-monitoring practices and strong community–school partnerships can enhance the positive influence of parenting behavior on a youngster. Youngsters from families in which a parent has a drug use disorder do better when there are more working adults in the local community, probably because these adults provide mentoring and enhance socialization. From a broader perspective, macrosocial conditions, as embodied in neighborhood characteristics and socioeconomic status, may be fundamental causes of the family, peer, and school contexts that underlie the multiple risk factors associated with substance use and misuse.

Intervention and Prevention Programs

Ongoing life settings and intervention programs are comparable in that both encompass aspects of social bonding and monitoring, modeling and peer norms, and behavioral choice; both establish a context for substance use or nonuse; and both involve self-selection and social causation processes.

Social Bonding and Monitoring

An emphasis on social bonding and monitoring is one of the key common aspects of intervention programs and may have as much or more of an impact on clients than does the specific content or type of intervention. In general, counselors who are better able to establish a supportive therapeutic bond, and those who maintain an appropriate level of social control and monitoring, enhance clients' substance use outcomes. Supportive group and residential treatment settings that are clear, well organized, and monitor clients' substance use tend to engage clients in treatment, strengthen their self-confidence, and contribute to a reduction in symptoms and substance use. In contrast, clients of counselors who are impersonal or confrontational consistently do poorly, probably because criticism and conflict discourage social bonding and elicit resistance and withdrawal.

Similarly, the positive effects of mutual help groups on substance use appear to be due in part to their emphasis on social bonding and monitoring. Members of mutual help groups that are more cohesive and well organized, and that include some monitoring, such as is provided by Alcoholics Anonymous sponsors, tend to have better substance use outcomes. These social contexts create and maintain participants' motivation for change, enhance self-efficacy and reliance on approach coping, and strengthen supportive friendship networks.

Modeling and Peer Norms

The power of modeling and peer norms is demonstrated most profoundly in therapeutic community and other sober-living and residential treatment programs, and is one of the hallmarks of 12-step treatment. Moreover, a primary reason that self-help and mutual support groups are associated with positive long-term outcomes is that they provide a cohesive social network that models abstinence and monitors individuals' substance use.

Most broadly, the benefits of intervention programs seem to depend on the same conditions that impel positive substance use outcomes in other life domains: high-quality relationships that provide a context for social bonding, a moderate level of structure and monitoring, and abstinence-oriented peer norms. In addition, these programs encompass activities that provide alternatives to substance use, such as engagement in work, active leisure, and spiritual pursuits. In this regard, the social processes that underlie the initiation and cessation of substance use and misuse may be common to everyday life domains, formal treatment, and informal help.

Robust Principles

Theoretical Perspectives

1. Common forces in family, friend and peer group, work, and neighborhood contexts influence youngsters' and adults' substance use and misuse. These forces involve social bonding and monitoring, behavioral choice or availability of activities that protect against substance use, modeling and norms, and life stress and coping factors.
2. Social contexts tend to maintain or accentuate individual characteristics that are congruent with their dominant aspects.

The Family

3. Disruptions in parenting lead to a lack of cohesion and control and to social stressors that impair the bonding process and heighten

the likelihood of a youngster's substance use and misuse. In contrast, parental support and monitoring enhances youngsters' bonding with family and social values and lessens the chance of youngsters developing deviant attitudes and using substances.

4. When parents and other family members approve of and engage in substance use, youngsters and adults are more likely to develop positive expectancies about substances and to model family members' substance use.

5. Parents' substance misuse is associated with more childhood stressors, such as parental neglect and conflict, disruption of family routines, and physical and sexual abuse, which foreshadow a higher likelihood of their children's substance use.

6. Stressful life circumstances, especially those associated with parental and family problems, may shake youngsters' beliefs in the predictability of events and the relevance of conventional norms, and lead to alienation and a loosening of social bonds, which heighten the likelihood of substance use.

7. There are mutual influence processes between parents and children: lack of family support and monitoring can trigger an increase in a youngster's substance use and, in turn, a youngster's substance use can trigger a decline in family support and monitoring.

8. Role transitions, such as getting married and becoming a parent, involve socialization in which young adults reduce their substance use to make it more compatible with their new role expectations. However, precocious transitions, such as marriage or parenthood before completing high school, are associated with more substance use and misuse.

Friends and Peer Groups

9. Social learning and modeling, especially exposure to friends and peers who use substances, peer approval and offers of substances, and the perceived prevalence of substance use among peers, are associated with an increased risk of youngsters' initiation of substance use and progression to substance misuse.

10. Youngsters who are extroverted, have a present time perspective, report low self-esteem, rely on avoidance coping, and prefer a submissive or follower role tend to be more susceptible to peer influence; this is also true of youngsters who are social outsiders or isolates.

11. Friends mutually reinforce each other for norms, values, and behaviors that are consistent with their own inclinations; thus friend-

ships can result either in an increase or in a decline in substance use.

12. Peers' involvement in conventional pursuits and disapproval of substance use can enhance social bonding and modeling and participation in activities that protect youngsters from exposure to and use of substances.

13. Schools may serve a social monitoring and social control function. Students in schools that emphasize student involvement and discipline are less likely to begin substance use or to transition into daily or heavy use.

14. There is a lifespan developmental continuity in the influence of modeling: friends' alcohol consumption and approval of drinking, positive drinking norms, and overt offers to use substances are associated with more substance use and misuse among young, middle-aged, and older adults.

Work

15. High-school students who engage in intensive part-time work show a decline in family bonding and more conflict with parents, lower academic aspirations, and more exposure to deviant peers, and are more likely to engage in substance use.

16. Among adults, employed status helps to keep substance use in check due to the monitoring, supervision, and social control imposed by a regular job. In contrast, unemployed or underemployed status increases the risk of heavy drinking, probably due to alienation and lack of monitoring.

17. In the workplace, lack of monitoring and social control, availability of substances, positive norms and coworker substance use, and work stressors that contribute to alienation are associated with employees' substance use.

18. Workplace social context risk factors for alcohol use are more closely associated with heightened alcohol use among individuals who endorse escapist reasons for drinking than among those who do not.

Neighborhoods

19. In neighborhoods, positive substance use norms and modeling, lack of monitoring and social control, and deprivation and stressors are associated with a heightened prevalence of substance use.

20. Neighborhood risk factors are associated with a decline in proximal protective factors, such as supportive family and peer relation-

ships; the lack of these supportive bonds may heighten the effect of neighborhood risk factors on substance use.

Intervention and Prevention Programs

21. Ongoing life domains and intervention programs are comparable in that both involve social bonding and social control, peer modeling, and behavioral choice, and both establish a context for substance use or nonuse.
22. The emphasis on social bonding, social control and monitoring, and peer modeling are common aspects of formal intervention programs and mutual support groups, and may have as much or more of an impact on clients as does the specific content or type of intervention.
23. The benefits of intervention programs depend on the same conditions that impel positive outcomes in other life domains: high-quality relationships that provide a context for social bonding, a moderate level of structure and monitoring, and modeling of abstinence-oriented norms and conventional behavior.

Acknowledgments

Preparation of this chapter was supported by the Department of Veterans Affairs Health Services Research and Development Service and by Grant No. AA12718 from the National Institute on Alcohol Abuse and Alcoholism. Ruth Cronkite, John Finney, and Christine Timko made helpful comments on an earlier draft of the chapter. The views expressed here are mine and do not necessarily represent the views of the Department of Veterans Affairs.

Suggested Readings

Aquilino, W. S., & Supple, A. J. (2001). Long-term effects of parenting practices during adolescence on well-being outcomes in young adulthood. *Journal of Family Issues, 22,* 289–308.

Aseltine, R. H., Jr. (1995). A reconsideration of parental and peer influences on adolescent deviance. *Journal of Health and Social Behavior, 36*(2), 103–121.

Audrain-McGovern, J., Rodriquez, D., Tercyak, K. P., Epstein, L. H., Goldman, P., & Wileyto, E. P. (2004). Applying a behavioral economic framework to understanding adolescent smoking. *Psychology of Addictive Behaviors, 18,* 64–73.

Bachman, J. G., Wadsworth, K. N., O'Malley, P. M., Johnston, L. D., & Schulenberg, J. E. (1997). *Smoking, drinking, and drug use in young adulthood: The impacts of new freedoms and new responsibilities.* Mahwah, NJ: Erlbaum.

Bauman, K. E., & Ennett, S. T. (1996). On the importance of peer influence for adolescent drug use: Commonly neglected considerations. *Addiction, 91*(2), 185–198.

Borsari, B., & Carey, K. B. (2001). Peer influences on college drinking: A review of the research. *Journal of Substance Abuse, 13*(4), 391–424.

Dishion, T. J., & Owen, L. D. (2002). A longitudinal analysis of friendships and substance use: Bidirectional influence from adolescence to adulthood. *Developmental Psychology, 38*(4), 480–491.

Ennett, S. T., Flewelling, R. L., Lindrooth, R. C., & Norton, E. C. (1997). School and neighborhood characteristics associated with school rates of alcohol, cigarette, and marijuana use. *Journal of Health and Social Behavior, 38*, 55–71.

Erickson, K. G., Crosnoe, R., & Dornbusch, S. M. (2000). A social process model of adolescent deviance: Combining social control and differential association perspectives. *Journal of Youth and Adolescence, 29*(4), 395–425.

Jessor, R., Donovan, J. E., & Costa, F. M. (1991). *Beyond adolescence: Problem behavior and young adult development.* New York: Cambridge University Press.

Kandel, D. B. (Ed.). (2002). *Stages and pathways of drug involvement: Examining the gateway hypothesis.* New York: Cambridge University Press.

Martin, J. K., Roman, P. M., & Blum, T. C. (1996). Job stress, drinking networks, and social support at work: A comprehensive model of employees' problem drinking. *Sociological Quarterly, 37*, 579–599.

Perkins, H. W. (2002). Social norms and the prevention of alcohol misuse in collegiate contexts. *Journal of Studies on Alcohol,* (Suppl.) (14), 164–172.

Petraitis, J., Flay, B. R., & Miller, T. Q. (1995). Reviewing theories of adolescent substance use: Organizing pieces in the puzzle. *Psychological Bulletin, 117*(1), 67–86.

Sher, K. J., & Gotham, H. J. (1999). Pathological alcohol involvement: A developmental disorder of young adulthood. *Development and Psychopathology, 11*, 933–956.

CHAPTER 13

Ethnography and Applied Substance Misuse Research

Anthropological and Cross-Cultural Factors

ROBERT G. CARLSON

Ethnographers, primarily from the disciplines of sociology and anthropology, have made contributions to understanding the role and use of alcohol and other drugs in different settings around the world since the early 1930s. As an applied field in substance use/misuse research, ethnography differs from other approaches to understanding the phenomena in several key respects.

Ethnographic research is *inductive*, meaning that we attempt to describe a group of people, their behaviors, and the meanings they attach to them from their perspectives *without* attributing preconceived ideas from our own culture or values to them. As such, the people we work with are the experts, or "teachers," and an ethnographer takes on a subordinate, or "student," role. The goal of an ethnographer is to present a holistic understanding of the culture, symbolic meanings, and patterned behaviors of a particular group of people from their own perspectives—perspectives that differ more often than not from professional models based in other disciplines. In this sense, ethnographers "give voice" to the "subjects" we are trying to learn more about and maybe even help in some way. The inductive approach is realized through relatively unique data collection and analytic methods.

One method that distinguishes ethnographic research from survey or quantitative data collection methods is *fieldwork*, a data collection process that combines participation in the daily lives of some people with simultaneous observation of their behaviors. An ethnographer might live among a cultural group and study the role of alcohol in their daily lives, for example, as I did among the Haya people of Tanzania in East Africa. In such cases, an ethnographer might observe and assist in the production of local brews and indulge in the drinking behaviors acceptable in the society to develop a greater sense of the role of alcohol in daily life. By contrast, an ethnographer working among heroin injectors might conduct fieldwork by observing injection practices or "hanging out" in drug-copping areas to get a sense of the flow of daily life; however, he or she would not engage in illegal behaviors for obvious ethical and legal reasons. As such, the extent of participant observation varies according to the psychoactive substances being studied and the research objectives. The results of participant observation are recorded in *fieldnotes*, a detailed account of experiences and initial insights.

A second distinguishing method is that ethnographers talk with people about their experiences, behaviors, values, and beliefs. Ethnographic (sometimes loosely defined as qualitative) interviews range from open-ended conversations, often conducted during fieldwork, to life histories and semistructured individual interviews that follow a guide covering various domains of interest. Ethnographic research is based on empathy, respect, and careful listening without projecting one's own beliefs or worldview onto the participants—to the extent this is possible. Through the indigenous language recorded by audiotape, ethnographers attempt to understand, and ultimately describe, how other people interpret their own behaviors, experiences, and surroundings, as well as how they negotiate the challenges of daily life.

Analyzing texts from ethnographic interviews or fieldnotes involves searching for patterns or themes that people attach to specific meanings and behaviors. Often using various data management software programs, ethnographers code sections of text referring to specific topics and then analyze them to identify recurring themes. Codes may refer to some predetermined topic, such as "barriers to treatment," or to emergent categories. Through their detailed analysis of themes and patterns recorded in texts, ethnographers describe some dimension or dimensions of a people's culture, including behavior. In these ways, the systematic nature of ethnographic data collection, analysis, and interpretation differs significantly from first-person, journalistic accounts of drug use or the treatment experience.

An example of the relevance of ethnographic research in reference to primary prevention is the revision of the needle-sharing myth among injection drug users. When I began research on HIV risk behaviors among heroin and cocaine injectors in Dayton, Ohio, in 1989, a common idea in the public health literature was that needle sharing was a ritualized behavior. As such, I expected to observe heroin and cocaine injectors passing used needles to one another and bonding in some way. However, when I interviewed injectors and asked them about needle sharing, they basically said, "You got it all wrong!" Injectors generally do not want to share needles because no one wants to wait to "get off" (inject), and the tips of used syringes are dulled quickly, thereby making it more difficult for a person to "get a hit" (penetrate a vein). Moreover, some injectors had learned about the dangers of needle sharing through earlier experiences with hepatitis B virus transmission. These findings were confirmed as I observed the individualistic nature of drug injection in "shooting galleries" (places where people obtain and inject narcotics) and the squabbles over who got the greatest share of a heroin solution. Such corrective understanding makes it clear that accessibility to new needles and legal sanctions that prohibit carrying injection paraphernalia have a tremendous influence on the spread of HIV and other blood-borne infections.

Another general area in which ethnographers have made contributions to substance misuse research is documenting the special terminology, or indigenous argot, people use to describe various dimensions of drug use, ranging from terms for injection paraphernalia, to various drugs, to perceived changes in altered states of consciousness. For example, among crack cocaine smokers in central Ohio, the verb *geeking* is used to describe the behavior of someone who is smoking crack and "is on a mission," or bingeing, that is, continually buying and smoking more of the drug. "Geeking" refers to the behaviors that some people engage in to obtain the resources needed to get more crack, such as shoplifting, stealing and pawning commodities, or exchanging sexual favors. In addition, "geeking" refers to the paranoia experienced by some people as they smoke crack. This is expressed when people constantly peek out of windows because they believe drug enforcement agents are outside or when someone searches all over the floor looking for small crumbs of crack. In short, the term "geeking" encapsulates a particular dimension of the crack life. Understanding indigenous terminology better prepares us not only to appreciate the lives of people we are working with, but also may contribute to the design of interventions. Such understanding can also help frame and interpret findings from quantitative surveys.

In summary, describing the culture and behavior of alcohol and other drug users from their perspectives is one of the hallmarks of ethnographic contributions to substance use/misuse research. Well-known studies in the 1960s and 1970s demonstrated that the life of a heroin user is not one of chaos or unstructured behavior, but one that is carefully planned in terms of strategies used to obtain an adequate supply of drugs and "getting off" or "getting well" (recovering from withdrawal). Ethnographic studies range from focused descriptions of drug-using behaviors and meanings among a particular population to broader explanatory studies that interpret alcohol and other drug use in a wider political–economic context, thereby linking micro- and macroperspectives. The ethnographic study of drug use, misuse, prevention, and treatment is one that can place the researcher as a mediator among domains ranging from neurochemical processes involved with the use of drugs to the general role of drugs in daily life, to the larger, political–economic context in which people live—although the implications of this mediator role have yet to be realized. A basic premise of applied ethnographic research is that understanding how other people view their drug-using behavior or attempts at recovery, for example, can complement other professional models, aid in improving prevention and treatment interventions, and perhaps inform policy. In addition, ethnographic studies can be used to inform treatment professionals and scientists in other fields about the daily lives of the people they are trying to help or better understand from a particular scientific perspective.

> *The life of a heroin user is not one of chaos or unstructured behavior, but one that is carefully planned.*

My goal in this chapter is to illustrate how ethnographic research can provide the fields of substance misuse prevention and treatment with a very different, yet complementary, way to understand and evaluate very complicated phenomena. What specifically can the ethnography of substance abuse treatment contribute? Most importantly, ethnographers can provide a complementary systemic perspective that takes into account not only the patient/client, but also his or her interactions with counselors, the treatment center program, other clients, the larger human and health services system, as well as his or her interactions with family and wider social networks over time. If substance use disorders are in part problems of motivation and decision making (see Miller, Chapter 9, this volume), ethnographic research can provide important insight into the process of change or stasis from the perspective of the patient/client. Ethnography can help us understand how a person moves through the process of problem recognition, to doing something about a problem, to actually engaging and linking with treatment, to becoming a part of the therapeutic milieu, and ultimately understanding how he or she relearns the ability to interact with family and friends and change his or her identity from "addict" to something else. If the addictions are chronic health problems that require long-term monitoring and management (see McLellan, Chapter 17, this volume), the ethnographic approach is one that can complement other professional models by helping to provide long-term observation and interpretation. Before describing some contributions that ethnographers have made to understanding substance use disorders and treatment experiences, I present a very brief and general cross-cultural overview of alcohol and other drug use. My premise is that to better understand substance use disorders and treatment, it is necessary to appreciate some of the practical roles of alcohol and other drugs in various cultures.

Symbolic Mediation: From Psychotherapeutic Agent to "Social Lubricant" to Sacrament

Ethnographers—at least in anthropology—generally accept a panhuman drive to alter consciousness that takes as many different forms as there are cultures and various psychoactive substances throughout the world. At the most obvious level, many psychoactive substances that can be misused can also make people feel very good, feel better, or induce another way of looking at the world. At another level, people in various cultures around the globe use psychoactive substances to accomplish something. For example, for thousands of years, shamans in the Old and New Worlds have used psychoactive substances to facilitate altered states of consciousness that allow them to communicate with spirits in a domain of reality usually obscured in daily life. As a shaman facilitates a journey with a participant, he or she interprets the visions and experiences of the patient to achieve healing in the broadest sense of the term. In such cases, very strong hallucinogens, such as *Banisteriopsis caapi* in some South American cultures, are carefully used to induce altered states and gain access to another dimension of reality.

Experimental use of hallucinogens to manage or even cure alcohol and other drug problems has been attempted in Western societies— even by Bill W., one of the cofounders of Alcoholics Anonymous who reportedly used LSD to fight depression. Currently, scientists are evaluating the potential benefits of using MDMA (ecstasy), an entactogen that produces stimulant and mild hallucinatory effects, as a therapeutic agent among people suffering from posttraumatic stress disorder (PTSD).

As psychotherapeutic agents, hallucinogens can be used to gain access to another domain of reality as well as to simply look at the world differently; in short, they can be used to mediate or link the domains of everyday life and a spiritual world (the profane and the sacred) in various ways. The same can be said of the use of peyote in some Native American religions as well as the use of wine in other religions.

Why Are Psychoactive Substances Good Symbolic Mediators?

To illustrate in a general sense why some psychoactive drugs are good symbolic mediators, I describe the role of banana beer among the Haya people of Tanzania. The Haya make a low-alcohol-content (4.5%) wine or "beer" using a particular variety of bananas that are ripened, mashed, and allowed to ferment. Traditionally, banana beer is used in various ways to mediate or link various domains of reality as well as to mark various kinds of transitions. For example, communal drinking of banana beer creates a sense of social bonding, linking people together in part through their shared experience of altered perception. Banana beer is also consumed and used in prescribed ways in all traditional life-status-transition ceremonies. Finally, banana beer is used to link people with their ancestors and other spirits by placing offerings of banana beer in sacred places. How does banana beer work as a symbolic mediator that can link the profane and the sacred domains, facilitate social bonding, or mark status-transition rituals? Here, I consider how the Haya characterize perceived alterations in consciousness.

Four hierarchical stages of altered consciousness are associated with the consumption of banana beer. The first stage satisfies a basic need, to refresh oneself; little alteration in consciousness is experienced. Traditionally, adult men sipped banana beer throughout the day. Such behavior was perceived as an essential dietary component that increased strength.

The second stage can be described as experiencing a slight alteration in consciousness. It is characterized as slightly feeling the effects of banana beer, feeling happy, "full," proud, and willing to express inner thoughts. Individuals still speak sensibly in this state.

The third stage may be described as just beginning to "lose control of the self" due to the effects of alcohol. It is described by indigenous verbs meaning "to go beyond," or "to bypass." While people in this state can be tolerated in the absence of disgraceful behavior, it is viewed as a condition indicating a lack of self-respect.

The fourth level of altered consciousness can be translated as "being very drunk." This state is marked by slurred, loud, incomprehensible speech; staggering; confusion; and perhaps violence.

From the perspective of traditional culture, Haya valued experiencing the first two levels of altered consciousness: quenching a thirst and "feeling high." Although the third level could be accepted in the absence of improper behavior, the fourth level, or "being drunk" was perceived as a pitiful state. The crucial factor demarcating the valued state of slightly altered perception from the devalued state of drunkenness is self-control of transition in states of consciousness. Unlike the role of alcohol or other psychoactive substances in some other cultures, intoxication in the Haya culture is not perceived as a means of communicating with ancestors or other spirits.

The analysis below is based on the premise that primary structures or patterns that can be used to create a shared cultural model of reality emerge from repetitive experiences based in the body. As such, the Haya schema of levels of altered consciousness may be viewed as a syntagmatic, or metonymic, chain of states of perception related by contiguity. The Haya value experiencing the first two levels of the chain only. However, by experiencing the first two levels of the domain, the third and fourth levels of altered perception are suggested through metonymy, thereby creating a sense of wholeness. As such, in one sense banana beer can be used as an apt symbolic mediator because its controlled consumption invokes a subjective sense of wholeness, both the culturally valued quality of self-control and slightly altered perception and its opposite: drunkenness or chaos. Moreover, this schema involving transition in subjective states of consciousness can be used to construct or invoke cultural patterns. In the case of ancestor propitiation, for example, placing an offering of banana beer in a sacred location symbolizes transition in state of consciousness, and thereby transition and linkage to the spiritual realm of the ancestors.

In summary, psychoactive substances are often used as symbolic mediators to help humans deal with a fundamental problem: our biological separateness from each other as well as our separateness from other culturally defined domains of reality. Psychoactive drugs are good symbolic mediators because their use results in relatively predictable, repetitive patterns of altered consciousness—patterns that can sometimes be used to symbolize and create more objective cultural patterns. In relation to psychoactive substances, symbolic mediation takes three general forms: (1) linking perceived domains of reality that are culturally defined as separate; (2) marking transitions or boundaries relative to some aspect of life, whether changes in life status (e.g., birth, marriage), the Sabbath and the rest of the week, or changes in prescribed behavior (e.g., the transition from work to relaxation); and (3) facilitating social bonding or connecting individuals through shared common experience.

Symbolic mediation is achieved through the relationship between patterns of alteration in consciousness induced by psychoactive substances and more objective, shared, cultural patterns. For example, transition in subjective state of consciousness may be "mapped" by analogy onto more objective social transitions, such as in the changing status of a couple in a marriage ceremony. Understanding how psychoactive substances sometimes function as symbolic mediators can help us understand substance use disorders and issues related to their treatment.

Alcohol and Other Drugs as Commodities

When psychoactive substances become commodities, they take on a powerful, potential new function. In addition to being potential symbolic mediators, they are fundamentally transformed into consumables that can bring profit. Psychoactive properties and, to some extent, legality establish the extent to which substances are transformed into commodities that potentially can be misused. Drugs that make people feel good and more energetic, and that also have other reinforcing properties, are the most likely to bring profit, regardless of their legality.

In a general sense, people are constantly monitoring and manipulating changes in subjective experience and perception as they negotiate the challenges of daily life. People use various psychoactive substances throughout the day to accomplish something. We only have to think of the role of caffeinated beverages or nicotine consumed first thing in the morning among people in many societies as a simple example. An altered state of stimulated consciousness is produced, thereby not only providing stimulation, but also marking a more objective transition from sleep and rest to wakefulness and readiness to begin the day's activities. Transition in internal state of consciousness is paralleled by a more objective transition in expected and required patterns of behavior. This monitoring of consumption has been referred to as the "chemical management" of daily life and extends beyond drugs that are misused to a wide array of herbal supplements, vitamins, and so on.

The four stages of altered consciousness recognized by the Haya are similar to Western concepts in a general sense. For example, just beginning to perceive an alteration in consciousness is similar to what is sometimes referred to as "social drinking." Similarly, much has been written about using alcoholic beverages to mark a transition between the normal work day and a period of relaxation ("happy hour"). Again, alcohol is used as a symbolic mediator. Here, ideally, a slight alteration in consciousness is mapped by analogy onto more objective realities: the transition from work to pleasure and relaxation.

When people misuse or become dependent on psychoactive substances as commodities, their potential role as symbolic mediators is obfuscated; instead of being used in creative ways to link various domains, to create a shared experience of social bonding, or to mark various kinds of transitions, their misuse isolates an individual from other people as well as from culturally defined domains of reality. Why?

At least to some degree, when psychoactive substances become commodities, the full range and diversity of potential altered states of consciousness become potential resources for the creation of profit. That is, instead of controlling alteration in consciousness, the entire range of stages of altered consciousness in the case of the Haya, for example, become targets for increasing consumption, thereby increasing profits. In the case of heroin, cocaine, methamphetamine, and other substances, for example, we might even think of receptor cells as potential targets that can be exploited for profit, in addition to the simple fact that they make people feel extremely good. The pharmacological reinforcing properties of cocaine, heroin, and methamphetamine, for example, make them ideal commodities that can be consumed in great quantity.

> When psychoactive substances become commodities, altered states of consciousness become potential resources for the creation of profit.

"Addiction," or drug dependence, becomes a lifestyle with its own structure and rewards, although these rewards increasingly isolate the self from other people and reality in general—as well as potentially have adverse health consequences. Useful forms of symbolic mediation through consuming psychoactive substances are relinquished. Increasing consumption of substances that make people feel good and have reinforcing neurochemical properties of their own (see Koob, Chapter 3, this volume) is further reinforced by commitment to, and familiarity with, a particular lifestyle—the often-discussed "career" of a heroin injector, for example. These lifestyles of addiction often include other behaviors that induce "highs" of their own—for example, the "rush" associated with shoplifting and other forms of "hustling," or the "rush" associated with the ritualized behavior one follows in preparing injection equipment.

In summary, psychoactive substances that can be misused are often put to good use as symbolic mediators, in addition to the fact that many of them make people feel very good or provide a means to look at the world differently. As commodities, the symbolic mediating roles of various psychoactive substances are often still realized. Yet, for some people, mechanisms for linking subjective experience with more objective cultural patterns through the use of psychoactive substances become weakened. Understanding the practical roles of psychoactive drugs as well as the underlying reasons for how they become misused can help us contextualize obstacles to substance abuse treatment and recovery.

Ethnographic Perspectives on the Prevention and Treatment of Substance Use Disorders

Ethnographic studies of substance misuse prevention are rare. Similarly, with the possible exception of Alcoholics Anonymous and the use of methadone, ethnographic studies of the treatment of substance use disorders as well as the process of recovery are relatively limited for reasons that are unclear. To a large extent, these areas remain open fields for future contributions. Nevertheless, some initial insights can be presented.

Barriers to Treatment Linkage, Engagement, and Outcome

Inconsistent Goals

Ethnographic studies have shown that there is often a mismatch between the goals of people seeking treatment and treatment program goals. From the perspective of counselors, the definition of "success" is most often long-term abstinence after a single treatment episode, rather than monitoring and helping a person manage a chronic condition where some continued drug or alcohol use is a common occurrence. For example, heroin users will sometimes begin methadone maintenance for reasons such as to rest and rebuild their strength when they are tired of hustling. A crack cocaine smoker may enter treatment determined to reduce or stop using crack but may have no immediate intentions of stopping alcohol or marijuana use.

When the goals of therapists and clients are dissimilar, the outcome is unlikely to be optimal—from the program perspective. When the goals of counselors are complete abstinence and the goals of the patient/client are something else, the therapeutic relationship is likely to be confrontational, thereby leading to dishonesty. For example, a recovering crack user in outpatient treatment drinks a 40-ounce beer and decides he or she cannot go to a session for two reasons. First, his or her counselor might scold him or her; second, he or she could tell his or her probation officer, thereby perhaps resulting in a return to prison. As discussed above, recovery is partly about reestablishing means of linking with people and other culturally defined domains without using a particular psychoactive substance or substances. As such, confrontational relationships will only impede a person's ability to relearn this fundamental aspect of being human. In the case of people who have not learned basic ways of linking with people, such as adolescents who develop substance use disorders, the problem is even greater because they cannot relearn to do what they have not had a chance to learn previously.

In summary, any kind of confrontational approach to treatment is unlikely to succeed. In this sense, the ethnographic interview may have a potential role to play because it is nonconfrontational and is based on empathy and respect. Several people with whom I have interacted over the last 16 years contact me regularly for additional interviews, particularly when they are experiencing problems. These interactions, under the guise of an interview, give a person the opportunity to assess his or her level of drug use in a nonthreatening way or the opportunity to validate and further evaluate his or her recovery by talking with someone who wants to understand his or her life from his or her perspective without evaluating him or her. As such, ethnographic and motivational interviewing may potentially be linked. After a motivational interviewing session, for example, do people talk about their experiences with others? What do they say? Would linking motivational interviews with subsequent ethnographic interviews over a long term contribute to success or better understanding of underlying patterns of behavior and meanings, thereby indicating what form of intervention might be productive? At a basic level, ethnographic research can complement other forms of outcome evaluation by describing the processes of change from the perspective of the patient/client.

Stigma

Substance misuse problems, in the United States at least, are still not widely perceived as a health condition requiring long-term care, but rather as a moral problem, a problem indicating a lack of self-control, or a potential legal problem. This was recently illustrated when a family member of a project participant who had an acute substance misuse episode said, "I don't want to call the police or paramedics—it will be all over the news." As such, stigma is still a tremendous obstacle to confronting substance use disorders. Moreover, the stigma associated with substance use disorders is often perceived to be greater among women because they often have higher expectations about being good mothers and caretakers of society in general.

Criminalization

The criminalization of people who misuse psychoactive substances is also a significant obstacle to identifying and addressing substance use disorders, although some substance misusers enter the criminal justice system on purpose as a means to rest and recover their strength in a controlled environment. In some sense, it is illegal to have a chronic disease when people are dependent on illegal drugs. No one has addressed how issues of legality are managed in treatment settings. In some ways, heroin, cocaine, or methamphetamine users in treatment in the United States are operating in a liminal space, somewhere between legal and illegal worlds. This may be one reason why methadone clinics are sometimes located in the marginal areas of cities, often with drug dealing prevalent in the nearby area in which individuals who seek profit illegally by selling heroin or cocaine, for example, compete with those selling methadone at treatment clinics.

> *The criminalization of people who misuse psychoactive substances is a significant obstacle to identifying and addressing substance use disorders.*

Waiting Lists

People with substance use disorders who make the decision to access treatment services are taking a tremendous risk. They risk admitting to others that they have a disorder that carries substantial stigma or even potential incarceration. They risk potential economic difficulties or losing their children. When such people are confronted with waiting lists, they can often use that as an excuse to continue with familiar behaviors—particularly when withdrawal is an issue. In short, waiting lists may result in the loss of a "teachable moment." This is maybe one reason why self-help sponsors are so important; they are ready to intercede relatively immediately to take advantage of potential opportunities to foster change.

Admissions Criteria

Another obstacle that people talk about in relation to accessing treatment services is not meeting the admission criteria. People then learn that acute alcohol intoxication or threatening suicide will enable them to gain treatment entry, and some may resort to this strategy. Another obstacle is previous treatment history. I have been told that people with multiple treatment experiences are sometimes turned away from treatment because they "already know it all," or they are viewed as "incurable" rather than helping them to manage a chronic illness.

Counselor Experience

Often people in treatment feel uncomfortable when counselors have not experienced similar problems themselves. Consequently, from the perspective of some people seeking help, counselors who cannot "speak their language" or understand their experiences may be discounted. In comparison, a cardiologist does not need to have experienced heart problems to be able to treat them. Similarly, sensitivity to cultural themes and patterns is often discussed as a substantial obstacle to treatment linkage, engagement, and outcome.

A "Street Culture" of Addiction

Among the crack and heroin users with whom I am most familiar, a "culture of addiction" exists on the streets. One of the most salient obstacles to problem recognition and, ultimately, recovery is the concept of "hitting bottom." A crack cocaine user, for example, may not feel his or her drug use has reached the point where intervention or change is needed because house and family are intact, or at least fairly so, bills are paid, food is in the house, and children are clothed. So why is change needed? Until one "hits bottom," the perceived benefits of addressing a substance misuse problem outweigh the perceived risks of doing so. In a related sense, the idea that change is not possible until a person has made a conscious decision to do so, or "is ready," is also a significant obstacle. This street culture of addiction is, of course, learned through experiences people have with others who have been through treatment and/or through their own treatment and self-help experiences.

Economics

Among many other things, drug misuse treatment is a business. As one recovering drug user recently commented in a focus group, "It's a money game, and we're the pawns, the junkies." Most crack and heroin users I know believe that if a person does not have money or adequate insurance, he or she will have difficulty accessing services, especially when he or she feels he or she needs them. As one crack user commented, "Well, it seems to me all these treatment centers, all they're worried about is money. If you ain't got no money or insurance, then you don't get no help."

Substance Use Disorders as Chronic Health Problems

It is often said that substance use disorders are chronic health problems, yet the immediate objective of most treatment programs is oriented toward a relatively immediate bivariate outcome: abstinence or failure. Rather than approaching occasions of substance use as potentially integral parts of a chronic health problem, they are often viewed with opprobrium or as "failure." Continued misuse of substances carries a stigma of its own, especially during or after a treatment encounter. As such, people are often unwilling to be honest with counselors. For example, an adolescent who smokes marijuana is referred to treatment, is labeled as an abuser, and is required to attend Alcoholics Anonymous meetings. From the youth's perspective, he or she does not think of him- or herself as an addict, but he or she is essentially defined as such, particularly in a legal sense.

The abstinence/failure dichotomy also contributes to the search for "magic bullets" to solve the problem of the addictions. There will be no single magic bullet, whether a new form of cognitive or of chemical therapy. Take the example of buprenorphine, recently approved for prescription by private physicians. Theoretically, this should result in a major advance in treating opioid dependence at a time when misuse of heroin and prescription opioids in the United States is increasing. Instead, buprenorphine is facing significant obstacles in its adoption. Why?

One reason may be because it is not economically rewarding to providers. Another may be that family physicians are generally untrained to identify and work with people who have substance misuse problems. Another may be that physicians do not have the time to become qualified to prescribe it. Still another reason may be that some physicians simply don't want "junkies" hanging around their offices. The point is that even if innovative, potentially more successful, approaches to treatment are identified, getting them to be adopted in practice is an extremely complicated sociocultural, economic, political, and health delivery system process. Ethnography can help us understand and evaluate processes like this. Moreover, an ethnographic approach can help us understand how changes in neurochemical processes associated with chemical therapy are interpreted in the course of reestablishing connections with people and readapting to the challenges of daily life.

I use the term "addictions" because although there may be underlying causes or processes common to substance use disorders, the process of recovery is idiosyncratic in many ways. Each individual must learn how to reestablish connections with people as well as cultural domains on the basis of his or her previous relationships, social networks, stage of life, physical health, socioeconomic status and education, religious background, genetics, and possible co-occurring disorders. It's no wonder why the success rate is low! But here, it may be prudent to reconsider what is meant by "success."

What does it mean when someone has been through treatment five times over a period of 10 years, has short periods of abstinence, and then begins a long period of abstinence after the sixth treatment experience? Understanding substance use disorders as chronic diseases, was the person an eventual success relative to his or her first five times in treatment or only the last?

How do people succeed? In my limited experience, this is often a self-fulfilling prophecy. "I got better when I was ready: I hit bottom." "Could anything have helped you to change earlier during one of the other times you were in treatment?" "No, I had to make the decision to do it myself." In some ways, if we do understand substance misuse as a chronic health problem with varying degrees of continued substance misuse being common, they may be right. Minimization of potential adverse consequences associated with chronic substance use disorders, in addition to abstinence, would be consistent with the recognition that any individual who has a substance use disorder is on a *potential* trajectory for abstinence or reduction in substance use. The key is identifying ways to enhance the trajectory.

The Political Economy of Substance Use, Misuse, and Treatment

Substance use, misuse, and treatment services operate in sociopolitical, economic, and cultural contexts that are global in scope. Trends in substance use patterns skip across the globe rapidly, as we have recently seen with the rave phenomenon. Relatively naive, largely middle-/working-class young people are relearning the dangers of heroin in the United States, in part because drug producers in South America have learned how to produce a very high-quality heroin that can be inhaled. The transshipment of illegal drugs has spread to new countries; inevitably, some of the product finds its way into new markets, thereby resulting in increases in misuse among various populations around the globe.

In the global economy, there appears to be virtually no limit to the new forms or combinations of drugs that can be marketed legally, like the new beers that contain large amounts of caffeine being sold in parts of the United States. Rural populations provide new markets for high-quality heroin, partly because people have had previous experience with pharmaceutical opioids. Heroin dealers realized they had a new market for their product after misuse of pharmaceutical opioids increased in some rural areas, because heroin is less expensive than diverted pharmaceutical opioids. Illegal distribution of pharmaceutical drugs on the Internet is yet another factor contributing to increasing availability. This is part of the context within which new patterns of drug use and misuse unfold, as well as the context within which prevention and treatment systems must be able to adapt.

Another dimension of the global context is the confluence of poverty, unemployment, racism, and violence within which some people use various psychoactive substances. Although the term "self-medication" often refers to the use of psychoactive drugs to manage another underlying mental or physical health problem, it can also be used to refer to drug use and misuse as a means of escaping from or coping with oppressive life conditions in which many individuals lack the material resources and social capital needed to participate successfully in the global economy. At the same time, people are constantly bombarded through the media with symbols of success.

People without access to things that symbolize participation in the good life may be at increased risk for substance use disorders. The resources they have to participate in the global economy are limited. Among those resources they do have are those repeating patterns of experience based on the body, including such things as potential altered states of consciousness and sexual response. By smoking crack, for example, one becomes a real consumer of globally produced commodities, among other things, when there are considerable obstacles to participate as "successful citizens" in the global economy. These issues create additional challenges for substance misuse management.

Conclusion

If substance use disorders are chronic health problems, long-term ethnographic studies of people are needed after they first enter treatment programs. At this time, we have very limited understanding of the ways in which people change or remain the same while in treatment or after they leave from their own perspectives. We have limited ethnographic understanding of how existent patterns of interaction in social networks influence the treatment experience or outcome with respect to age, gender ethnicity, socioeconomic status, comorbidity, or different drugs. We have very little understanding of the local "culture" of individual treatment centers or the problems experienced by counselors. We have limited understanding of the therapeutic process from the perspectives of clients and counselors. We have very limited understanding of how people successfully change their identities from "junkie," "crackhead," or "alcoholic" to lifestyles without drugs in different settings. These are some of the research questions that can be addressed, in part, using ethnographic methodologies.

More immediately, ethnographic research can help provide an important perspective to complement different ways of understanding and treating substance use disorders, as have been discussed in this volume. In contrast to evaluation studies per se, ethnographic research is largely descriptive, rather than a field with a specific research agenda. If there is any agenda to ethnographic research, it is to present a faithful description of how different people view, experience, and negotiate the challenges of daily life. As such, ethnography can help to describe and evaluate the diverse processes of problem recognition, help seeking, and transformation from the perspective of individuals in diverse social settings. Moreover, the ethnographic approach in substance abuse research is open to help frame and answer questions posed by professionals in other fields. For example, our current study on barriers to treatment is designed to better understand and improve treatment linkage and engagement in the local community. As substance use and misuse trends change and as new populations become involved, new ethnographic studies of the treatment process and rehabilitation will be needed.

Robust Principles

1. Anthropologists generally accept a panhuman "drive" to alter consciousness.
2. Alcohol and other drugs associated with substance use disorders make people feel good, feel better, or simply view the world differently, however temporary that may be.
3. The prescribed role and use of psychoactive substances across cultures is extremely diverse, ranging from medicinal/psychotherapeutic agents, to agents that induce sociality to sacraments, to symbolic mediators, to commodities.
4. From a cross-cultural perspective, psychoactive substances are often used as symbolic mediators. Their roles as symbolic mediators vary significantly but include facilitating social bonding, linking domains of reality such as the profane and the sacred, or marking status transitions, such as birth, marriage, or death, among other things.
5. Various psychoactive substances work as symbolic mediators because subjective changes in altered states of consciousness induced by various psychoactive substances are analogous to changes in more objective cultural patterns.
6. When psychoactive drugs become commodities, the entire range and diversity of states of altered consciousness becomes targets for increasing production and consumption. The symbolic mediating roles of psychoactive substances are therefore sometimes diminished; rather than being used to link people to one another and with other cultural domains, their misuse contributes to isolation and disconnection.
7. Recovery from substance use disorders involves learning new ways

of linking with other people and culturally defined domains of reality without the misuse of psychoactive substances.

8. Recognition of substance use disorders, engagement in treatment services, and therapeutic outcome are impeded by:
   a. stigma associated with substance use/misuse;
   b. criminalization of illicit substance use/misuse;
   c. difficulty accessing services, including long waiting lists and lack of insurance;
   d. societal approaches to substance use disorders as moral problems, rather than as chronic health problems; and
   e. a "street culture of addiction" heavily influenced by concepts such as "hitting bottom," or that treatment will not work until one is "ready" for change.

9. The obstacles indicated above create an environment of risk in confronting a substance use disorder, rather than an open approach to long-term management of a chronic health problem.

10. When the objectives of people seeking treatment and program goals are inconsistent, the outcome is unlikely to be positive. Honesty in the therapeutic environment is vital for success.

Acknowledgments

This chapter was written while being funded by the National Institute on Drug Abuse (NIDA), Grant Nos. R01 DA14488 (Robert G. Carlson, Principal Investigator), R01 DA14340 (Harvey A. Siegal, Principal Investigator, Robert G. Carlson, Co-Principal Investigator), R01 DA 10099 (Harvey A. Siegal, Principal Investigator), R01 DA15363 (Brenda M. Booth, Principal Investigator), and R01 DA15690 (Harvey A. Siegal, Principal Investigator). Special thanks to the late Harvey A. Siegal, Russel S. Falck, and members of the CACTUS group for their comments on earlier drafts. The findings do not necessarily reflect the views of the NIDA or any other government agency.

Suggested Readings

Agar, M. (1977). Going through the changes: Methadone in New York. *Human Organization, 36*, 291–295.

Agar, M. H. (1985). Folks and professionals: Different models for the interpretation of drug use. *International Journal of the Addictions, 20*, 173–182.

Battjes, R., Onken L. S., & Delany, P. J. (1999). Drug abuse treatment entry and engagement: Report of a meeting on treatment readiness. *Journal of Clinical Psychology, 55*, 643–657.

Brooks, C. R. (1994). Using ethnography in the evaluation of drug prevention and intervention programs. *International Journal of the Addictions, 29*(6), 791–801.

Carlson, R. G. (1992). Symbolic mediation and commoditization: A critical examination of alcohol use among the Haya of Bukoba, Tanzania. *Medical Anthropology, 15,* 41–62.

Carlson, R. G. (1996). The political economy of AIDS among drug users in the United States: Beyond blaming the victim or powerful others. *American Anthropologist, 98,* 266–278.

Carlson, R. G., Siegal, H. A., Falck, R. S., & Wang, J. (1996, December 3–4). *Exploring the cultural logic of addiction: Drug abuse treatment and engagement in the Midwest.* Invited paper presented at "Treatment Readiness: Factors Influencing Entry and Engagement," Robert Battjes, organizer, National Institute on Drug Abuse, Rockville, MD.

Duroy, T. H., Schmidt, S. L., & Perry, P. D. (2003). Adolescents' and young adults' perspectives on a continuum of care in a three year drug treatment program. *Journal of Drug Issues, 33,* 801–832.

Koester, S., Anderson, K., & Hoffer, L. (1999). Active heroin injectors' perceptions and use of methadone maintenance treatment: Cynical performance or self-prescribed risk reduction? *Substance Use and Misuse, 34,* 2135–2153.

Miller, W. R., Walters, S. T., & Bennett, M. E. (2001). How effective is alcoholism treatment in the United States? *Journal of Studies on Alcohol, 62,* 211–220.

Reisinger, H. S. (2004). Counting apples as oranges: Epidemiology and ethnography in adolescent substance abuse treatment. *Qualitative Health Research, 14,* 241–258.

Reisinger, H. S., Bush, T., Colom, A., Agar, M., & Battjes, R. (2003). Navigation and engagement: How does one measure success? *Journal of Drug Issues, 33,* 777–800.

Skoll, G. R. (1992). *Walk the walk and talk the walk: An ethnography of a drug abuse treatment facility.* Philadelphia: Temple University Press.

Stephens, R. C., & Weppner, R. S. (1973). Legal and illegal use of methadone: One year later. *American Journal of Psychiatry, 130,* 1391–1394.

Part V

Interventions

CHAPTER 14

Behavioral Therapies
The Glass Would Be Half Full If Only We Had a Glass

KATHLEEN M. CARROLL
BRUCE J. ROUNSAVILLE

Background and Overview

Until fairly recently, behavioral therapies[1] for substance use problems, while universally available in the treatment system, had either thin or nonexistent evidence regarding their effectiveness. Treatment typically involved extended stays in inpatient or residential facilities where the individual was offered, often on a daily basis, self-help groups as well as group and individual counseling, education, family sessions, and occupational therapies, integrated with strong admonitions to remain involved in self-help groups following discharge. These approaches did interrupt substance use (at least while the individual was in the facility), but attrition and relapse after treatment were common.

Moreover, treatment programs and their components were rarely subject to systematic evaluation. Hence, much of what was known regarding the effectiveness of treatment emerged from large-scale epi-

---

[1]The term "behavioral therapies" is used here to encompass psychotherapy and counseling but also more broadly nonpharmacological interventions of many kinds that seek to change specific behaviors.

demiological and program evaluation studies. These suggested that (1) many individuals with substance use problems did not seek or access formal treatment; (2) of those that applied for treatment, many never kept their initial appointments and many others dropped out after only a session or two; and (3) the subgroup of individuals who sought and remained in treatment over longer periods had reasonably good outcomes (at least compared to individuals who did not receive treatment), but relapse and recurrence of problems was frequent.

During the past 20 years, much has changed. Outpatient and intensive day treatment approaches have become the dominant model of treatment delivery. Inpatient treatment is much less frequently available and hospital stays have been drastically curtailed. Systematic assessment of outcomes in clinical programs (particularly retention and abstinence) are increasingly emphasized by policymakers and third-party payors. Clinical research has identified a number of well-defined, theoretically driven behavioral therapies demonstrated to be effective with a wide range of substance users and in a wide range of settings; these are described in the sections below.

With few exceptions, however, progress in the development of effective behavioral therapies has not been met by adoption of these approaches in clinical practice. The treatment system, with some exceptions, is dominated by the delivery of approaches of unknown efficacy and often by treatments demonstrated to be of little or no benefit. As described in more detail by McLellan (Chapter 17, this volume), the existing treatment system is poorly suited and poorly disposed to deliver empirically supported therapies. It is notable that few or no programs can give precise rates or information regarding the outcomes an individual seeking treatment in the program might expect (i.e., information regarding the proportions of individuals who show improvement across programs or clinicians).

A significant impediment to dissemination of empirically supported therapies for substance use problems is the practice by clinical researchers who devise and test the efficacy of a bewildering number of highly specialized therapies aimed at comparatively narrow groups of substance abusers. The existing treatment system is highly unlikely to be able to adopt a large number of novel treatments, with one for every subvariant of substance use, much less implement them effectively.

An alternative strategy would be to identify the fundamental processes of problem substance use that might be amenable to behavioral interventions. That is, to identify those processes that while not necessarily unique to are at least basic to addiction, and to organize treatment development and dissemination more efficiently within that framework. In this chapter, we assert that both treatment development and treatment dissemination may be fostered through articulation of a small set of core principles for changing substance users' behavior and the identification of a manageable set of key skills that can be conveyed to clinicians or even directly implemented with patients using interactive computer technology. In the sections below we briefly outline these core principles, relate them to existing effective behavioral approaches, and suggest directions for improving treatment of substance use problems.

Fundamental Principles

As described in the other chapters in this volume, addiction and the troublesome use of substances can be conceptualized via a wide range of models (e.g., sociological, genetic, neurobiological, interpersonal, spiritual). For those individuals whose substance use is severe enough to warrant treatment, we believe many aspects of these behaviors can be characterized as an *impulse control disorder with two general, socially defined dysfunctional elements*: (1) the excessive desire to use or craving for substances, and (2) insufficient impulse control associated with neuroadaptation and neurocognitive impairment. These processes, analogous to a car driven by someone who pushes the gas pedal to the floor and rarely brakes, are described only briefly below, as they constitute underlying themes of a number of chapters in this volume.

Excessive Drive Based on Associative Learning via Classical and Operant Conditioning

Factors associated with the excessive drive for drugs include the development of conditioned craving for and the increased valence of substances, as well as poor or weakened behavioral controls through failure to learn coping strategies or to seek and value alternative socially sanctioned rewards that are incompatible with drug abuse. Principles of operant and classical conditioning and behavioral pharmacology are fundamental to understanding substance abuse and dependence and the development of excessive desire to use substances that persists in the face of serious negative consequences. An extensive literature in behavioral pharmacology has established that those substances that are abused by humans are those that are self-administered by animals, and that substance use is repeated and becomes ingrained in affected individuals because abused substances are powerful and reliable reinforcers. Substance use tends to be more likely among individuals with fewer countervailing reinforcers and protective factors (families, jobs, social standing, pursuits in which they are invested). Loss, or threats of loss, of those countervailing reinforcers tends to encourage change and treatment seeking. Repeated pairing of substance use with social, environmental, affective, and physiological cues leads to often powerful craving or reinitiation of substance use when individuals are exposed to those cues, even after fairly extended periods of abstinence.

Neuroadaptation, Neurotoxicity, and/or Preexisting Deficits in the Brain's Reward Circuitry

Poor behavioral controls, or "bad brakes," can result from preexisting or substance-induced impairment in the brain regions responsible for impulse control and emotion regulation. These processes contribute to excessive drive through changes in the structure and function of brain nerve cells that lead to withdrawal symptoms when drug use stops; they are described in detail by George Koob (Chapter 3, this volume). Repeated exposure to most abused substances produces predictable alterations and impairments in neurocognitive functioning (with memory, attention, and other executive functions among the most consistently affected), neurotransmitter levels, and brain activity. Some of these effects may be permanent, but others are at least partly reversible after periods of abstinence. Individuals with preexisting disorders that have a neurocognitive component (e.g., attention-deficit/hyperactivity disorder, anxiety, schizophrenia, conduct disorder, and some aspects of impulsivity) are particularly vulnerable to developing substance use problems. Individuals whose neurocognitive functioning is impaired to begin with and/or further damaged by chronic substance use are likely to present special challenges for treatment, and may have particular problems with remembering or adhering to treatment recommendations, conceptualizing long-term goals, and organizing or temporizing behavior. Taken together, these processes contribute to excessive drive through development of conditioned craving and to bad brakes through failure to learn effective coping and emotional regulation strategies or to seek and value socially sanctioned rewards that are incompatible with drug use.

Shoring Up Brakes and Reducing Drives: The Effectiveness of Behavioral Therapies

In the sections below we briefly review the major categories of behavioral interventions that have achieved consistent empirical support for substance use problems through randomized controlled trials. The summary is highly simplified, as our intention is only to describe those major categories of behavioral intervention that have been demonstrated to be effective in multiple controlled trials and in a range of substance-using populations. Beyond an overview of "what works," we hope to highlight broader principles of behavioral change that might be drawn from this literature and to link these principles to the fundamental processes of reducing drives and enhancing behavioral controls among individuals with substance use problems.

Brief and Motivational Models

One of the surprising revelations of the past 20 years of treatment research in the addictions has been the findings regarding the efficacy and durability of brief behavioral therapies for many individuals with substance use problems. Relatively brief, focused interventions consisting of as little as a single session have not only been demonstrated to be effective, but have in several studies been shown to be as effective as lengthier, more intensive, and more expensive approaches. Described in greater detail by Miller (see Chapter 9, this volume, on motivation and motivational approaches), these brief approaches typically include provision of assessment and feedback on substance use and consequences; an empathic, nonjudgmental stance by the clinician that emphasizes individual choice and autonomy; acceptance of client ambivalence about changing his and her problem behavior; and emphasis on a range of possible clients goals that may or may not include formal treatment or abstinence. Furthermore, it should be noted that *these approaches are also marked by the absence of elements that have characterized many traditional specialty treatment programs.* For example, substance users are not pressured to subscribe to a goal of complete abstinence nor required to attend daily self-help meetings and education groups. "Denial" is not seen as an underlying issue that must be ferreted out, acknowledged, and confronted before meaningful change can occur.

Brief interventions have not only been demonstrated to be effective, but have in several studies been shown to be as effective as more intensive and expensive approaches.

Not only have rigorous clinical trials indicated that brief motivational approaches are associated with durable change in individuals with smoking, alcohol, marijuana, and other substance use problems, these approaches have also substantially broadened our conceptions of how and where interventions can be offered—that is, not just in specialty substance abuse treatment clinics but also in primary care settings, in emergency rooms, in social service agencies, and in criminal justice settings. Similarly, the literature on brief motivational approaches has also broadened our view of the types of substance users who many be amenable to brief behavioral intervention strategies, that is, not only those individuals with highly severe or chronic substance use disorders with significant impairments in functioning that have made intervention unavoidable, but also those individuals at earlier stages of addiction who have fewer substance-related problems.

Contingency Management Models

Another major development in the treatment of substance use problems has been the findings regarding the efficacy of contingency management interventions. Based on principles of behavioral pharmacology and operant conditioning, contingency management approaches acknowledge that abused substances are powerful reinforcers, and demonstrate that reinforcement of abstinence (or other behaviors incompatible with substance use) can reliably, and comparatively easily, interrupt substance use for a large number of individuals. For example, individuals enrolled in methadone maintenance programs who continue to abuse illicit drugs will reliable reduce their use of illicit drugs when offered tangible incentives, such as "take-home" methadone doses or access to employment, contingent on producing drug-free urine specimens. Similarly, cocaine, marijuana, and alcohol users will remain in treatment longer and be much more likely to initiate abstinence when provided incentives (e.g., vouchers redeemable for goods or services or inexpensive prizes) contingent on submitting drug-free urine specimens.

The emerging literature on contingency management approaches has demonstrated that substance users' behavior can be changed by altering the consequences of substance use; that targeting, monitoring, and reinforcing abstinence reliably increases abstinence; and that reinforcement of other target behaviors (e.g., treatment attendance, meeting other treatment goals) reliably increases the specific behaviors targeted by the contingencies while the contingencies are in place. Moreover, changes in targeted behaviors tend to occur very quickly after contingencies are instituted, highlighting the apparent ease with which many substance users can change their behavior when effectively motivated to do so. Although contingency management approaches do have weaknesses (e.g., substance use tends to rebound to some extent when the contingencies are terminated, the translation of these approaches into clinical practice is not straightforward), and while not all individuals respond uniformly well to these approaches, it is notable that contingency management approaches have been shown to be effective in populations of comparatively severe substance users with substantial comorbidity (including those who have not responded to other, less intensive interventions).

Thus the introduction of contingency management approaches into the substance abuse treatment repertoire has made it theoretically possible to retain large numbers of individuals in treatment and to initiate abstinence in a large proportion of them, a remarkable achievement in the behavioral therapies literature. In many ways, the introduction of contingency management principles into substance abuse treatment could have an influence akin to how the introduction of methadone maintenance in the 1960s revolutionized the treatment of opioid dependence. That is, the availability of methadone maintenance programs offered for the first time a viable approach for retaining heroin-dependent individuals in outpatient treatment, interrupting cycles of drug acquisition, drug use, and recovery from drug use; reducing criminal behavior; and stabilizing individuals and setting the conditions under which other problems could be assessed and treated.

Principles of contingency management could be applied, with similar goals, to a broad range of substance-using populations, particularly those in programs where treatment adherence is essential to good outcome. For example, contingency management has been used to improve compliance with naltrexone treatment of opioid dependence, a pharmacological approach with great promise that was rendered largely a failure by compliance problems. Similarly, contingency management approaches could be used to improve outcomes in a range of other populations where treatment effectiveness has been undercut by poor compliance, including fostering improved compliance with antiretroviral medications for substance users with HIV or with antipsychotic medications for substance users who also have severe mental illness. Moreover, because so many outcomes are directly related to sustained abstinence (e.g., medical, psychological, interpersonal, legal, and employment functioning), use of contingency management principles to retain substance users in treatment and increase abstinence has many important implications for improving treatment effectiveness in general.

Social Learning, Skills Training, and Cognitive-Behavioral Models

These approaches are grounded in social learning models and generally emphasize patterns or habits associated with the maintenance of substance use or relapse to substance use after initial periods of abstinence. Strategies for identifying patterns of behavior that sustain substance use (e.g., using substances in response to strong affect, conditioned cues, and other relapse determinants) and strategies for temporizing behavior are emphasized, with the goal that the individual will, over time, learn and implement effective behavioral alternatives that facilitate his or her ability to tolerate abstinence and cope more with issues and problems that play a role in sustaining his or her substance use.

Skills training and cognitive-behavioral approaches encourage behavioral change through exposure to and practice of coping behaviors, that is, practical strategies for dealing with problems that are frequently encountered in early abstinence that often lead to relapse. Cognitive-behavioral approaches usually include a broad menu of skills and principles (e.g., coping with craving, understanding patterns of substance use, problem solving, identifying and changing cognitive distortions, social skills training) that are intended to be selected and tailored to address the strengths and weaknesses of the individual and to help him or her achieve greater control over substance use, but can also be generalized to other co-occurring problems. These approaches posit that, through systematic practice, the individual will learn and implement important skills such as avoidance of situations associated with substance use, strategies for delaying and temporizing impulsive behaviors, coping with uncomfortable internal states, reducing stress, and broadening social support. These skills are often absent or inadequate among substance users—for example, they may not have been acquired due to lack of suitable role models or initiation of substance abuse during adolescence and early adulthood when these skills are usually mastered, or they may be inaccessible because of cognitive limitations or impairment. While these approaches are complex and require extensive training for clinicians and are comparatively demanding of patients, cognitive-behavioral and skills training approaches have been shown to have comparatively durable effects in several populations of substance users, with some studies showing continued improvement even after treatment ends.

Social Support, Social Network, and Family Models

Another broad category of intervention that has achieved substantial empirical support are those that seek to strengthen the individual's involvement with social networks that discourage substance use (described in greater detail by McCrady, Chapter 11, this volume). Although there are substantial variations among the various family and social network treatment models, in general, there has been consistent support in the literature for interventions that include family members and significant others in treatment, reinforce social networks that promote abstinence, reduce interactions with associates that support substance use, and improve family functioning and communication. Involvement of non-substance-using family members and significant others promotes help seeking and fosters better retention in treatment. In particular, inclusion of parents and social support systems may be critical in retaining adolescent substance users in treatment and in encouraging normative behavior. Another important benefit of those interventions that involve families and significant others is that although the children of substance users may not be specifically targeted by the intervention, there is some evidence that the children's functioning may improve as well. Hence, such interventions may play a role in prevention of substance use problems in the children of substance users. Interventions that foster meaningful involvement of substance users in social networks that encourage abstinence, such as self-help and support groups, have also been shown to be effective.

Behavioral Therapies and Basic Processes in Substance Dependence

As noted above, a significant impediment to the dissemination of empirically supported behavioral therapies for substance use problems is the sheer number of them. For example, a task force of the American Psychological Association recently identified over 140 highly specific behavioral therapies that were judged to be "empirically validated" through support by at least two randomized clinical trials. The existing drug abuse treatment system and its constituent clinicians are ill-equipped to master such an array of treatments. Our position is that effective treatment dissemination and delivery is at least in part dependent on communication of a small number of basic principles of change and a manageable set of key skills associated with fundamental elements of substance dependence, specifically, constructing interventions around reduction of drives and enhancement of controls. Many of the available empirically supported behavioral approaches described in the sections above fit at least in part into this framework.

Shoring Up Brakes

At this fundamental level, all four of the general categories of addictions behavioral therapies are strongest at "shoring up brakes" by helping substance users achieve better behavioral control, interrupting and changing learned pathways, altering reinforcing aspects of abused substances, and strengthening countervailing reinforcers. Motivational interviewing can be seen as enlisting executive function through clarification of values and goals. Cognitive-behavioral interventions can be conceived as those that fos-

Addictions behavioral therapies are strongest at "shoring up brakes."

ter executive control (planful, goal-directed behavior) by targeting affect regulation, tolerance of unpleasant internal states, and temporizing of impulsive behaviors. Contingency management approaches
provide incentive to one's available brakes and behavioral controls and
can be used to shape other behaviors that are incompatible with substance use and to provide alternative, ongoing sources of reward. Because substance use tends to rebound to some extent when the external
reinforcers are terminated, it may be essential that incentives used in
contingency management approaches are implemented over longer periods of time and are linked clearly to natural reinforcers (e.g.,
strengthening of interpersonal ties, helping achieve occupational stability), or conceived of as platforms for the introduction of other interventions. Social learning and cognitive-behavioral models focus almost
entirely on developing efficient braking systems through interrupting
connections between substance cues, patterns, and drug use; fostering
executive control (planful, goal-directed behavior), as well as targeting
affect regulation, tolerance of unpleasant internal states, and temporizing of impulsive behaviors. Family therapy models likewise provide the
promise of alternative rewards through reengagement with the family,
strengthening of countervailing reinforcers, and attention to the cost of
continued substance use, with provision of an external locus of efficiently applied brakes.

Cognitive remediation strategies, aimed at strengthening brain
function, may also have some potential in their application to this fundamental process of addiction. These strategies have attracted renewed interest due to recent evidence for the brain's surprising capacity for neural plasticity in adulthood. For example, there is some evidence that
cognitive remediation strategies (e.g., repeated intensive exposure to
computerized exercises intended to strengthen memory, attention, planning, and other aspects of executive functioning) not only improves
neurocognitive functioning in schizophrenics but also improves their
general social and occupational functioning. There is emerging but preliminary evidence that computerized cognitive remediation improves
cognitive functioning in substance users with neuropsychological deficits and also improves treatment engagement and outcome. Cognitive
remediation techniques, the neuropsychological equivalent of "mental
pushups," may be a novel way to bring about structural and functional improvement in the brain's braking systems among substance users.

Reducing Drives

The role of behavioral therapies in drive reduction is important but
less direct. Deconditioning of cue-induced craving can take place with

any treatment that fosters abstinence in the context of normal social routines. Hence, while the capacity to experience craving may not be affected, the frequency of craving can be dramatically reduced. Similarly, substance abuse-associated neuroadaptation is at least partially reversible and withdrawal symptoms fade substantially even after relatively brief periods of abstinence. Hence, any behavioral treatment that can foster abstinence initiation can provide the brain with some time to recover from the multiple insults of chronic substance use. In fact, given the negative impact of many types of substances on cognitive functioning, attention, and memory, initiation of behavioral treatments that are based on learning new skills may need to take place only after an initial period of abstinence and cognitive recovery.

Perhaps the most potent avenue for behavioral therapies to foster drive reduction is through combination with pharmacological treatments for drug abuse, most of which have their primary impact on drive reduction. Agonist treatments (such as methadone for heroin/ opioid addiction) help the individual avoid withdrawal symptoms and reduce craving. Craving reducers (e.g., bupropion for smoking, naltrexone for alcohol dependence) are not direct substitutes like agonists but do provide some of the desired effects of the drug. Pharmacotherapies directed at comorbid psychopathology may reduce craving by eliminating symptoms that drug abusers are attempting to self-medicate. Antagonists (e.g., naltrexone for opioids) that effectively block the reinforcing effects of drugs and medications that yield aversive responses to use (e.g., disulfiram for alcohol) provide fairly potent pharmacological braking.

Drive reduction strategies may thus lead to renewed emphasis on combined behavioral/pharmacological approaches, which invoke both the "top-down" approach of behavioral therapies and the "bottom-up" approach of pharmacotherapies. The literature has repeatedly indicated that, for those classes of substance use where effective pharmacotherapies exist, their effects are routinely strengthened, broadened, and made more durable when delivered in combination with behavior therapies. This occurs not only because behavioral therapies play an important role in enhancing adherence (as compliance problems undercut the effectiveness of virtually all existing pharmacotherapies for substance use problems), but because behavioral therapies and pharmacotherapies target very different and complementary aspects of substance use. Behavioral therapies can foster compliance with available pharmacotherapies, which, in turn, can yield periods of freedom from substance use that facilitate the ability of behavioral therapies to have an effect on coping skills, building supportive social networks, and solidifying motivation to continue abstinence.

To summarize, behavioral therapies (along with potentially complementary pharmacological treatments) can be characterized as targeting one or both of two major goals: improving impulse control and reducing craving. This is not to imply that the process is simple, as seeking these fundamental goals entails interventions that act at multiple, complex, interdependent levels (social, cognitive, behavioral, neurobiological) to help the patient maximize his or her own valences toward recovery and growth.

> Behavioral therapies target one or both of two major goals: improving impulse control and reducing craving.

Where Do We Go from Here?

A drawback to the current strategy for development of behavioral therapies for substance use disorders is the highly specific, piecemeal nature of the treatments (and manuals) developed, as well as the bewildering multiplicity of disorders (or subgroups within disorders) for which the treatments are "empirically validated." Effective dissemination of effective treatments for substance use problems can be fostered through identifying common treatment goals and a core set of change induction principles and techniques. Greater confluence of different behavioral therapies on the shared goal of improving behavioral controls raises issues about the potential redundancy or complementary nature of the four major classes of behavioral therapy.

In particular, we need to learn much more regarding issues such as the optimal sequencing, patient–treatment matching, and combinations of effective behavioral approaches along with their interrelation with pharmacological therapies. It is noteworthy that many of the highly successful treatments (be they behavioral or pharmacological) focus on a single aspect of the system such as enhancing motivation or providing contingent rewards for a single targeted behavior while leaving the rest of the recovery process up to healing influences in the patient's own person or social setting. These more focused treatments have the attraction of conceptual clarity and/or brevity, features that bode well for efficient dissemination. These strong (contingency management) and/or brief (motivational interviewing) treatments would appear to be useful strategies for stepped-care approaches that begin with widely applied minimal treatments and follow up with more intensive efforts only for those who do not respond to initial efforts. Alternatively, they may provide an efficient and success-enhancing entré into a more efficient sequence of treatment delivery with, for example, contingency management used to initiate abstinence followed by more cognitively demanding cognitive-behavioral therapy that is facilitated by the reduced craving and improved cognition that result from abstinence initiation.

The articulation of core behavior change principles and core techniques is particularly useful in devising strategies for dissemination of effective behavioral therapies. As noted above, it is highly unlikely that even a subset of substance abuse treatment programs or treatment settings could effectively provide the specific versions of even the four major classes of currently available empirically supported behavioral therapies for substance abuse disorders and problems, let alone the many variants currently under development. Currently available experience from research on behavioral therapies training and dissemination of standardized diagnostic systems would suggest that there may be trade-offs in organizing large-scale training programs around teaching either a small set of specific techniques or a comparable set of principles. For example, in the realm of diagnosis of mental disorders, instruments that feature very limited interviewer judgment consistently yield higher reliability than those that rely on clinician judgment guided by general diagnostic guidelines. In the behavioral therapies realm, it is noteworthy that different contingency management reward schedules have dramatically different efficacy at, for example, reducing cocaine use, even though all of the methods are based on investigators' correct understanding of basic behavioral principles.

We would suggest that an effective dissemination strategy would focus on providing a core set of overlearned, easily understood behavioral skills to the broadest group of clinicians (e.g., urine-monitoring principles, specific contingency management protocols, motivational interviewing techniques, core cognitive-behavioral skills). Newly developed, computer-administered or Internet-based training techniques are promising venues for this technology transfer because they are inexpensive, widely accessible, and amenable to allowing trainees to work at their own pace to achieve fluent mastery of skills. The amenability to simplification for computerized clinician training may also facilitate the development of motivational interviewing, contingency management, and cognitive-behavioral therapy treatment packages that can be directly used by patients. Arguably, family and couple therapy approaches may be less amenable to automated training and treatment delivery. Nonetheless, these would be best disseminated to a smaller group of more highly trained, specialized clinicians along with other more complex and specialized approaches, such as dialectic behavioral therapy for substance abusers with borderline personality disorder. In

a stepped-care or patient–treatment matching model, these more re-
source-intensive treatments would be reserved for nonresponders to
initial treatments or for those whose initial assessments indicate the
need for more intensive care.

Robust Principles

Efficacy of Behavioral Interventions

1. The four broad categories of behavioral interventions summarized
   above (brief motivational, contingency management, cognitive-
   behavioral, family and social network) have been generally shown
   to be effective across the major classes of substance use (alcohol,
   cocaine, marijuana, opioids, and to some extent smoking). This is
   clinically important, as "pure" forms of substance use are rare. It is
   also significant that these behavioral approaches do not necessarily
   target phenomena that are unique to specific classes of substance
   use, but rather the commonalities across the many types of substance use.

2. These approaches also tend to have firm support for their efficacy
   for treating other psychological problems. Again, this is important
   due to the high levels of comorbidity among substance users and
   also because of the commonalities across many behavioral disorders (e.g., the importance of supportive social networks in preventing relapse).

3. The identification of a range of empirically supported behavioral
   therapies is a notable accomplishment of recent clinical research in
   the addictions. Nevertheless, outcomes remain variable and none
   of these approaches are universally effective (i.e., associated with
   durable, long-term abstinence and the resolution of related problems in the majority of treated individuals).

4. Outcomes are generally better for individuals who have less severe
   or less chronic substance use (especially those who can initiate abstinence early in treatment or in the process of seeking treatment),
   intact and supportive families and social networks, fewer psychological symptoms or disorders, less involvement with the criminal
   justice system, better occupational functioning, and fewer medical
   problems. The effectiveness of these approaches tends to decrease
   with increasing severity of substance use and related problems.

5. While these general classes of behavioral therapies vary in their
   theoretical basis and the specific interventions they employ, they
   share several common principles of behavior change. These include heightening motivation (by enhancing recognition of the

problems associated with and the consequences of substance use, clarification of goals, and self-efficacy), encouraging behavioral controls (reinforcing behaviors incompatible with substance use, encouraging use of strategies to reduce impulsive responding, exercising interpersonal influence), and changing reinforcement contingencies so that abstinence is facilitated and rewarded (through interpersonal support, delivery of tangible incentives, increased emphasis on and access to other reinforcers and alternatives to substance use, and introduction of normative comparisons). One approach that encompasses all these change principles and effective elements of many existing empirically supported therapies is the community reinforcement approach, which has a very high level of empirical support.

6. Similarity of change processes across treatments may in part underlie existing data that suggest the comparability of long-term outcomes across different types of behavioral approaches. It may also be a factor in "nonspecificitis," the finding that efforts to evaluate process differences theoretically associated with the specific type of treatment delivered have generally yielded findings showing comparable changes across different types of treatment. Moreover, individuals who change substance use without formal treatment also appear to make use of these strategies (see DiClemente, Chapter 6, this volume).

7. Several general classes of effective behavioral therapies exist for substance use disorders, with brief motivational therapies, contingency management approaches, cognitive-behavioral approaches, and family/couple and interpersonal approaches having the highest current level of empirical support. These approaches are rarely available in clinical treatment settings. The current treatment system is unsuited either to adopt a large number of empirically supported therapies or to deliver them effectively.

8. Existing empirically validated treatments tend to emphasize one or two particular salient aspects of substance abuse and dependence. There are inherent limitations in any approach that addresses single elements of any phenomenon as complex as substance abuse and dependence and hence none is universally effective.

9. An emphasis on fundamental processes of addiction that may be amenable to behavioral intervention may lead to a more integrated model of treatment. Candidates for those processes include learning and habit strength as well as neurocognitive impairment and dyscontrol.

10. We would suggest that an effective dissemination strategy would focus on providing a core set of overlearned, easily understood be-

havioral skills and principles to the broadest group of clinicians (e.g., urine-monitoring principles, specific contingency management protocols, motivational interviewing techniques, core cognitive-behavioral therapy skills).

Acknowledgments

Support was provided by in part by National Institute on Drug Abuse Grant Nos. K05-DA0089 (to Bruce J. Rounsaville), K05-DA00457 (to Kathleen M. Carroll), P50-DA09241, U10 DA13038, and R37 DA15969 and by the U.S. Department of Veterans Affairs VISN 1 Mental Illness Research, Education, and Clinical Center.

Suggested Readings

Babor, T. F., & Del Boca, F. K. (Eds.). (2003). *Treatment matching in alcoholism.* Cambridge, UK: Cambridge University Press.

Carroll, K. M., & Onken, L. S. (2005). Behavioral therapies for drug abuse. *American Journal of Psychiatry, 162,* 1452–1460.

DeRubeis, R. J., & Crits-Christoph, P. (1998). Empirically supported individual and group psychological treatments for adult mental disorders. *Journal of Consulting and Clinical Psychology, 66,* 37–52.

Goldapple, M., Segal, Z., Garson, C., Lau, M., Bieling, P., Kennedy, S., et al. (2004). Modulation of cortical–limbic pathways in major depression: Treatment-specific effects of cognitive behavior therapy. *Archives of General Psychiatry, 61,* 34–41.

Goldstein, R., & Volkow, N. D. (2002). Drug addiction and its underlying neurobiological basis: Neuroimaging evidence for the involvement of the frontal cortex. *American Journal of Psychiatry, 159*(10), 1642–1652.

Griffith, J. D., Rowan-Szal, G. A., Roark, R. R., & Simpson, D. D. (2000). Contingency management in outpatient methadone treatment: A meta-analysis. *Drug and Alcohol Dependence, 58,* 55–66.

Higgins, S. T., & Silverman, K. (1999). *Motivating behavior change among illicit-drug abusers.* Washington, DC: American Psychological Association.

Institute of Medicine. (1998). *Bridging the gap between practice and research: Forging partnerships with community-based drug and alcohol treatment.* Washington, DC: National Academy Press.

Kazdin, A. E. (2001). Progression of therapy research and clinical application of treatment require better understanding of the change process. *Clinical Psychology: Science and Practice, 8,* 143–151.

Miller, W. R. (2000). Rediscovering fire: Small interventions, large effects. *Psychology of Addictive Behaviors, 14,* 6–18.

Miller, W. R., Brown, J. M., Simpson, T. L., Handmaker, N. S., Bien, T. H., Luckie,

L. F., et al. (1995). What works?: A methodological analysis of the alcohol treatment literature. In R. K. Hester & W. R. Miller (Eds.), *Handbook of alcoholism treatment approaches: Effective alternatives* (pp. 12–44). Boston: Allyn & Bacon.

Petry, N. M., Petrakis, I., Trevisan, L., Wiredu, L., Boutros, N., Martin, B., et al. (2001). Contingency management interventions: From research to practice. *American Journal of Psychiatry, 20*, 33–44.

Rotgers, F., Morgenstern, J., & Walters, S. T. (Eds.). (2003). *Treating substance abuse: Theory and technique* (2nd ed.). New York: Guilford Press.

Roth, A., & Fonagy, P. (2004). *What works for whom?: A critical review of the psychotherapy literature* (2nd ed.). New York: Guilford Press.

Sammons, M. T., & Schmidt, N. B. (2001). *Combined treatments for mental disorders: Pharmacological and psychotherapeutic strategies for intervention.* Washington, DC: American Psychological Association Press.

Stanton, M. D., & Shadish, W. R. (1997). Outcome, attrition, and family-couples treatment for drug abuse: A meta-analysis and review of the controlled, comparative studies. *Psychological Bulletin, 122*, 170–191.

CHAPTER 15

Pharmacotherapy of Addictive Disorders

STEPHANIE S. O'MALLEY
THOMAS R. KOSTEN

The role that pharmacotherapy has played in the treatment of substance use disorders varies considerably depending on the drug of abuse. Pharmacotherapy is a mainstay of treatment for nicotine dependence, which typically incorporates minimal behavioral interventions, while for stimulants such as cocaine and amphetamine behavioral interventions are the mainstay and no pharmacotherapies approved by the U.S. Food and Drug Administration (FDA) exist. Pharmacotherapy for the treatment of marijuana dependence is an emerging concept, fueled by the development of cannabinoid antagonists, but in contrast to cocaine pharmacotherapy, for which more than 50 medications have been tested, few cannabinoid pharmacotherapies have even been proposed. Pharmacological interventions are central to the treatment of opiate addiction in combination with relatively comprehensive behavioral interventions in recognition of the wide-ranging effects that addiction has on other lifestyle issues. Since the approval of naltrexone 10 years ago, pharmacotherapy has shown growing acceptance in the treatment of alcoholism. This acceptance has been improved by understanding the neurobiological underpinnings of addiction, accruing clinical research, and the promise of new and more effective medications. The epidemiology of alcoholism, a highly prevalent disorder that affects individuals from all facets of society, makes it likely that pharmaceutical companies will step up to the drug development plate.

Pharmacotherapies for substance abuse have been used to address two broad objectives in treatment: (1) management of acute withdrawal or initial attainment of abstinence, and (2) prevention of relapse to either any use or heavy use. Although some new immunotherapies actually prevent the entry of abused drugs into the brain, most pharmacotherapies target the brain receptors or neurotransmitters/neuromodulators that are dysregulated in addiction to a particular drug of abuse. Toward this end, four main classes of drugs have been tested. *Agonist drugs* directly stimulate the receptor—for example, methadone binds to the opiate receptors—and are often used as replacements for the abused drug. Other medications can act as *indirect agonists* by increasing levels of the transmitter indirectly by (1) decreasing breakdown of the transmitter, (2) by increasing its release, or (3) by blocking its reuptake into the neuron that released the transmitter. *Partial agonists* act like agonists but do not stimulate the receptor to the same degree. *Antagonists* bind to the receptor but do not stimulate it and prevent agonists from binding.

> *Pharmacotherapies address two broad objectives: initial attainment of abstinence and prevention of relapse.*

In this chapter, we briefly review the agents that are currently in use as well as agents on the horizon for addiction to nicotine, alcohol, opiates, cocaine, and marijuana, and we describe the mechanism by which the medications are thought to work. The role of medication compliance and behavioral treatments in combination with medications is also discussed.

Nicotine

Pharmacotherapy is a mainstay of treatment for smoking cessation, with five different forms of nicotine replacement therapies and bupropion currently approved by the FDA. Nicotine replacement therapies (NRT) are designed to replace the nicotine obtained from smoking in order to prevent withdrawal symptoms and improve smoking cessation outcomes. Approved formulations include the transdermal nicotine patch, nicotine gum, nicotine vapor inhaler, nicotine spray, and most recently the nicotine lozenge. Typically, a person is counseled to quit smoking, provided with brief advice about how to do this, and helped to establish a quit date. On the quit date, the person ceases other forms of tobacco use and begins the NRT. Success in quitting on the quit date is highly predictive of end-of-treatment success.

NRT is generally recommended as a short-term therapy; however, longer term treatment is being investigated for particularly hard-to-treat smokers. NRTs are considered first-line therapies for smoking cessation and have been demonstrated efficacious compared to placebo in numerous studies on measures of abstinence (not even a puff) at the end of the trial and at later time-points (e.g., 6 and 12 months).

Bupropion, an atypical antidepressant agent, has also been shown to improve quit rates compared to placebo in short-term and long-term follow-up. The mechanism of action is not proven, but it is thought to work through modest blockade of dopamine and norepinephrine uptake and antagonism of the high-affinity nicotinic acetylcholine receptor, which is the target brain receptor underlying nicotine's reinforcing effects. Unlike NRTs, bupropion is taken for 1–2 weeks prior to the quit date and then continued following the quit date. During the period prior to the quit date, many smokers experience a reduction in their urges to smoke and may reduce their smoking, thereby facilitating success on their target quit date. For some individuals, side effects including insomnia, headache, and jitteriness are troublesome and limit bupropion's effectiveness.

There are a number of nonapproved clinically available treatments for nicotine addiction that are recommended as second-line therapies, including clonidine and nortriptyline. Clonidine, an alpha2 adrenergic agonist, modestly increases quit rates compared to placebo, probably through its effects on reducing nicotine withdrawal symptoms. Clonidine has a number of side effects, such as dry mouth, sedation, constipation, and orthostatic hypotension. Nortriptyline, a tricyclic antidepressant, has been shown to be efficacious, but has significant adverse effects, some of which limit its safety (e.g., risk of lethality in overdose). It is thought to work by increasing norepinephrine and serotonin levels by inhibiting their reuptake.

Another strategy for indirectly increasing important neurotransmitter levels is by inhibiting the enzymes that break down or metabolize these neurotransmitters. One such approach that shows promise is inhibition of monoamine oxidase B by selegiline. This enzyme breaks down dopamine, and thus its inhibition tends to increase dopamine levels and reduce nicotine craving. This enzyme is also specifically inhibited by some component of tobacco smoke (not nicotine) and selegiline restores this inhibition, potentially further contributing to the relief of craving and withdrawal symptoms.

The possibility that new treatments will be marketed for smoking cessation in the near future is high. One agent that seems particularly promising is a partial agonist of the nicotinic acetylcholine receptor under development by Pfizer. Partial agonists are similar to full agonists in that partial agonists bind to and activate receptors. At lower doses, the full agonists and the partial agonists produce effects that are essentially indistinguishable. However, increasing the dose of a partial agonist does not produce as great an effect as does increasing the dose of a full agonist. Partial agonists have the potential to reduce withdrawal symptoms due to the drug's agonist properties and to reduce smoking satisfaction if there is a lapse occupying the nicotinic receptors, thereby decreasing the likelihood of relapse.

A selective cannabinoid receptor antagonist is currently being investigated as treatment for obesity and smoking cessation. Data presented from a company-sponsored study indicates that this class of medications can substantially limit the weight gain typically associated with smoking cessation and modestly improve smoking cessation rates. This side benefit of treatment may be particularly attractive to weight-concerned smokers or obese smokers who might not otherwise attempt to quit or who might relapse in response to weight gain following quitting.

Some of the other medications under investigation for smoking cessation include naltrexone, drugs that modify gamma-aminobutyric acid (GABA) and glutamate levels, and vaccines. Vaccines result in the production of drug-specific antibodies, which bind to the drug, thereby reducing its distribution into the brain. In animal studies, for example, nicotine vaccines have been shown to reduce several actions of nicotine including the induction of nicotine dependence, locomotor activation, the discriminative stimulus characteristics of nicotine, nicotine-induced dopamine release, and the reinstatement of nicotine responding following nicotine exposure. They also appear to reduce distribution of nicotine to the fetus in pregnant animals.

Alcohol

The first advance made in the pharmacotherapy of alcoholism was the discovery that benzodiazepines could be used to manage alcohol withdrawal. Chronic use of alcohol interspersed with periods of withdrawal can result in a withdrawal syndrome marked by autonomic hyperactivity, anxiety, and in severe cases seizures, delirium, and even death. This withdrawal syndrome is related in part to counteradaptive responses to alcohol potentiation of the major inhibitory neurotransmitter GABA, resulting in hyperreactivity when alcohol is removed. Benzodiazepines act at $GABA_A$ receptors to stimulate GABA release and are used to more gradually detoxify the patient from alcohol in order to avoid these withdrawal symptoms. The use of benzodiazepines in this manner revolutionized the treatment of alcohol withdrawal and unequivocally reduced the risk of death associated with detoxification. Benzodiazepine treatment, however, does not make an effective long-term strategy because tolerance to benzodiazepines occurs and potentially dangerous interactions can occur with alcohol.

Other anticonvulsants have been studied for their efficacy in the treatment of alcohol withdrawal, including valproate and carbamazepine. Of particular note, in one clinical trial comparing carbamazepine to lorazepam for alcohol withdrawal, both medications were effective in reducing withdrawal symptoms, but carbamezepine-treated patients showed less posttreatment drinking. Additional research is needed to confirm these findings and also to examine the efficacy of carbamazepine in severe alcohol withdrawal. The possibility that other treatments that increase GABA levels (e.g., topiramate) can be used to facilitate long-term recovery is under investigation.

Of course, helping patients safely stop drinking is just the beginning of treatment for alcohol dependence. Maintenance of abstinence and prevention of relapse to heavy drinking are other important targets. In this regard, there are three pharmacotherapies approved for use in the United States, including disulfiram, naltrexone, and most recently acamprosate. Disulfiram, approved in the 1940s, is an alcohol-sensitizing agent and is used to deter a patient from drinking by producing an aversive interaction with alcohol. Specifically, disulfiram inhibits the liver enzyme that breaks down acetaldehyde, a toxic by-product of ethanol metabolism. The resulting buildup of acetaldehyde yields a reaction characterized by facial flushing, headache, nausea and vomiting, and a number of other aversive signs and symptoms. Not all patients actually experience this interaction at the doses that are typically prescribed, and adverse events limit the safety of higher doses. In addition, disulfiram works primarily through the patient's knowledge of the potential ethanol–disulfiram interaction rather than by reducing the urge to drink or addressing the underlying neurobiology of the disorder. As a result, problems with compliance and patient acceptance abound. Controlled clinical trials suggest that unless disulfiram administration is supervised in some way (e.g., by a family member or staff member), disulfiram does not significantly improve abstinence rates compared to placebo.

Naltrexone, an opiate antagonist approved for use in 1994 for the treatment of alcoholism, was first tested in humans based on the knowledge that alcohol stimulated the release of endogenous opioids and animal studies showing that opiate antagonists decreased alcohol drinking reliably under a variety of circumstances. Approximately 2,300 alcohol-dependent patients have been studied in at least 15 published controlled studies of naltrexone, with the majority of the studies showing improved efficacy relative to placebo. While naltrexone is an opiate antagonist and is thought to antagonize some of the effects of alcohol, it does not block the effects of alcohol in the same way that it completely blocks the effects of opiates. In fact, one hypothesis for the ability of naltrexone to reduce drinking following a lapse in abstinence is that it unmasks some of the sedating effects of alcohol that limit alcohol consumption. Naltrexone has been shown to reduce the risk of relapse to heavy drinking and to increase the percentage of days abstinent. The effect size observed is similar to that seen with nicotine replacement therapies for smoking cessation but substantially smaller that that reported for antidepressant therapies for depression. The most common side effects of naltrexone include nausea and headache. At higher doses than typically prescribed, naltrexone can be hepatotoxic.

Acamprosate (calcium acetylhomotaurine) is a structural analogue of taurine, and has modulatory effects at N-methyl-D-aspartate (NMDA) receptors. Acamprosate, by reducing neuronal hyperexcitability during alcohol withdrawal, may reduce the physiological and psychological distress and desire to drink that results from protracted alcohol withdrawal and thereby promote maintenance of abstinence. Acamprosate has been extensively studied in Europe, where it has been approved for many years. These studies were conducted primarily in patients who had been detoxified from alcohol prior to beginning acamprosate. The primary outcomes on which the drug has been shown to be superior to placebo are measures of abstinence. A meta-analysis of 17 studies, which included 4,087 individuals, found that continuous abstinence rates at 6 months were significantly higher in the acamprosate-treated patients. Acamprosate also had a modest effect on retention in 13 of 16 European studies. One study in the United States, which did not require abstinence prior to beginning acamprosate, did not find efficacy in the intent-to-treat sample, but showed an advantage in a highly motivated and compliant subsample. Based on submission of efficacy data from three European studies, the FDA recently approved acamprosate for treating alcohol-dependent individuals seeking to remain alcohol-free after they have stopped drinking. The FDA notes that acamprosate may not be effective in patients who are actively drinking at the start of treatment, or in patients who abuse other substances in addition to alcohol. Diarrhea is the primary adverse event associated with acamprosate.

Several other medications, which are available by prescription for other indications, have been studied for use in the treatment of alcoholism. In this regard, increasing attention is being paid to pharmacological interventions that are designed to enhance inhibitory controls on dopamine release, an "accelerator" implicated in many forms of drug dependence. In the treatment of alcoholism, for example, topiramate, a medication that is approved for the treatment of epilepsy, is being studied in a range of disorders characterized by impulsivity.

Topiramate has been evaluated because of its ability to augment GABA function and inhibit excitatory glutamatergic pathways, which together can decrease dopamine activity and perhaps alcohol's reward. In one study, a novel approach was employed in which abstinence was not required and minimal counseling emphasizing compliance was utilized. Following an 8-week titration period, drinking outcomes including drinks per day, drinks per drinking day, percentage of heavy-drinking days, and the percentage of abstinent days improved for the active compared to the placebo group. Topiramate has a number of side effects, including modest cognitive impairment, and requires slow titration over 5–8 weeks before a fully effective dose is reached. Other mood stabilizers are also under investigation.

Based on the hypothesis that alcoholism is associated with serotonergic deficiencies and preclinical data and human laboratory studies suggesting that selective serotonin reuptake inhibitors (SSRIs) could reduce alcohol drinking, a relatively large number of clinical trials have tested the efficacy of this class of medications. In the end, there is little support for the use of SSRIs as first-line therapy for alcoholism in unselected patients. Secondary analyses of these clinical trials suggest that patients with milder late-onset alcoholism may benefit. For those with early-onset severe alcoholism, an initial study found that ondansetron, a 5-HT$_3$ antagonist, may be helpful. Additional prospective randomized studies of these agents in the groups hypothesized to benefit are needed.

Opiates

The most effective pharmacotherapies for opiate addiction have involved agonist therapies. Agonists are drugs that occupy the receptor and turn it on; this approach typically involves administration of drugs with actions similar to those of the abused drug (agonists), but which have different pharmacokinetic profiles such that they are longer acting and less reinforcing and/or have fewer drug-like effects (e.g., intoxication, euphoria). In the case of opiates, opiate-addicted individuals, who are using short-acting opiates (e.g., heroin), are placed on methadone, which has a much longer duration of action. Once stabilized on methadone, the patient no longer experiences peaks of euphoria or the aversive effects of withdrawal, is no longer preoccupied with drug seeking, and is able to participate more fully in other aspects of life. When adequate doses are used, methadone replacement also reduces the reinforcing effects of shorter acting opiates through cross-tolerance, a phenomenon in which the diminished intensity of drug responses to a particular drug (e.g., methadone) transfers to other drugs from the same class (e.g., heroin). This combination of alleviation of withdrawal and prevention of reinforcement makes methadone replacement therapy extremely effective as measured by opiate-free urines. In addition, methadone treatment appears to normalize many aspects of the hormonal disruptions found in addicted individuals. While methadone maintenance has been used on a short-term basis to detoxify from opiates, most researchers and clinicians argue that methadone maintenance should be considered a long-term treatment for this chronic disorder.

> *Methadone treatment appears to normalize many aspects of the hormonal disruptions found in addicted individuals.*

One of the important limitations of methadone is the potential for diversion and the risk of overdose, which has resulted in a number of regulatory requirements for programs and patients (e.g., observed daily dosing during the beginning of treatment). Buprenorphine, an opioid partial agonist, which was approved in 2002, has been shown to be safer than methadone on measures of respiratory depression and other overdose risks. Furthermore, a formulation that combines buprenorphine, which is administered sublingually, with oral naloxone was designed to prevent the drug from being diverted to injection drug use. A major advantage of buprenorphine is that it can be obtained by prescription from the patient's primary care physician or psychiatrist who has completed specialized training rather than through attendance at a specialty clinic.

Finally, naltrexone, a competitive opiate antagonist, is approved for the treatment of opiate addiction. Antagonists bind to receptors, but instead of activating the receptors antagonists effectively block the receptors. By doing so, they prevent the receptors from being activated by an agonist compound. The analogy that is frequently used to explain this effect is that of a key that fits in a lock but doesn't open it. In the case of opiates, naltrexone occupies brain opiate receptors without stimulating them, and in doing so prevents opiates from stimulating the receptor. Since the addict cannot get high from opiates while on naltrexone, it was thought that this would improve abstinence rates. Although naltrexone is extremely effective in blocking the effects of opiates, its utility in treatment has been disappointing due to substantial problems with treatment retention, even in the context of supervised administration. Another limitation is that opiate-dependent individuals must be detoxified from opiates prior to beginning naltrexone in order to prevent a severe withdrawal syndrome. Whether longer acting formulations, such as once-a-month injections, improve efficacy by reducing compliance problems remains to be demonstrated. Naltrexone has also been studied as a tool for rapidly detoxifying opiate-addicted individuals in combination with clonidine and other agents to manage the withdrawal syndrome that is precipitated by naltrexone.

Stimulants

Over 50 medications have been tried for the treatment of cocaine or amphetamine addiction, but to date no medications have FDA approval for this indication. Although there is clear evidence that psychostimulants have their effects through dopaminergic mechanisms, studies of direct dopamine agonists have been disappointing. Other agents that raise dopamine levels through indirect mechanisms may have more promise. For example, disulfiram can increases dopamine levels by inhibiting the activity of an enzyme called dopamine beta-hydroxylase (DBH) that converts dopamine to norepinephrine and has been shown to be effective in the treatment of cocaine dependence. Interestingly, the original rationale for studying disulfiram was based on the common association between alcohol and cocaine use, and posited that by preventing alcohol use, disulfiram would reduce the risk of cocaine use since alcohol is a strong cue for cocaine use and can lead to impairments in judgment that may reduce the patient's ability to resist cocaine. A controlled clinical trial, however, has since shown that the benefits of disulfiram are most pronounced in patients who are not alcohol-dependent at baseline and those who abstain from alcohol. These data suggest that other mechanisms are responsible, including inhibition of DBH, thereby increasing dopamine availability. In an abstinent person, disulfiram may increase dopamine levels sufficiently to reduce the drive to use cocaine. In combination with cocaine, which also boosts dopamine activity in the brain, the resulting dopamine levels may produce an unpleasant reaction, such as anxiety and paranoia that limits continued use.

Another class of medications that have been extensively studied is antidepressants, which are thought to down-regulate synaptic catecholamine receptors, an action opposite to the presynaptic up-regulation caused by chronic stimulant use. Desipramine, an older agent that inhibits reuptake of norepinephrine, has the most evidence in support of its use for cocaine dependence.

Several other pharmacological strategies hold some promise for the future, including agents that alter GABA levels such as baclofen (a GABA agonist) and tiagabine (a GABA reuptake inhibitor) and cocaine vaccines. Cocaine vaccines work by preventing the drug from entering the brain and have been shown to reduce cocaine self-administration in rodents. The ability of these vaccines to prevent the drug from entering the brain is incomplete; therefore, a person could override these effects by taking larger amounts of cocaine. As a result, behavioral counseling is likely to be an important component of treatment.

Marijuana

Pharmacological interventions for marijuana dependence have not received a lot of attention, although a cannabinoid antagonist that partially blocks the effects of marijuana at the doses tested has been developed. However, based on the limited effectiveness of opiate antagonists in opiate dependence, even if effective doses are determined, compliance with a cannabinoid antagonist may limit its effectiveness in treating marijuana dependence.

Combination Pharmacotherapy

Given that drugs of abuse affect multiple neurotransmitter and/or hormonal systems, the possibility that combinations of therapy will be more effective than monotherapy seems plausible. One strategy is the combination of agonist agents to reduce withdrawal symptoms and antagonist agents to reduce rewarding drug effects; examples include mecamylamine and nicotine replacement therapy for smoking cessation. Partial agonists may be a more effective strategy as they become available. Another strategy is to combine treatments that target different aspects of the drug-dependence syndrome. For example, in alcoholism protracted withdrawal might be relieved by acamprosate and reinstatement of alcohol drinking might be attenuated by naltrexone. For tobacco dependence, tobacco withdrawal might be addressed by a nicotine patch and acute exacerbations of tobacco craving by nicotine gum. Alternatively, tobacco relapse might be addressed by a nicotine vaccine following initial treatment with nicotine replacement therapies for withdrawal. Thus, these strategies may be sequenced such that a patient begins one treatment and is then switched to an alternative or to an augmentation strategy if they do not respond. The appropriate sequence of therapy may be determined by an understanding of the drug's mechanisms, cost issues, and patient preference. Ultimately, informing the patient that additional options are available may help address the problem of retention in substance abuse treatment.

Patient–Treatment Matching

The majority of pharmacotherapy trials have not been completed in samples of participants who were selected on the basis of their potential to respond to the medication. Secondary analyses have identified factors that may predict differential response to the treatments. For example, studies of antidepressants (e.g., SSRIs) in alcohol dependence have failed to consistently demonstrate an advantage over placebo in the overall sample, although there is some evidence that these medications may be helpful to those with late-onset alcoholism, which is characterized by anxiety and other affective symptoms. In contrast, SSRIs may be counterproductive in early-onset alcoholics. Naltrexone therapy appears to be particularly effective for those with high levels of craving at baseline and those who have a family history of alcoholism, while both of these factors are associated with poorer response to placebo and behavioral counseling. Of interest, secondary analyses of naltrexone clinical trials have suggested that a functional variant of the mu opiate receptor gene, which leads to a 10-fold greater affinity of the opiate receptor for its endogenous ligand—beta endorphin—predicts differential response to naltrexone.

In the smoking cessation literature, there is evidence that women are not as responsive as men to NRTs, whereas the disadvantage conferred by female gender does not generalize to bupropion therapy. One potential advantage of bupropion therapy is that it limits weight gain during treatment. The possibility that this will translate into improved smoking cessation outcomes for weight-concerned smokers is under prospective investigation. Weight also predicts response to different forms of NRT, with obese smokers responding better to nicotine spray than to nicotine patch.

Ultimately, research that identifies who is most likely to respond favorably to a particular pharmacotherapy will improve the clinical care of patients by reducing exposure to ineffective treatments that are associated with adverse events and offering the best chance for improvement from the outset of treatment.

Does Pharmacotherapy Have a Place for Individuals without Long-Term Dependence?

In general, most pharmacotherapy research has focused on dependent individuals. However, the potential of using pharmacological treatments for those who are engaging in hazardous use is compelling. By intervening early, it may be possible to interrupt the development of a long-term dependence syndrome, or, to borrow an analogy used by Carolyn Knapp in *Drinking: A Love Story*, it may be easier to prevent a cucumber from becoming a pickle than to turn a pickle back into a cucumber. Vaccines certainly represent one pharmacological intervention that fits within this strategy. Other potential examples include naltrexone for young opiate users who do not meet federally mandated eligibility criteria for maintenance therapies or naltrexone for reducing hazardous drinking among nondependent drinkers.

Adherence

For medications to be effective, they must be taken. As a result, considerable attention has been paid to the issue of compliance with or adherence to treatment. Adherence to a medication regimen is a product of several factors. First, the characteristics of the drug include efficacy or lack thereof, adverse events, ease of dosing, and the costs of the medication. Second, the characteristics of the patient may include cognitive impairment, motivation for change, environmental supports for compliance, attitudes and beliefs about his or her illness and treatment, and perceptions of medication efficacy, among many others. Third, the interventions of the provider to enhance adherence include teaching patients about the medications and the need for compliance, as well as providing more targeted interventions to enhance patient compliance, such as contingency management procedures or supervised medication administration. Future research building upon models of health protective behaviors should help us to further understand the factors that influence the desire to use and to adhere to treatment and how we can effectively motivate behavior change.

Motivation to adhere to a medication schedule can vary over time. The classic example of this is antibiotic compliance. When a person is acutely ill he or she is highly motivated to comply with antibiotic therapy, but as the sore throat resolves compliance drops off, leaving the patient susceptible to a relapse caused by bacteria that are still present. A similar phenomenon can be imagined for substance use disorders in which early compliance is high when the person is distressed but trails off as his or her situation improves; however, many challenges are still to be faced and the potential safety net provided by pharmacotherapy will be weakened.

In the case of problem alcohol or drug use, desire to use the drug of choice and the belief that the medication will interfere with the drug experience may be a unique factor that can influence medication compliance. For example, adherence with disulfiram for cocaine dependence is reduced in those participants who find it difficult to abstain from alcohol. These participants may stop taking the disulfiram in order to drink, thereby undermining the efficacy of disulfiram for cocaine dependence.

There are a number of methods related to drug formulation that can result in improved adherence, including new formulations or dosing strategies that reduce the risk of adverse events (e.g., gradual drug taper) and those that reduce the frequency of dosing. A number of companies have been developing long-acting versions of naltrexone, including implants and injections that can be administered once a month.

Behavioral or environmental interventions that can enhance compliance include developing a routine for taking medications, packaging medications in a way that promotes compliance (e.g., blister packs, pill bottles that display when the bottle was last opened), counseling about the importance of compliance, as well as more intensive interventions. In the case of medications that work by interfering with drug use (e.g., naltrexone for opiate use, disulfiram for alcohol dependence), behavioral methods for improving adherence seem particularly important. Supervised administration by either a family member or the treatment program is the most common and most easily implemented method. Contingency management in which medication adherence is rewarded can dramatically improve compliance and treatment outcome.

Interactions with Behavioral Therapies

All studies of pharmacological treatments have incorporated some component of counseling, ranging from minimal education about the expected effect of the pharmacotherapy and about the nature of the disorder in the case of over-the-counter nicotine replacement products to comprehensive behavioral therapies. The potential for behavioral interventions to influence the ultimate success of treatment is critical. Behavioral interventions can increase the number of individuals who are successful by increasing their compliance and retention in treatment (e.g., medication compliance therapy, contingency management). These interventions can also impart new skills and knowledge that could help sustain improvements after treatment ends (e.g., cognitive-behavioral therapy). Similarly, an effective pharmacotherapy may help retain a patient in treatment, thereby increasing his or her ability to make use of behavioral interven-

Behavioral interventions can increase compliance and retention.

tions. Finally, behavioral interventions could be specifically designed to take advantage of the pharmacological effect of the medication (e.g., drinking-reduction strategies in combination with naltrexone).

The combination of a particular behavioral intervention and a particular pharmacotherapy does not always increase the number of successful participants over that seen with either approach alone. For example, a study in which participants received either disulfiram or placebo and either cognitive-behavioral therapy or interpersonal therapy for cocaine dependence found that disulfiram improved outcome relative to placebo and that cognitive-behavioral therapy improved outcome relative to interpersonal therapy. However, there was no additional advantage to the combination of cognitive-behavioral therapy and disulfiram. A finding like this might result because the patients who respond to each treatment overlap. A negative interaction is also possible, if the mechanisms of action of each treatment are at odds with each other. For example, 12-step facilitation therapy that promotes abstinence may reduce the likelihood that naltrexone will provide additional benefit, since an important component of naltrexone's effect is in preventing relapse following a lapse in abstinence. This hypothesis might account in part for the negative findings with naltrexone in the U.S. Veterans Administration Cooperative Naltrexone Study. Another potential mismatch may have occurred in the U.S. acamprosate study in which participants did not have to be abstinent nor have an abstinence goal, whereas the strongest effects of acamprosate appear to be on maintaining abstinence through a hypothesized effect on protracted withdrawal. A final example of a potential negative interaction could involve less active participation by the patient in the behavioral intervention due to his or her reliance on the medication as the answer to his or her problems.

The intensity of the behavioral intervention to be provided in combination with pharmacotherapy should be a function of the characteristics of the patient and the setting in which treatment is being conducted. While some studies have shown that the addition of more intensive treatment to a pharmacological intervention such as methadone maintenance can improve success rates, pharmacological interventions and concurrent brief counseling methods that can be used by primary care providers have the potential to extend the settings in which substance abuse treatment can occur. This has been one important rationale for the development of buprenorphine for opiate addiction. Research on naltrexone for alcoholism suggests that naltrexone also can be used effectively in a primary care model compared to a specialty model using cognitive-behavioral therapy, although those who initially responded to cognitive-behavioral therapy and naltrexone were better able to maintain their improvement without continued naltrexone.

A medication can be used in the absence of direct provider intervention. For example, nicotine replacement products have been available without a prescription since shortly after their development. Over-the-counter medications have the potential advantage of reducing health care costs, increasing availability, and having a larger public health benefit. For a medication to be approved for over-the-counter use, it must be safe and effective without the supervision of a licensed practitioner; it should have low potential for misuse; the condition treated should be benign and self-diagnosable by the average person; and labeling instructions must be understandable to the average person who will use the product. Whether medications for other substances will meet these criteria in the future remains an open question.

Robust Principles

1. Agonist replacement therapies have shown consistent efficacy for some drugs, such as methadone for heroin and nicotine patches for tobacco. In these cases, agonist therapies have a number of advantages in that they do not require detoxification, can prevent withdrawal, and at adequate doses can reduce the reinforcing effects of the abused drug by occupying the involved brain receptor. Partial agonists such as buprenorphine for opiates, which have milder agonist properties, less abuse liability, and greater safety, can be very useful for office-based practice.

2. Although pharmacologically efficacious, antagonists of specific receptors, which are also the principal target of the abused drug, generally have been ineffective in clinical practice due to problems with adherence, the need for detoxification, and side effects. Antagonists may be more useful with drugs like alcohol, which have multiple effects, because the antagonist blocks only a subset of the drug's actions (e.g., naltrexone blocks opiate-receptor-mediated effects) and are therefore less likely to precipitate a withdrawal syndrome or to result in the patient discontinuing the medication for the specific purpose of using the drug.

3. Indirect methods of inhibiting a drug's reinforcing potential (either positive or negative reinforcement) that appear promising include medications that enhance the function of the GABA system (e.g., topiramate for alcoholism) or increase tonic levels of dopamine (e.g., disulfiram for cocaine).

4. Drugs that primarily make the drug of choice aversive (e.g.,

disulfiram for alcoholism) are likely to be associated with compliance problems.

5. Pharmacotherapy can play a role at different stages of the recovery process including initial abstinence and relapse prevention. The type of pharmacotherapy needed at each stage may vary.

6. The intensity and nature of the behavioral treatment component can influence the overall outcome of treatment for an individual patient as well as the number of patients who ultimately receive the treatment. Combining medications such as buprenorphine with supportive treatments that can be implemented by primary care providers or even over-the-counter medications such as nicotine patches requiring no professional supportive treatments have the potential for a great public health impact.

Acknowledgments

Support was provided by Grant Nos. P50-DA12762, P50-DA18197, K05-DA00454 (to Thomas R. Kosten), P50-AA015632, and K05-AA014715 (to Stephanie S. O'Malley) from the National Institute on Drug Abuse and the National Institute on Alcohol Abuse and Alcoholism.

Suggested Readings

Carroll, K. M., Fenton, L. R., Ball, S. A., Nich, C., Frankforter, T. L., Shi, J., et al. (2004). Efficacy of disulfiram and cognitive behavior therapy in cocaine-dependent outpatients: A randomized placebo-controlled trial. *Archives of General Psychiatry, 61*, 264–272.

Cramer, J. A. (1995). Optimizing long-term patient compliance. *Neurology, 45*(2, Suppl. 1), S25–S28.

Fuller, R. K., & Gordis, E. (2004). Does disulfiram have a role in alcoholism treatment today? *Addiction, 99*, 21–24.

George, T. P., & O'Malley, S. S. (2004). Current pharmacological treatments for nicotine dependence. *Trends in Pharmacological Sciences, 25*(1), 42–48.

Gonzalez, G., Oliveto, A., & Kosten, T. R. (2004). Combating opiate dependence: A comparison among the available pharmacological options. *Expert Opinion on Pharmacotherapy, 5*, 713–725.

Johnson, B. A., Ait-Daoud, N., Bowden, C. L., DiClemente, C. C., Roache, J. D., Lawson, K., et al. (2003). Oral topiramate for treatment of alcohol dependence: A randomised controlled trial. *Lancet, 361*, 1677–1685.

Kosten, T. R., & O'Connor, P. G. (2003). Management of drug and alcohol withdrawal. *New England Journal of Medicine, 348*(18), 1786–1795.

McCaul, M. E., & Petry, N. M. (2003). The role of psychosocial treatments in pharmacotherapy for alcoholism. *Journal on Addictions, 12*(Suppl. 1), S41–S52.

O'Malley, S. S., & Foehlich, J. C. (2003). Advances in the use of naltrexone: An integration of preclinical and clinical findings. *Recent Developments in Alcoholism, 16*, 217–245.

O'Malley, S. S., Rounsaville, B. J., Farren, C., Namkoong, K., Wu, R., Robinson, J., et al. (2003). Initial and maintenance naltrexone treatment for alcohol dependence using primary care vs. specialty care: A nested sequence of 3 randomized trials. *Archives of Internal Medicine, 163*(14), 1695–1704.

Tobacco Use and Dependence Clinical Practice Guideline Panel, Staff, and Consortium Representatives. (2000). A clinical practice guideline for treating tobacco use an dependence: A U.S. Public Health Service report. *Journal of the American Medical Association, 283*, 3244–3254.

CHAPTER 16

Religion, Spirituality, and the Troublesome Use of Substances

KEITH HUMPHREYS
ELIZABETH GIFFORD

Religious and spiritual organizations are an extremely influential force in the substance control field. At the individual level, religious involvement remains the strongest protective factor in the prevention of troublesome substance use initiation among children and adolescents. At the public policy level, religious movements have inspired and shaped major legislative efforts to combat substance use problems in the United States. The temperance movement, for example, was inspired and led by the social gospel faction of evangelical Protestantism, which combined an optimistic view of improving human society with a moral imperative to care for those in need. Temperance and related religious social movements produced social tributaries that permanently shaped the landscape of addiction recovery, treatment, and prevention programs in the United States and in some European nations as well. Among the most important of these tributaries are spiritual and religious mutual help organizations, which provide assistance to more addicted people than all professional treatments combined.

Religious involvement remains the strongest protective factor in the prevention of substance use initiation among children and adolescents.

This chapter presents an overview of scientific information on the role of religion and spirituality in the troublesome use of substances. After defining our key terms and providing background information about religion, spirituality, and substance use, we discuss the role of religion in the prevention of troublesome use of substances. We then turn to how religion and faith-based treatments affect addicted individuals. Next, we discuss the effectiveness of spiritual self-help organizations as initiators and supporters of recovery from addiction. We close by abstracting principles from the research base that might inform efforts to alleviate troublesome use of substances.

Introduction and Background

Definitions

We adopt a definition of *religion* widely used in theological studies: a religion is an organization that comprises a set of cumulative traditions (e.g., rituals, scriptures, physical structures) and a set of beliefs about some transcendent reality in which its participants have faith. Defining the overused term "spiritual" is a challenge, because members of the addiction field and the general public employ it in myriad ways. Our definition of *spirituality*, a word that stems from a Latin root meaning "breath" or "wind," is an individual's personal sense of the sacred and its relationship to ultimate concerns, namely, the meaning of existence, morality, suffering, and death. Spirituality may be tied to or independent from a religious tradition.

What is the definition of *a spiritual mutual help organization*? Mutual help organizations are peer-led fellowships of individuals who share a problem or status (e.g., drug dependence, depression, diabetes, cancer). They are free of charge, do not have professional leaders, and should not be equated with treatment services. Members turn to each other for support, guidance, understanding, practical advice, and a sense of belonging. Every developed society has mutual help organizations (sometimes also called "self-help organizations") that focus on addictions. Many (but not all—e.g., Moderation Management, Vie Libre) of these organizations conceptualize recovery as an inherently spiritual process. The best-known examples in the United States are 12-step organizations such as Alcoholics Anonymous (AA). Spiritual mutual help organizations do not qualify as religions because they have no specific required beliefs in a transcendent reality (e.g., AA members can define "Higher Power" in any fashion, including in entirely material and prosaic terms). European mutual help associations such as Croix Bleue and Croix d'Or exist in the gray area between religious and spiritual organizations: they were founded by the Protestant and Catholic Churches, respectively, and make reference to Scripture, but they no longer require members to be affiliated with any particular faith tradition.

Religions and Their Views on Substance Use

The United States is the most religious country in the developed Western world, with most adults (92%) reporting affiliation with a religion. The most prevalent affiliations reported are Protestant (55%) and Catholic (28%), followed by Jewish (2%) and Muslim (2%; although this number is debated). Gallup Poll data show that about 95% of the U.S. population believe in God, about 90% believe in heaven, about 80% believe that God is still performing miracles today, about 35% report having personally experienced or witnessed a divine miracle, and a similar percentage report that God speaks to them directly. Over the past 25 years, an average of 40% of the population has responded affirmatively to a Gallup Poll question asking whether they have been "born again." U.S. religious beliefs and practices have been fairly stable in the past 15 years, but to the extent they have been changing it has been in the direction of greater religiosity.

Proscriptive and prescriptive tenets about substance use differ across and within religions. Christian denominations, for example, vary in their attitudes toward alcohol, from the traditional Catholic tolerance for moderate use of alcohol to the traditional Methodist endorsement of total abstinence. Islam repudiates all use of intoxicants. This prohibition comes directly from the Koran, where the prophet Mohammed describes the use of alcohol and other intoxicating substances as a sin. According to Islamic scholars, Islam holds that alcohol use causes social problems and interferes with prayer and remembrance of Allah. The Jewish religion emphasizes moderation in the use of alcohol. Wine is incorporated into some religious rituals, but intoxication is generally viewed as antithetical to one's religious practices, one's obligation to the community, and one's relationship with the divine (with the exception of certain Hasidic sects who see drinking at religious community celebrations as a *mitzvah*—a good deed—helping to awaken the light of God hidden within all things through joyful celebration). In spite of the aforementioned differences, all three of the major monotheistic religions emphasize the importance of maintaining the health of the body.

Spiritual Mutual Help Organizations and Their View on Substance Use

Worldwide membership in 12-step organizations is probably around 5–7 million people, with about half of those members residing in the

United States and Canada. Each 12-step organization endorses abstinence for the specific substance it addresses, but does not have a consistent position on whether abstinence from all substances is necessary
for recovery (e.g., Is an AA member who does not drink alcohol but
smokes cigarettes really in recovery?). Importantly, 12-step organizations by tradition take no official position on how the availability of
substances may affect substance use problems and engage in no activ-
ism to change laws or develop social policies related to the troublesome
use of substances.

Organizations like Croix Bleue and Croix d'Or are much smaller
than their 12-step cousins, and indeed have been losing members to
AA in some European countries. A rough estimate of their size extrap-
olated from the limited available data would be 25,000–50,000 members across Europe. Unlike 12-step organizations, Croix Bleue and
Croix d'Or live out temperance ideals, including making public statements on the importance of reducing the availability of alcohol and increasing the availability of alcohol treatment (note that membership in
these organizations is not anonymous). These organizations may have a
particular potent type of political clout because, like the temperance
movement, their membership includes nonaddicted family members
and other supporters who can enter the advocacy arena without the
stigma attached to being an alcoholic.

Social Science and Religious/Spiritual Organizations

Universities and research institutions are one of the few settings in U.S.
life where nonreligious people are often in the majority. Psychiatrists
and psychologists in particular are among the least religious groups in
the United States, and have been so for many decades. Religion may in
fact serve as a selection factor out of social science, as positive attitudes
toward psychology among undergraduates are correlated with negative
attitudes toward religion, and directors of psychology internship programs report on some surveys that they are less likely to accept highly
religious internship candidates. Negative views of religion are interwo-
ven into many influential social science theories, including Freud's psychoanalytic theory, Marx's analysis of class structure, and Ellis's rational–
emotional therapy.

Within social science disciplines that have an associated helping
profession (e.g., clinical psychology), guild issues may exacerbate negative attitudes about religion and mutual help groups. Clergy and mutual help organizations are sought out for help with mental health and
addiction problems at much greater frequency—and at much lower
financial cost—than are mental health professionals, which creates a
natural tension. Feelings of competitiveness sometimes surface in dis-

cussions of research evidence. For example, a study showing the effectiveness of a nonprofessional helper is likely to endure more criticism from professionals than is a study using the same method showing the effectiveness of a professional helper.

Many U.S. treatment professionals are enthusiastic about 12-step concepts and mutual help groups. However, this does not necessarily mean they are enthusiastic about the spiritual aspects of 12-step groups. For example, a study by Jon Morgenstern and Barbara McCrady found that professionals who considered themselves experts in the 12-step disease model rated spiritual change as unimportant in treatment.

This intellectual context may help explain, to use William Miller's turn of phrase, spirituality's role as the "silent dimension" of addiction social science. To be sure, the research base in this area is growing, but it is not large and may never be taken as seriously as would comparable evidence in other areas. It will also at times evoke strong negative reactions—for example, one prominent addiction researcher stated with commendable candor that the content of this chapter "made my skin crawl." Nonetheless, we believe the research base is advanced enough to merit an evenhanded appraisal of evidence that might inform prevention and intervention efforts.

Preventing the Development of Troublesome Substance Use

The Protective Effects of Religious Affiliation

In a research review chapter, Richard Gorsuch described the negative relationship between religiosity and heavy alcohol use as "major, strong and well-replicated." Ample research supports the same conclusion for other substances; the results that follow are more fully described in major reviews of the field. African American young adults who attend church are less than half as likely to use marijuana as nonattenders. In the National Comorbidity Survey's adolescent sample, personal religious devotion was associated with a 33–41% decrease in the likelihood of using marijuana, use of any contraband drugs, and substance dependence or abuse. In another study, spiritually minded youths were 150% less likely to use marijuana, 130% less likely to use alcohol, and 190% less likely to use hard drugs than their nonspiritually oriented peers. A review of the 40 studies on religiousness and delinquency published in criminology, sociology, and psychology journals between 1985 and 1997 reports that *all* studies that adopted reliable measures and/or multiple indicators showed an inverse relationship between delinquency and religiosity. These findings appear to hold true for adults as well. Adults who do not consider religious beliefs important are over 150% more likely to use alcohol and cigarettes, over 300% more likely to use an illicit drug other than marijuana, and over 600% more likely to use marijuana than adults who strongly believe that religion is important.

The relationship between religiosity and reduced risk for troublesome use of substances is not only large, it is also probably the best replicated relationship in the field that has important implications for primary prevention policy (e.g., it appears more important than education, income, or family structure). Some prevention programs also have impressive effect sizes, but public health impact is a function of effect size multiplied by scope, and no prevention program could ever hope to reach as many people as do organized religions.

Religion and Prevention Policy

Religion has exerted enormous influence on substance control policy. The temperance movement, which focused on public education and prevention, was actively supported by Christian denominations including Methodists, Presbyterians, Protestant Evangelicals, the Society of Friends, the Seventh-Day Baptists, the Universalists, and the Church of Latter-day Saints. This movement successfully limited alcohol's availability in many states before achieving national influence with Prohibition. Passage of the 18th Amendment, the so-called noble experiment that prohibited the manufacture, transport, or sale of alcoholic beverages in the United States, precipitously lowered population-level alcohol consumption and liver cirrhosis mortality. The movement's focus on abstinence from other intoxicants, including the opiates and cocaine freely sold as pharmaceutical cures throughout the 1800s, facilitated the passage of the federal Pure Food and Drug Act of 1906—the forerunner of the U.S. Food and Drug Administration.

An important feature of the temperance movement was the recognition that people with drinking problems needed help, and that helping them would benefit society as a whole. Although alcohol abuse was regarded as a moral vice, and the responsibility of the individual, such responsibility did not abnegate society's responsibility to "reclaim the drunkard." The realization that such reclamation was important, difficult, and required the support of the community created a cultural context in which many mutual help societies and other remedial environments flourished.

There are risks in incorporating religious/moral imperatives into substance control policy. Although Prohibition reduced alcohol consumption, it also promoted the development of a large underground market in alcohol and associated criminal activity. Furthermore, although recovery has a moral dimension (e.g., the recognition that ceasing substance abuse helps make one a better spouse, parent, and citizen), a common hazard of moralizing addiction is a resultant incorrect assumption that we can "punish the sin out of the offender." No scientific evidence supports the proposition that an effective social policy for promoting recovery from addiction should comprise belittling, shaming, and castigating addicted people; taking away their children and social benefits; and incarcerating them for extended periods. Such policies are usually ineffective, and in some cases may have paradoxical effects by alienating addicted people further, thereby giving them more incentive to bury themselves in their substance of choice.

> *No scientific evidence supports belittling, shaming, and castigating addicted people; taking away their children and social benefits; and incarcerating them for extended periods.*

Religious Organizations and Scientists as Prevention Partners

Religions affect adherents by preaching particular transcendent beliefs, and by offering a social context with powerful peer- and authority-based influences on behavior. Although the former are outside the purview of science (e.g., a scientific study can't and shouldn't try to tell us whether Dalai Lamas really are reincarnations of the Bodhisattva of Compassion), the latter are amenable to scientific study and are able to support the transmission of scientific information. For example, at the World Health Organization Meeting on Tobacco and Religion, numerous religious leaders took the position that tobacco use violated the sanctity of the human body. This is a religious statement, but for most of the history of the religions participating, the effects of tobacco on human health were not well understood. Indeed, many considered tobacco use healthful and therefore not a violation of the sanctity of the body. The documentation by modern medical science of the destructive effects of tobacco use on health has influenced what religions preach, and in so doing has spread a scientifically informed message to large numbers of people (even more than peruse some of our best journals!).

Although it has been insufficiently studied, preventive interventions developed by scientists might be effective in religious settings. For much of the U.S. population, religious and moral arguments are simply more persuasive than science- and health-based arguments. In turn, prevention programs in secular settings (e.g., public schools) may be able to learn from how religious organizations skillfully create a moral, caring, emotionally powerful community environment that decreases people's interest in using substances.

Spiritual Mutual Help Organizations and Prevention

Established addictions are the focus of almost all substance-related mutual help organizations, so their possible contribution to primary prevention is limited to the family members of addicted people. One noncontrolled study of adolescents with alcoholic parents showed that those who participated in Alateen mutual help groups had comparable psychological functioning to adolescents from nonalcoholic families, which may mean that membership in Alateen lowers the risk of developing alcoholism. However, that is a speculation based on a single, cross-sectional study. One might speculate also that family members and supporters of problem drinkers who join organizations like Croix Bleue might be less likely to develop an alcohol problem themselves, but we are aware of no data on this point.

Turning to secondary prevention, the only mutual help organizations to attempt early intervention with high-risk substance users have not been spiritually oriented (e.g., Moderation Management and Drinkwatchers). Why are there no spiritual mutual help organizations for nonaddicted heavy users? Substance use problems may be more likely to raise spiritual questions when individuals are severely affected, for example, when they feel helpless and out of control, have a brush with death or suffer grievous injury, or engage in behavior that grossly violates their moral values. Perhaps some people question their relationship with God when they score a 2 on the Alcohol Use Disorders Identification Test, but it is not a phenomenon we have observed.

Religious and Spiritual Treatments for Addiction

Does Religion Arrest Active Addiction?

Longitudinal research indicates that once an individual is actively alcoholic or drug-dependent, religious involvement per se is rarely sufficient to initiate recovery. A few cases of religiously inspired, sudden, and lasting remission have been documented, but they appear to be quite rare. As William James noted in *The Varieties of Religious Experience*, anecdotes about conversion experiences abound; however, there are barriers to integrating these anecdotes into scientifically based treatments. The low incidence of conversion creates a base rate problem that may preclude establishing empirical relationships. Even if these relationships between variables were determinable, there is no evidence that treatment facilities could "mandate miracles" for their clients. There are, however, a number of areas in which religion and spirituality have determinable, and demonstrated, effects.

Religious and Spiritual Treatment Evaluations

Having concluded that faith alone does not generally arrest addiction, we turn now to the question of "faith plus works," that is, Could religious activities and values facilitate an addicted patient's recovery if they were accompanied by a package of addiction treatment services in a faith-based program? Faith-based addiction treatment programs are sometimes stereotyped by their critics as not offering any real services—for example, all they do is try to "pray away addiction"—so it is worth noting that research does not support this view. For example, McCoy and colleagues found that Christian Evangelical addiction treatment programs offer psychosocial services similar to those in other parts of the public sector, and specifically renounce the idea that religious activity would reverse addiction on its own ("We don't believe in abra cadabra Christianity," as one respondent put it).

Research on the effectiveness of faith-based treatment programs is limited. Furthermore, some strong claims made about particular programs have not been subjected to careful empirical test. For example, in recent political debates about faith-based substance abuse treatment, an astonishing 80% success rate for the fundamentalist Christian program Teen Challenge has often been cited. Upon investigation, we found that this number actually refers to the success rate of the highly selected subset of individuals who completed this lengthy and demanding treatment program, which other reports indicate only 18% of entrants manage to do.

Starting with the criteria that a good outcome study has a longitudinal design, comparison groups, a high follow-up rate, and reliable and valid measures, we were able to identify three high-quality studies of spiritually oriented addiction treatment programs. The first was conducted by Rudolf Moos and colleagues, who compared a Salvation Army program for "skid row" alcoholics with a halfway house and a hospital-based program treating the same population. The Salvation Army program incorporated group therapy, job training, religious counseling, worship services, and AA meetings. After treatment, patients' alcohol consumption decreased 57% and their employment rate increased by 55%. These outcomes were similar to those attained in the comparison programs.

About 15 years after his Salvation Army study, Moos and one of us (KH) conducted a study of 1,774 addicted veterans treated either in 12-step-oriented treatment programs or in cognitive-behavioral-oriented programs. In the 12-step-oriented programs only, patients interacted extensively with chaplains, read the Bible, discussed God and spirituality, went to AA and other mutual help groups, and "worked" the first four AA steps. One year after treatment, abstinence rates were 28% higher in the five 12-step spiritually focused programs than in the five cognitive-behavioral programs; other substance use and psychiatric outcomes were comparable across programs.

Project MATCH, the largest randomized controlled trial of alcohol treatment ever conducted (with 1,726 patients), examined the efficacy of an Alcoholics Anonymous–oriented Twelve-step facilitation (TSF) treatment compared to cognitive-behavioral and motivational enhancement therapy. The TSF condition emphasized participating in AA and working the 12 steps. The outcomes for the TSF condition were as positive, and in some cases more so, than for the nonspiritual treatments. Outpatients in TSF were significantly more likely to remain continuously abstinent than outpatients in the other treatments (by a difference of 11 percentage points), and this effect persisted 3 years after treatment. TSF outcomes were particularly strong for severely dependent drinkers in aftercare programs, and for those aftercare patients who were in search of more meaningful lives. In short, like the other studies just described, Project MATCH showed that spiritually oriented treatments perform at least as well as treatment programs that have no religious or spiritual content.

Spiritually oriented treatments perform at least as well as treatment programs that have no religious or spiritual content.

Contributions of Religion and Spirituality to Treatment Outcomes

A number of findings in the addiction and health care field help to explain why religious patients might have particularly good outcomes in faith-based treatment programs. Most notably, shared values and language between counselor and patient help foster treatment retention, which in turn can foster good substance use-related outcomes. For many substance-dependent patients, faith is essential to the values and language they wish to share. Half of a sample of methadone patients reported that it would help "a lot" or "extremely" to have a treatment that addressed their spiritual or religious faith. In particular, participants felt that such treatment would help reduce their cravings for drugs, increase their motivation for reducing harm to self or others through unsafe practices such as having unsafe sex or sharing needles, and be "extremely helpful" in increasing their feelings of hopefulness. Of patients in an acute-care dually diagnosed inpatient unit, 97% reported belief in God, and 59% ranked God among the three most helpful factors in remaining drug-free. Sixty percent of patients in treatment ranked providing more faith-oriented treatment groups as either the first or second most important way to improve services. All of this indicates that religious patients may feel more comfortable in and may stay longer in religiously responsive treatment programs, which would help such patients on the path to recovery.

The literature on religion and health shows that religion and spirituality may help to maintain other health-promoting behaviors such as self-care, medical care, and adherence to treatment. Religious faith and spirituality is associated with positive mental health outcomes including increased positive coping, greater resilience, more hope for the future, greater perceived social support, and lower levels of anxiety. These mental and physical health outcomes may also have direct or indirect effects on the recovery process.

Religion and Spirituality Once Abstinence Is Initiated

Once abstinence from alcohol and drugs is initiated, religious involvement and recovery appear to have a synergistic relationship. At the very least, religious expression and spirituality may co-occur with recovery. Project MATCH, for example, found that religious/spiritual involvement increased after treatment and seemed to contribute to long-term abstinence.

Because pretreatment religious background and behaviors are associated with better outcomes and with greater spirituality after treatment, such findings might mean that recovery from addiction leads some individuals to return to the religion in which they were raised. According to a report by the National Center on Addiction and Substance Abuse, "the more affirming and positive one's childhood religion, the stronger one's spirituality in recovery."

Religious Organizations and Professionals as Partners in Treatment and Recovery

Given that African and Hispanic Americans are among the most religious populations in the United States, cultural competence training would seem a natural avenue for the largely secular members of the mental health professions to increase their understanding of their relatively religious addicted clients. *Cultural competence* refers to behaviors, attitudes, and policies that enable a program or provider to work effectively with culturally diverse clients and communities. There are multiple domains for increasing cultural competency including training staff, promoting workplace diversity, and collaborating with community health providers and organizations such as faith-based groups. In one study of 618 outpatient substance abuse treatment units, programs meeting other criteria for culturally competent treatment were also more likely to identify "achieving spiritual health" as a goal of treatment.

Even though cultural competence is officially endorsed as a goal by major professional associations (e.g., the American Psychological Association, the American Medical Association), cultural competency training typically provides little information on patients' religious or spiritual values. Indeed, only 10% of new PhDs in psychology report adequate training in this area, and these are primarily from religiously oriented programs such as those at Brigham Young University and Fuller Theological Seminary. What training there is typically fails to meet the basic standards for clinical training in other areas, for example, how to integrate client's spirituality and value traditions into clinical assessment, conduct effective interviews on these topics, define the limits of competence and professional ethics in this domain, and so on.

In parallel fashion, although churches, temples, and mosques provide naturalistic settings for access to treatment services, clergy seldom receive training in pastoral counseling for substance use. This is true even in African American churches in the southeastern United States, some of which are the primary providers of health and social services in their communities. Although 94% of clergy report that substance use is a major concern in their congregation, only 12.5% ever received any training on the topic, and few clergy report referring congregants to mental health professionals for addiction treatment.

Spiritual Mutual Help Groups as Initiators and Maintainers of Addiction Recovery

A large number of outcome studies of spiritually oriented mutual help organizations have been conducted in recent years. Selected 12-step organizations are the focus of this discussion because Croix Bleue and Croix d'Or do not appear to have been the subject of longitudinal evaluation.

Outcomes of Al-Anon Participation

Al-Anon, a large 12-step organization for family members (most often wives) of alcoholic people, has been studied in randomized trials as well as in matched comparison group studies. These studies collectively show that Al-Anon delivers essentially what it promises to members, namely, reduced anger, resentment, depression, and family conflict. Members often construe the process of achieving these outcomes in spiritual terms, as it involves accepting the limits of human control and being grateful for what good things one does have. Al-Anon, again true to its expressed intention, does not usually produce any change in the alcoholic's behavior, and in this sense may be less appealing to family members who desire that outcome, which is more readily produced by interventions such as behavioral marital therapy and community reinforcement approaches.

In addition, one study found that if an alcoholic husband is in AA, his odds of staying sober are about 50% better if his wife attends Al-Anon. This study requires replication, but does at least suggest that Al-Anon may influence the behavior of the alcoholic family member in the subset of cases where that individual is taking steps to recover.

Alcoholics Anonymous

To summarize an extremely large and complex research literature in a few sentences, the scientific evidence supporting AA's ability to reduce problem drinking is comparable to that for other ambulatory interventions. If the sole outcome of interest is abstinence, AA may well be the most effective ambulatory intervention for alcoholism. In contrast, one of the best outcome studies of AA showed that AA alone is not as effective as is inpatient treatment combined with AA, particularly for those alcoholic individuals who are also addicted to illegal drugs.

With regard to outcomes such as self-esteem, psychiatric symptoms, anxiety and depression symptoms, and the like, AA appears to have some benefit on average, but at a lower level than it has on drinking. The qualifier "on average" is important here because as the average benefit of an intervention gets smaller, it means the range of individual differences around that average are more likely to include people who do not benefit at all, or even get worse.

Finally, the effect of court-ordered AA has been the subject of two randomized trials, both of which are unfortunately of poor methodological quality and therefore hard to interpret. However, we would point out that court-ordered AA sounds more attractive to cash-strapped criminal justice systems than it often looks in practice, most notably in some districts where a literal busload of jailed alcoholics are dumped into AA meetings that may have only a handful of voluntary members present. This tends to result in a poor-quality AA meeting, which is punishment rather than rehabilitation for the prisoners as well as for the nonincarcerated people who voluntarily attend a community organization because they want to recover from alcoholism. A number of AA meetings have decided not to accept court-mandated individuals; because AA is a voluntary civic organization and not an arm of the state, they clearly have that right.

Cocaine Anonymous and Narcotics Anonymous

Research on drug-related 12-step groups is less advanced than research on alcohol-related groups, but early reports are encouraging. A number of large, nonrandomized, prospective studies of these groups have shown that participation in them predicts reduced anxiety, increased self-esteem, and reduced use of illicit drugs. Although spiritual change has not been the subject of many Narcotics Anonymous (NA) studies, one interesting report found that accepting a "Higher Power" did not lead, as some might believe, to failure to take responsibility for drug relapses.

Positive findings on NA/Cocaine Anonymous (CA) were originally generated in London, and have since been replicated in U.S. cities such as Detroit and Los Angeles. Those studies that have examined moderator effects of NA and CA have found similar impact on men and women, and on African Americans and Caucasians. All that said, the size and methodological quality of this literature must be augmented before researchers can draw conclusion about CA and NA with the same confidence as they can about AA.

Mediators of the Effects of 12-Step Groups on Substance Use

AA is the only 12-step organization whose mechanisms of change have been extensively examined. Among the mediators identified are increased self-efficacy, greater commitment to abstinence, greater acceptance of alcoholic identity, and increased abstinent-specific social support from friendship networks. Mediational pathways between AA involvement and outcomes are not mutually exclusive so it is possible that people might benefit from any number of these processes at different times and in different ways. Particularly apposite here are studies that link spiritual practices—broadly conceived—with better outcomes in AA. Put simply, those who engage in the most altruistic behaviors by spending more time helping others recover and doing other "12th-step work" are the most likely to achieve long-term sobriety in AA. In short, in AA it may be less spiritual beliefs than the living out of those beliefs in practical action that benefits members, which is probably what the organization's designers hoped.

Spiritual Outcomes of 12-Step Group Participation

The above discussion summarized the impact of 12-step organizations on what might be called "traditional clinical outcomes," for example, drinking, drug use, and psychological functioning. These are, of course, important changes in the lives of members, but in the present context the potential spiritual effects of 12-step groups also deserve comment. Spiritual change is conceptualized as central to recovery in AA's literature, reflecting the ideas of its founders, one of whom had a spiritual peak experience while in a detoxification ward. However, spiritual change is not universal among 12-step participants today, with anywhere from one-third to four-fifths of members reporting no significant changes in spirituality. Studies examining group members who attend regularly, using spirituality specific questionnaires and having stronger research designs, find higher rates of spiritual change.

Could 12-step groups serve as a productive substitute for religion for religiously alienated people or as an interim step on the pathway back to the religion in which addicted people were raised? The importance of this issue becomes clear if one recognizes the natural tension in the relationship between religions and addicted people of faith. Although being raised religious is probably the best protection against becoming addicted, once an addiction has taken hold people often feel alienated from and rejected by their religious traditions. Even addicted affiliates of less proscriptive faith traditions may feel ambivalent about their deity or religious community, that is, divided between their need for support and personal meaning and their fear of judgment. Just like policymakers and prevention professionals, religions (unlike mutual help organizations) are caught in the inherent conflict between prevention and treatment messages: when you tell children something is wrong over and over as a form of prevention, you inadvertently stigmatize those who were told but developed the problem anyway.

Project MATCH offers one of the few long-term empirical windows on this issue. Over a 10-year period, participants with sustained AA attendance after treatment showed increased "God consciousness" and religious practices (e.g., prayer). Such effects may be present across a range of faith traditions because the spirituality of 12-step organizations is flexible in interpretation. To wit, a cross-cultural study found that Israeli Jews addicted to heroin in Tel Aviv describe their spiritual life in 12-step groups in terms virtually indistinguishable from those used by alcoholic Christians in the midwestern United States.

Conclusions

Society has much to gain if scientists and other addiction professionals take religion and spirituality seriously. In terms of intervention, many addicted people tell us that their spiritual and religious values are important to their recovery. Religion and mutual help organizations clearly achieve a level of penetration in society far beyond that of an individual treatment or prevention program. If we can harness the power of these social forces to empirically supported prevention and treatment, we could develop truly novel and powerful pathways to reduce the suffering caused by troublesome use of substances. In terms of knowledge generation, behavioral scientists could, for example, ask scientific questions about the role of religion and spirituality in recovery from addiction or about the role of religious institutions in motivational health communication. Religious leaders may educate clergy in substance abuse treatment and delivery, and network with mental health providers to facilitate treatment access and service delivery. For these partnerships to form, certain prejudices must be overcome: scientists must be willing to ask scientific questions about the role of religion/spirituality in addiction and recovery, and religious leaders must value the scientific process and its rigorous humility.

Clarity in role definition may help surmount these prejudices. Science may be applied to any scientific subject matter, even, in the present case, the empirical phenomena of religious and spiritual human behavior. Yet scientific principles cannot be used to judge religious values and beliefs, as the scientific process restricts itself to the material world. Maintaining the integrity of these boundaries may permit scientists and religious/spiritual organizations to work together even while serving distinct social functions.

Robust Principles

1. Religious beliefs and practices are highly important to much of the U.S. population, including many people with substance use problems.
2. Mental health professionals are relatively nonreligious and may underestimate the importance of faith in their addicted clients' lives, as well as the strength of evidence supporting the protective effects of religious involvement.
3. Religious involvement greatly reduces risk for troublesome use of substances by children, adolescents, and adults.
4. Religious organizations may be potent vehicles for policy-oriented primary prevention efforts (e.g., laws reducing the availability of alcohol).
5. Scientifically sound substance use prevention information and religious organizations can coexist and enrich each other.
6. Spiritual mutual help organizations probably make only a modest contribution to primary and secondary prevention of substance use.

7. Religious involvement per se rarely alters the course of established addictions.
8. Many patients, particularly patients of color, express a desire for addiction treatment that incorporates their religious and spiritual values.
9. Faith-based substance use treatments appear to produce outcomes at least as impressive as comparison treatments that have no religious or spiritual content.
10. Health care provider training programs do a poor job of helping clinicians understand clients' religious beliefs and values; similarly, members of the clergy rarely receive training in substance use disorders.
11. Spiritually oriented mutual help groups such as AA promote abstinence from alcohol as well or better than any other ambulatory intervention. NA and CA participation appears to predict reduced drug consumption.
12. Spiritual and religious activities tend to increase in people who are successfully recovering from addiction, particularly those who are in AA.

Acknowledgments

Preparation of this chapter was supported by the Department of Veterans Affairs Health Services Research and Development Service and Mental Health Strategic Healthcare Group. Views expressed in this chapter do not necessarily reflect official policy positions of any of the funders.

Suggested Readings

Babor, T. F., & Del Boca, F. K. (2002). *Treatment matching in alcoholism*. Cambridge, UK: Cambridge University Press.

Gallup, G. (1995). Religion in America: Will the vitality of churches be the surprise of the next century? *The Public Perspective, 6*, 1–8.

Gorsuch, R. L. (1993). Assessing spiritual variables in Alcoholics Anonymous research. In B. S. McCrady & W. R. Miller (Eds.), *Research on Alcoholics Anonymous: Opportunities and alternatives* (pp. 301–318). Piscataway, NJ: Rutgers Center of Alcohol Studies.

Howard, D. L. (2003). Are the treatment goals of culturally competent outpatient substance abuse treatment units congruent with their client profile? *Journal of Substance Abuse Treatment, 24*(2), 103–113.

Humphreys, K. (2004). *Circles of recovery: Self-help organizations for addictions*. Cambridge, UK: Cambridge University Press.

Humphreys, K., & Moos, R. (2001). Can encouraging substance abuse patients to participate in self-help groups reduce demand for health care?: A quasi-experimental study. *Alcoholism: Clinical and Experimental Research, 25*(5), 711–716.

Johnson, B., Jang, S., Larson, D. B., & Li, S. D. (2001). Does adolescent religious commitment matter?: A reexamination of the effects of religiosity on delinquency. *Journal of Research in Crime and Delinquency, 38*(1), 22–44.

Johnson, B., Tompkins, R. B., & Webb, D. (2002). *Objective hope: Assessing the effectiveness of faith-based organizations: A review of the literature.* Philadelphia: Center for Research on Religion and Urban Civil Society, University of Pennsylvania.

McCoy, L. K., Hermos, J. A., Bokhour, B. G., & Frayne, S. M. (2004). Conceptual bases of Christian, faith-based substance abuse rehabilitation programs: Qualitative analysis of staff interviews. *Substance Abuse, 25*(3), 1–11.

Miller, W. R. (1999). Spirituality in professional training. In W. R. Miller (Ed.), *Integrating spirituality into treatment: Resources for practitioners* (pp. 253–263). Washington, DC: American Psychological Association.

Moos, R. H., Mehren, B., & Moos, B. (1978). Evaluation of a Salvation Army alcoholism treatment program. *Journal of Studies on Alcohol, 39*(7), 1267–1275.

Morgenstern, J., & McCrady, B. S. (1993). Cognitive processes and change in disease-model treatment. In B. S. McCrady & W. R. Miller (Eds.), *Research on Alcoholics Anonymous: Opportunities and alternatives* (pp. 153–166). New Brunswick, NJ: Rutgers Center of Alcohol Studies.

National Center on Addiction and Substance Abuse. (1998). *Religion plays key role in preventing teen drug, alcohol and tobacco use.* New York: Columbia University Press.

National Center on Addiction and Substance Abuse. (2001). *So help me God: Substance abuse, religion and spirituality.* New York: Columbia University Press.

White, W. L. (1998). *Slaying the dragon: The history of addiction treatment and recovery in America.* Bloomington, IL: Chestnut Health Systems.

CHAPTER 17

What We Need Is a System

Creating a Responsive and Effective Substance Abuse Treatment System

A. THOMAS MCLELLAN

While alcohol and drug abuse are readily acknowledged by the public as being partly or fully responsible for such serious public health and public safety problems as traffic accidents, street crime transmission of infectious diseases, child abuse and neglect, and excessive use of medical services, to name just the most prominent, it is also true that many segments of society are skeptical about the effectiveness of substance abuse treatments as a viable means of dealing with those "addiction-related" problems. Contemporary media portrayals of addiction treatment scoff at their methods and their effectiveness. Even a review by the *Wall Street Journal* questioned the effectiveness and value of substance abuse treatment, saying that "the success rate of treatment programs is highly uncertain."

Perhaps more importantly, there is substantial evidence that many of those for whom the treatment system was supposedly designed do not want to participate in it. Consider, for example, the reality that only a small fraction of those meeting criteria for substance dependence in this country seek treatment. Moreover, the great majority of those who do go to treatment have been pressured or forced into that treatment by their spouse, employer, the legal system, or the welfare system. Even with the threat of punishment hanging over their heads, the great majority of those who enter substance abuse treatments leave prematurely. Finally, more than half of those who complete the recommended duration of addiction treatment relapse to alcohol and drug use within 6 months following their discharge.

This broad indictment of the system is frustrating and puzzling given the facts that over the past two decades funding for addiction treatment research has more than doubled and with that funding has come many significant, basic, clinical accomplishments toward the better understanding, diagnosing, and treating of substance use disorders. Particular advances have been made in the areas of screening and diagnosis, development and testing of new medications, and creation and testing of new behavioral therapies. How can public skepticism be so pronounced at a time when scientific advances have been so significant? One reason may be that what we know about diagnosing and treating addiction from research may not have yet come into practice in contemporary treatment—the consequence of the so-called research-to-treatment gap that has been widely discussed in other areas of health care.

To explore this gap, the present chapter first reviews what has been learned from research studies investigating the major parameters of treatment such as length of treatment, the setting and modality under which treatment is provided, the role of the therapist who provides or coordinates treatment, and the role of various treatment components such as medications, therapies, and medical/social services. This type of review is important in that those aspects of care that have shown evidence of efficacy or effectiveness through scientific examination comprise the "evidence-based practices" recommended for broad use in the national treatment system.

The second section of the chapter reviews findings from recent studies of the national treatment system, specifically examining the capacity of that system to adopt these evidence-based practices. The results of this review do reveal a significant and disturbing gap between what is known to be effective and what is currently practiced—a gap so wide that it casts doubt on the viability of our current treatment system.

The chapter concludes with a summary of research-based findings that may be useful in efforts to create an attractive, accessible, efficient, and effective national treatment system.

Review of Findings from Research on Treatment Components

Prior to our review of research evidence on the effective components of treatment, it is important to differentiate three phases of treatment because they have distinctly different goals and may apply different methods. The three phases are detoxification/stabilization, rehabilitation, and continuing care.

1. The *detoxification and/or stabilization phase of treatment* is designed for people who experience frank withdrawal symptoms or significant physiological or emotional instability following a period of prolonged abuse of alcohol or drugs. True withdrawal occurs only from alcohol, opioid, or sedative/tranquilizer dependence, where a characteristic rebound physiological withdrawal syndrome is experienced usually around 8–30 hours following the last dose of the drug (depending upon the drug, dose, and period of use). While not considered subject to true physiological withdrawal, users of amphetamines and cocaine often also experience substantial emotional and physiological symptoms and sometimes require a period of stabilizing treatment.

The purpose of this phase of treatment is not to produce cure or lasting sobriety, but rather to prepare an unstable patient to do well in the subsequent rehabilitation phase of treatment. One of the major components of this phase of care is medications to relieve physiological and emotional symptoms and to reduce craving for the abused substance(s). These medications are typically accompanied by rest and motivational forms of therapy—usually in the context of a residential or hospital setting. On its own, detoxification is unlikely to be effective in helping patients achieve lasting recovery; this phase is better seen as a preparation for continued treatment aimed at maintaining abstinence and promoting rehabilitation.

2. *Rehabilitation* is appropriate for patients who are no longer suffering from the acute physiological or emotional effects of recent substance abuse. In turn, the goals of this phase of treatment are to prevent the patient's return to active substance abuse; to assist the patient in developing control over his or her urges to abuse drugs; and to help the patient regain or attain improved personal health and social functioning.

Professional opinions vary widely regarding the underlying reasons for the loss of control over alcohol and/or drug use typically seen in treated patients. In turn, there is an equally wide range of treatment strategies and treatment components designed to correct or ameliorate the hypothesized underlying problems and to provide continuing support for the targeted patient changes. Strategies have included such diverse elements as medications for psychiatric disorders; medications to relieve drug craving; substitution medications to attract and rehabilitate patients; group and individual counseling and therapy sessions to provide insight, guidance, and support for behavioral changes; and participation in peer-led, mutual support groups (e.g., Alcoholics Anonymous [AA], Narcotics Anonymous [NA]) to provide continued support for abstinence.

Short-term residential rehabilitation programs are typically delivered over 30–90 days; residential therapeutic community (TC) programs usually range from 3 months to 1 year; outpatient, abstinence-oriented counseling programs run from 30 to 120 days; and methadone maintenance programs can have an indefinite time period. Many of the more intensive forms of outpatient treatment (e.g., intensive outpatient and day hospital) begin with full or half-day sessions five or more times per week for approximately 1 month. As the rehabilitation progresses, the intensity of the treatment reduces to shorter sessions of 1–2 hours delivered twice per week and then tapers to once per week.

Regardless of the specific setting, modality, philosophy, or methods of rehabilitation, all forms of rehabilitation-oriented treatments for addiction have the following four goals: (a) to maintain physiological and emotional improvements initiated during detoxification/stabilization; (b) to enhance and sustain reductions in alcohol and drug use (most rehabilitation programs suggest a goal of complete abstinence); (c) to teach, model, and support behaviors that lead to improved personal health, improved social function, and reduced threats to public health and public safety; and (d) to teach and motivate behavioral and lifestyle changes that are incompatible with substance abuse.

3. *Continuing care* is the final stage of the substance abuse treatment process. It is appropriate for patients who have achieved the major goals of rehabilitation and is designed to provide continuing support for the behavioral changes achieved during detoxification and rehabilitation, as well as monitoring to detect early threats to relapse. All aftercare is delivered in outpatient settings, typically in tapering doses of group or individual counseling sessions (weekly to monthly) over a period of approximately 1 year, typically in association with parallel activities in self-help groups. Continuing care is less formalized than earlier stages of substance abuse treatment and has only recently received research attention. Most of the medications, therapies, and services that have been applied and studied in the rehabilitation phase of treatment are also applied in the aftercare phase of treatment, but telephone and even Internet forms of continuing care and monitoring are under investigation.

In the text that follows, we focus on the research findings from studies of rehabilitation rather than those that address detoxification or aftercare. Without demeaning the importance of the other two phases of treatment, we have elected to concentrate this review on the rehabilitation phase of treatment because of its traditional importance in initiating behavioral change and because of the far greater body of research on this phase of care.

Treatment Setting

A large number of studies have investigated potential differences in outcome between various forms of inpatient and outpatient treatment in the treatment of both alcohol and drug dependence. For example, there have been more than 30 studies in which alcohol- or drug-dependent patients have been randomly assigned to an equal length (usually 30–60 days) of some form of residential or inpatient treatment, or to some form of outpatient or day hospital treatment. While virtually all of these studies have shown significant improvements in substance use from admission to posttreatment outcome (usually 6–12 months postdischarge), it has been surprising to many that the great majority of these studies have shown essentially no significant differences in effectiveness between different settings of care, in either alcohol- or drug-dependent patient groups.

This body of research suggests that across a range of study designs and patient populations, there appears to be no significant advantage provided by inpatient or residential care over traditional outpatient care in the rehabilitation of alcohol or drug dependence—despite the substantial difference in costs (usually 10-fold cost difference). It should be noted, however, that in virtually every study of treatment setting, premature dropout was significantly higher in the outpatient condition than in the inpatient condition. While this is pertinent to the relative attractiveness of these two settings of care, it is not relevant to the relative effectiveness comparisons because most studies examined both intent-to-treat and fully treated groups, finding no evidence of differential effectiveness.

Of course, these findings were widely cited over the past two decades by those charged with reducing costs of care. In the absence of a significant difference in outcome, both public and private health care purchasers and managed care organizations reduced funding for residential care. In turn, the rush to reduce costs by essentially eliminating admission to inpatient or residential care led to serious attempts to formalize clinical decision processes regarding criteria for admission to inpatient and outpatient settings of care. The American Society of Addiction Medicine (ASAM) developed and tested a set of these decision criteria (ASAM Criteria) through a retrospective comparison of patients who had been randomly assigned to either inpatient or outpatient care. It was reasoned that if the ASAM Criteria were important and valid, then there should be significant differences in the 6-month outcomes of those whose admission was and was not consonant with the recommendation based upon the ASAM Criteria. In fact, several such studies have shown greater program retention and better posttreatment improvements among those whose placement was consonant with the ASAM Criteria.

Length of Treatment/Compliance with Treatment

Virtually all naturalistic field studies of alcohol or drug abuse treatment have shown that patients who voluntarily stay in treatment longer and/or attend the most treatment sessions have the best posttreatment outcomes. Specifically, there has been the suggestion based on the examination of outcomes from these naturalistic studies that outpatient treatments of less than 90 days are more likely to result in early return to drug use and generally poorer response than treatments of longer than 90 days duration. Despite the commonsense appeal of this finding, the meaning of the relationship is still ambiguous. Clearly, one possibility is that patients who enter treatment gradually acquire new motivation, skills, attitudes, knowledge, and supports over the course of their stay in treatment; that those who stay longer acquire more of these favorable attributes and qualities; and that the gradual acquisition of these qualities or services is the reason for the favorable outcomes. A less attractive but equally plausible possibility is that "better motivated and better adjusted patients" come into treatment ready and able to change; that the decisions they made to "change their lives" were made in advance of their admission; and that because of this greater motivation and "treatment readiness" they are likely to stay longer in treatment and to do more of what is recommended. There are several experimental studies where patients were assigned to different lengths of treatment and invariably there were no differences in their posttreatment outcome.

Participation in Alcoholics Anonymous and Other Peer Support Forms of Treatment

While there has always been consensual validation for the value of Alcoholics Anonymous (AA) and other peer support forms of treatment, the past few years has witnessed new evidence showing that patients who participate in AA, Narcotics Anonymous (NA), or other forms of peer support group, who have a sponsor, and who participate in the fellowship activities have much better abstinence records than patients who have received rehabilitation treatments but have not continued in peer support groups. There are over a dozen studies of AA participation and virtually all have shown that participation in posttreatment self-help groups is related to better outcome among cocaine- or alcohol-dependent individuals. Often this relationship pertains regardless of the type of treatment that was received prior to the AA participation.

It is important to note that in contemporary substance abuse treatment, AA has become synonymous with continuing care. Virtually all alcohol dependence rehabilitation programs and most cocaine dependence rehabilitation programs refer patients to AA programs with instructions to get a sponsor, to "share and chair" at meetings, and to attend 90 meetings in 90 days as a continued commitment to sobriety. Research studies done to date have generally suggested that while only about 25% of those who try one meeting of AA go on to active participation (e.g., attend 90 meetings, acquire a sponsor), for those who do attend there is every indication that this peer support component of rehabilitation is valuable for maintaining rehabilitation.

The Therapist or Counselor

Research suggests that particular characteristics of drug or alcohol abuse counselors can make an important contribution to the engagement and participation of the patient in treatment and to his or her posttreatment outcome. Within every setting and modality of care, there have been studies where patients have been randomly assigned to receive or not receive counseling as part of their care. In almost all of these studies patients who received counseling (even those who initially did not want it) had better treatment and posttreatment outcomes. Moreover, in field studies of those who attended counseling, those who had greater frequency of both group and individual counseling sessions typically had lower rates of relapse. Once again, however, it is difficult to determine whether the counseling was responsible for the improved outcomes or whether those with greater potential for better outcomes were more likely to self-select greater participation in treatment. In this regard, it is noteworthy that the relationships shown between more counseling and lower likelihood of relapse were seen even among patients who completed treatment—that is, among those having approximately the same length of stay in the programs. Thus, it may be that beyond the simple effects of attending a program, greater involvement in counseling activities is important to improved outcomes.

There are many important questions remaining to be answered in this area. While there is clear evidence that patients who meet with a counselor during treatment have better outcomes than those who have no counselor, and that there are significant differences in outcome for patients treated by different counselors, there is little indication regarding which types of qualities (e.g., personal, educational, philosophical) are important in determining who should and should not be a counselor or whether a particular counselor is likely to have good or bad outcomes with assigned patients. It is important to note that these relationships have been examined primarily for individual therapy and counseling; it is not known whether these relationships will be shown in group therapy settings.

Though it is relatively clear that therapists and counselors differ considerably in the extent to which they are able to help their patients achieve positive outcomes, it is less clear what distinguishes more effective from less effective therapists. One important variable is therapist style. Specifically, research has shown that a client-centered approach emphasizing reflective listening is more effective than a confrontational approach. It should be noted that there are a variety of certification programs for counselors (Committee on Addiction Rehabilitation [CARF] and Certified Addictions Counselor [CAC]), as well as for other professions treating substance-dependent patients (American Society of Addiction Medicine; American Academy of Psychiatrists in Addiction; recent added certification for psychologists through the American Psychological Association). These added qualification certificates are offered throughout the country, usually by professional organizations. While the efforts of these professional organizations to bring needed training and proficiency to the treatment of addicted persons are commendable, there are no published studies validating whether patients treated by "certified" addictions counselors, physicians, or psychologists have better outcomes than patients treated by noncertified individuals. This is a significant gap in the existing literature. Results from such studies would be quite important for the licensing efforts and health policy decisions of many states and health care organizations.

Medications

Great progress has been made in the development of new medications and in the application of existing medications for the treatment of particular conditions associated with substance dependence and for particular types of substance-dependent patients. A review of the now more than 200 randomly controlled trials of various types of addiction treatments is beyond the scope of this chapter. Here we present a brief overview of the most widely used medications.

Medications for Opioid Addiction

Agonist medications are prescribed acutely as part of an opioid detoxification protocol or chronically in a "maintenance" regimen (to reduce drug craving, maximize the patient's tolerance, and eliminate the effects of lower potency "street" opiates). Methadone has been used effectively as a maintenance medication because of its slow onset of action and long half-life. Twenty years of studies on the effectiveness of methadone were validated by a panel of impartial physicians and scientists in a National Institutes of Health consensus conference that confirmed major reductions in opiate use, crime, and the spread of infectious diseases associated with methadone maintenance.

A partial agonist, buprenorphine, was approved in 2002 by the U.S. Food and Drug Administration (FDA) for treatment of opioid dependence in general practice settings. Buprenorphine is administered sublingually and is effective in reducing opiate craving for 24–36 hours). The partial agonist actions of buprenorphine has advantages over methadone, such as few or no withdrawal symptoms upon discontinuation and lower risk of overdose even if combined with other opiates.

Opioid receptor antagonists such as naltrexone produce neither euphoria nor dysphoria when prescribed to abstinent opiate addicts. They have been on the market since 1984. Naltrexone is orally administered and blocks opioid effects through competitive binding for 48–72 hours. Like methadone, naltrexone is a maintenance medication but compliance has been generally poor, with most field studies showing retention rates of less than 20%. It may be most useful, therefore, in selected populations, when combined with social, employment, or criminal justice sanctions to increase compliance. For example, naltrexone has been used effectively in the monitored treatment of physicians, lawyers, nurses, and other professionals where maintaining a license to practice is contingent upon maintaining abstinence, and in opioid-dependent federal probationers who were under the threat of reincarceration if they returned to opioid use.

Medications for Alcohol Dependence

Disulfiram (trade name Antabuse) has been used in the treatment of alcohol dependence for three decades. It produces vomiting, facial flushing, and headaches following a drink of alcohol. Because of the severity of these effects disulfiram has been used with only a relatively select group of well-supervised patients.

In 1999, the opiate antagonist naltrexone was approved by the FDA for reducing drinking among alcohol-dependent patients. It blocks alcohol-mediated stimulation of endogenous opioids, thus blunting some of alcohol's "high" effects. Naltrexone also has some side effects (nausea, headaches) in a minority of patients but will not produce unpleasant physiological effects if alcohol is drunk. In 2004 a new alcohol-blocking agent called acamprosate was approved by the FDA to block craving and return to alcohol abuse. While acamprosate acts on different receptors than naltrexone, the clinical results are remarkably similar. Alcohol-dependent patients who take either medication have shown significantly lower relapse rates than those randomly assigned to placebo.

Medications for Stimulant Dependence

Over the past 10 years many medications have been tried in the treatment of cocaine and/or other stimulant dependence. Most agents tested have not shown benefit compared with placebo. One exception is disulfiram, the medication traditionally used in the treatment of alcohol dependence. It was initially thought that the reduction of cocaine use seem among those prescribed disulfiram was an indirect effect of reduced alcohol drinking. More recent evidence now suggests that disulfiram has an independent, direct, and significant effect on cocaine use. Research continues in this important area.

A General Note Regarding Medications

While the use of opiate and alcohol antagonists or blocking agents is increasing as addiction medicine physicians become more comfortable in prescribing adjunctive medications and as more substance dependence is treated by physicians in office settings, there are still relatively few patients who receive or physicians who prescribe medications. The responsible and appropriate use of medications in the treatment of substance dependence disorders may be among the most important topics for future research in the treatment field. There is a need for long-term studies of patients who have been prescribed these medications, as well as of the most appropriate and efficient mix of psychosocial and pharmacological services to maximize the effects of rehabilitation for various types of substance-dependent patients.

Provision of Specialized Services

The majority of patients admitted to substance abuse treatment have significant problems in one or more other areas of life function such as medical status, employment, family relations, and/or psychiatric function. The severity of these "addiction-related" problems generally is predictive of response during treatment, and also of posttreatment outcome. Studies have documented that strategies designed to direct and focus specialized services to these addiction-related problems can be applied in standard clinical settings and can be effective in improving the results of substance abuse treatment. For example, the addition of professional marital counseling, individual psychotherapy, and/or medical care have been shown in various randomized studies to produce significantly better outcomes than substance abuse treatment alone.

It is also true that the improved outcomes shown in most of these studies were seen in the personal health and social function domains and not typically in reduced relapse rates. Also, there are many studies where the addition of health and social services has not produced better outcomes. It appears that at least two conditions are required to show a significant difference: (1) the additional service components should be both needed and desired by the target group; and (2) the additional services should be delivered at an intensity and for a duration that is likely to be effective at reducing target problem symptoms.

Many investigators in this area have suggested that *both* potent and well-implemented addiction-focused interventions (e.g., drug counseling, aftercare, AA) and health- and social problem–focused services (e.g., drug-free housing, self-support skill training, psychiatric care) are necessary for effective treatment, but that neither one alone is sufficient.

Matching Patients and Treatments

The past two decades witnessed substantial research attempting to match patients with specific types, modalities, or settings of treatment. The approach to patient–treatment matching that has received the greatest attention from treatment researchers involves attempting to identify the characteristics of individual patients that predict the best response to different forms of treatment. Another approach to matching is to assess the nature and severity of patients' problems at intake and then to add specific, problem-focused treatment services to address those particular problems.

It is fair to say that neither approach has produced unambiguous findings. In general, there has not been much evidence to suggest that a particular setting, modality, or form of treatment is significantly better for any specific type of patient. There is better evidence to suggest that patients with particular constellations of health and/or medical problems benefit from specific forms of adjunct services targeted to those problems—but again, apparently only when the services are desirable to the target population and are provided in sufficient intensity and duration to effect improvement in the target problem area; and apparently only under conditions where there is concurrent treatment or counseling for the substance use disorder.

The primary limitation of the problem–services matching approach concerns the potential lack of resources in a time of health care cost containment. Funding is often not available for adjunctive services in areas such as medical care, employment help, housing aid, and psychiatric care. Also, not all services may be potent enough to make a significant impact on a target problem area. For example, despite the importance of employment-related problems in predicting treatment outcomes and despite the range of interventions that have been developed to improve employment and self-support among substance-dependent patients, there is little evidence that this type of specialized service is effective in improving the employment of the patients or in improving their abstinence from drugs.

A Review of the Contemporary Addiction Treatment System

The Specialty Sector Addiction Treatment System for Adults

The great majority of the settings and components of the substance abuse treatment previously described is provided by specialty sector programs funded primarily through federal state block grants, the U.S. Department of Veterans Affairs, Medicaid, private medical insurance, and other sources. Most of this care is "carved out" from general health plans and is provided by these specialty programs through a myriad of reimbursement arrangements. Indeed, substance abuse treatment may be the only area of medical care where there is *specialty care* without corresponding *primary care*. That is, substance abuse patients are very rarely referred to specialty care from a primary care physician (less than 2% of all substance abuse admissions); and almost none of those who complete specialty care addiction treatment are referred for continuing care management through their primary care physician.

Two sets of forces have combined to affect the national substance abuse treatment system over the past two decades. The wide recognition that alcohol and other drug abuse are associated with serious public health and public safety problems has led to increases in substance abuse treatment referrals from agencies that have been affected by addiction-related problems. For example, the criminal justice system accounts for 50–60% of all patients referred to substance abuse treatment, the welfare system and employers or employment organizations each account for about 15% of referrals, and mental health and infectious disease clinics combined account for an additional 12% of referrals to the specialty sector system.

A second force that has affected the substance abuse treatment system has been the rising costs of health care over the past two decades. Because of these costs employers and government purchasers of health care have turned to managed care organizations to reduce those costs. While cost reduction and treatment streamlining efforts have affected all areas of health care, it is widely acknowledged that the addiction and mental health treatment systems have been disproportionately affected. For example, in 1990 there were over 16,000 substance abuse treatment facilities operating in the United States; approximately 55% of those were residential or inpatient hospitals, approximately 15% were methadone maintenance programs, and about 30% were outpatient programs. Figures from 2002 show a radical shift in substance abuse treatment: of 14,000 programs, only 10% were residential or inpatient hospitals, about 12% were methadone maintenance programs, and approximately 78% were abstinence-oriented outpatient programs. Thus, as an industry, the substance abuse treatment field is shrinking. Despite a widely perceived growth in the need for substance abuse treatment, there are fewer programs in operation and fewer patients in treatment today than there were in 1990.

Despite growth in need, there are fewer programs and fewer patients in treatment today than there were in 1990.

In addition to outright closure, administrative restructuring is also quite prevalent. About 20–30% of programs undergo some form of organizational takeover each year, leaving them under a different administrative structure—usually a mental health firm or agency. Perhaps because of this high level of reorganization, directors of these programs also change regularly. Less than half of program directors surveyed in a national sample had been in their jobs for even a year. This does not mean that they are new employees. Indeed, at least 80% of program directors had been working within their program prior to their appointment as director, usually in a clinical position. About 20% of those program directors had no college degree, half to two-thirds had bachelor's degrees, and about 20% had master's degrees. Less than 2% were physicians.

Beyond their administrative structure, it is important to note the nature of their staffs and the composition of their treatments as one indication of their readiness to adopt and ability to provide evidence-based treatments. The modal treatment program in the United States employs 6–10 counselors to treat an active caseload of 150–500 clients. Apart from counselors, there are very few other professional disciplines represented in most of these programs. For example, only about 50% of the nation's treatment programs have even a part-time physician on staff. If methadone maintenance programs are excluded from this group, the proportion drops to about 35%. In fact, only about 50% of U.S. addiction treatment programs even perform an on-site physical examination at intake. Outside of methadone programs, less than 15% of programs employ a nurse, and even fewer employ so much as a part-time social worker or psychologist. Annual turnover rates for these staff are in the 50% range—approximately the same as in the fast-food industry.

One of the significant burdens associated with working in this field is the "paperwork," starting with admission intake forms and continuing through the reporting of patient progress to the various referral agencies from which most patients have come. In this regard, there are few electronic aids that can reduce the burden of the paperwork or increase the information value from that effort. Again, national reviews reveal that about 20% of programs had no electronic information services of any type, e-mail, or even voice mail for their phone system. In contrast, approximately 30% of programs had access to well-developed clinical information systems and Internet services. The remaining 50% had some form of computerized administrative information system dedicated to billing or administrative record keeping, but these information services were typically only available to the administrative staff. Almost none of the treatment programs sampled had an integrated clinical information system for use by most of their treatment staff.

As might be expected from the staffing complement in these programs, the great majority of what goes on in treatment programs is some form of group counseling. Essentially all treatment programs in the United States employ group counseling, but only about 40% provide individual counseling. Typical types of groups include orientation groups (where patients introduce themselves and learn about group therapy), relapse prevention groups, and general drug education groups. While some reports focusing on national surveys of drug abuse treatment program directors have suggested that a wide range of services are available at the programs, most studies of patients in treatment reveal that very few patients actually receive medical or social services beyond general counseling.

Very few patients actually receive medical or social services beyond general counseling.

The Specialty Sector Addiction Treatment System for Adolescents

The situation is arguably worse for the specialty sector substance abuse treatment programs designed for adolescents. There are far fewer of these adolescent programs. They comprise only about 12% of all substance abuse treatment programs. Of course, additional adolescent-specific treatment slots would initially increase system capacity, and more evidence-based interventions by a properly trained and credentialed staff could improve treatment, but there are other fundamental problems associated with substance abuse treatment for adolescents.

Lack of Credentialed Staff

No state in the United States offers adolescent-specific provider certification and only five states require adolescent-specific knowledge for licensure. While the National Association of Alcoholism and Drug Abuse Counselors (NAADAC) offers competency-based credentials for counselors, there are no adolescent-specific knowledge requirements for any level of NAADAC certification. Since knowledge of adolescent development is of paramount importance in treating adolescents, it is reasonable to wonder whether the few staff who do treat adolescents are sufficiently skilled to do so.

Restricted Funding for Services

Approximately 4 million youth in this country do not have any form of health insurance. Many adolescents have insurance that does not cover behavioral health treatment, and many programs will not accept some of the insurance coverage that is available. For example, less than 50% of adolescent programs accept Medicaid, less than two-thirds accept private insurance, and less than two-thirds have a sliding fee scale.

Thus, while the national addiction treatment system for adults suffers from many flaws, the situation for adolescents is arguably much worse due to inadequate numbers of adolescent treatment programs, lack of insurance coverage, and insufficiently trained counselors.

Summary and Discussion

Our review of the research on treatment interventions (medications, therapies, and services) and the United States specialty sector designed to deliver those interventions suggests the following three points.

1. Research findings suggest there are many potent and efficacious treatments for alcohol, opioid, stimulant, and marijuana dependence. The treatment variables associated with better outcomes include: (a) longer periods of *outpatient* treatment; (b) reinforcement (via vouchers, removal of legal sanctions, etc.) contingent upon verifiable prosocial behaviors (e.g., negative urines, employment); (c) *individual* counseling; (d) proper medications (antiaddiction medications and medications for adjunctive psychiatric conditions); (e) supplemental social services for medical, psychiatric, and/or family problems; (f) participating in AA, some other mutual self-help group, or aftercare following treatment.

2. Research in this field is quite active. Findings from basic, clinical, and services research are converging on better understanding of the onset, course, and mechanisms for intervening against addiction. Thus more evidence-based interventions can be expected.

3. The substance abuse treatment infrastructure in this country is not capable of delivering these emerging "evidence-based practices." This situation is particularly worrisome within the addiction field because, unlike other areas of health care, there is no primary care for substance use disorders. Only the specialty sector programs provide any care for addiction. The number of these programs is inadequate and many are on the brink of closing. The clinical workforce is turning over at the same rate as that in the fast-food industry. Though very serious within the adult treatment sector, the situation is even worse within the adolescent treatment sector.

> *Unlike other areas of health care, there is no primary care for substance use disorders. The number of specialty programs is inadequate and many are at the brink of closing. The clinical workforce is turning over at the same rate as the fast-food industry.*

Thus our review suggests that the gap is widening between what we know can work in the treatment of addiction and what we are able to deliver. For substance-dependent patients to receive evidence-based care, and for the field to advance within the health care field, it is imperative that patients have access to proven forms of medication and psychosocial interventions. If this is not possible within the existing specialty sector, then this capability will have to be developed elsewhere. Indeed, the contemporary phenomenon of drug courts can be reasonably interpreted as the court system's abandonment of community-based addition treatment to create a form of care, reporting, and communicating that met its special needs for dealing with addiction-related crime problems.

Robust Principles

1. To be perceived as useful, effective, and worthwhile to the parts of society that now pay for addiction treatment, new addiction interventions will have to address the "addiction-related problems" that society finds so troubling.
   a. Reductions in social harms and medical costs.
   b. "Customer service."

2. To be perceived as useful and worthwhile to the affected individual, new addiction interventions will have to be perceived as attractive, easy to access, potent, rapid, and delivered at a price that is affordable.

3. To be perceived as an attractive opportunity to those who might be able to develop and deliver new addiction interventions, there will have to be greater financial rewards in the addiction intervention business.

Acknowledgments

This work was supported by ongoing National Institute on Drug Abuse Health Services Research grants and by an unrestricted grant from the Robert Wood Johnson Foundation to A. Thomas McLellan.

Suggested Readings

Addiction and addiction treatment. (1999, July 18). *Wall Street Journal*, p. A12.

Finkelstein, R., & Ramos, S. L. (Eds.). (2002). *Manual for primary care providers: Effectively caring for active substance users*. New York: New York Academy of Sciences Press.

Gastfrriend, D. R., & Mee-Lee, M. D. (2003). The ASAM Patient Placement Criteria: Context, concepts and continuing development. *Journal of Addictive Diseases, 38*, 136–141.

Humphreys, K., Wing, S., McCarty, D., Chappel, J., Gallant, L., Haberle, B., et al. (2004). Self-help organizations for alcohol and drug problems: Toward evidence-based practices and policies. *Journal of Substance Abuse Treatment, 26*(3), 151–159.

McLellan, A. T., & Meyers, K. (2004). Contemporary addiction treatment: A review of systems problems in the treatment of adults and adolescents with substance use disorders. *Biological Psychiatry, 28*, 345–361.

Moos, R. H. (2003). Addictive disorders in context: Principles and puzzles of effective treatment and recovery. *Psychology of Addictive Behaviors, 17*(1), 3–12.

National Academy of Sciences, Institute of Medicine. (2001). *Crossing the quality chasm: A new health system for the 21st century*. Washington, DC: National Academy Press.

O'Brien, C. P. (1996). Recent developments in the pharmacotherapy of substance abuse. *Journal of Consulting and Clinical Psychology, 64,* 677–686.

Prendergast, M. L., Podus, D., Chang, E., & Urada, D. (2002). The effectiveness of drug abuse treatment: A meta-analysis of comparison group studies. *Drug and Alcohol Dependence, 67*(1), 53–72.

Prendergast, M., Podus, D., & McCormack, K. (1998). Bibliography of literature reviews on drug treatment effectiveness. *Journal of Substance Abuse Treatment, 15*(3), 267–270.

Simpson, D. D. (2002). A conceptual framework for transferring research to practice. *Journal of Substance Abuse Treatment, 22*(4), 171–182.

CHAPTER 18

Drawing the Science Together

Ten Principles, Ten Recommendations

WILLIAM R. MILLER
KATHLEEN M. CARROLL

Suppose it were literally true that we had at our disposal the wealth of scientific knowledge represented in this volume, but had no organized system for addressing the troublesome use of substances. The first of these two conditions *is* true, of course. We do have available an impressive range and depth of science regarding the nature, causes, course, and resolution of drug problems.[1] That breadth of information is not often gathered together and synthesized, and certainly society has not adequately applied even a fraction of this science in practice. Yet the knowledge, the fruit of decades of scientific research funded by billions of taxpayer dollars, is there. Giving people and communities access to this science base is a primary purpose of this book.

What about the second proposition: Suppose that society had no organized system for addressing drug problems? In many respects, that is the actual state of affairs in the United States at present (see McLellan, Chapter 17, this volume). Cutbacks in funding for health

---

[1]As elsewhere in this book, we are using "drug problems" to describe the full range of personal and social difficulties that arise in relation to alcohol and other drug use, including but not limited to the current diagnostic categories of substance abuse and dependence.

and social services have been dismantling the minimal infrastructure that existed to care for people with drug problems. Rather than being integrated within a system of care, specialist programs tend to compete for survival. There is often little or no coordination among or between prevention and treatment efforts. Interventions are rarely even nominally based on scientific knowledge, and the concept of delivering evidence-supported prevention or treatment services is a relatively new and contentious standard of care. Other nations are experiencing similar disintegration of their substance abuse specialist care infrastructure, if ever they had one in the first place.

The challenge given to the authors of the preceding chapters pressed this issue still further. Suppose that we had no brand-name treatments, no addiction specialists, no programs intended to prevent or treat drug problems. Suppose we were literally starting from scratch, and were committed to using the available science to inform and guide efforts to address these problems. Where would we place our bets? What kinds of interventions would we design and implement based on the scientific knowledge base? Each author was charged to summarize what is known and to derive some general principles that can be asserted with reasonable confidence in his or her particular sector of addiction science.

This closing chapter posed the still more vexing task of drawing together the hard-won knowledge that is summarized in the preceding chapters, and considering its implications for practice. What follow are, of course, *our* own integration of and extrapolations from evidence-based principles. Other readers may derive different conclusions from the same knowledge base.[2] This is our best distillation of how current science could be applied to decrease the enormous suffering and social costs related to problematic drug use. We first offer 10 crosscutting principles derived from the wealth of scientific knowledge synthesized in the preceding chapters, then reflect on their implications with 10 recommendations for intervention.

Broad Principles of Drug Use and Problems

Principle 1. Drug Use Is Chosen Behavior

For half a century strong emphasis has been placed on external control in understanding and addressing drug problems, reflecting more gen-

---

[2]A compilation of the reflections of other participants in the conference that gave rise to this volume can be found at http://casaa.unm.edu/cactus.html.

eral trends in popular culture and psychology. Deterministic models of addiction have highlighted causal factors that override conscious control. Viewing affected individuals as incapable of rational choice, interventions have often featured external control elements including coercion, confrontation, institutionalization, breaking down defenses, and mandated treatment. Drug policy has emphasized and differentially funded costly law enforcement, incarceration, and supply-side interdiction, in spite of clear evidence of the ineffectiveness of these efforts and the availability of more cost-effective approaches.

One consistent theme that runs through the chapters of this volume is that drug use is behavior, chosen from among behavioral options. It is influenced by the same principles of learning and motivation that shape other human behavior. Even the aspects of drug use that become self-perpetuating (see Principle 3) are not unique, but are shared with other compulsive behavior patterns where no drug use is involved (e.g., pathological gambling, sexual compulsions, overeating). This willful-choice aspect of drug use has sometimes been denied or downplayed, perhaps in hopes of inspiring compassionate care rather than harsh and moralistic treatment of those affected. That society holds people personally responsible for drinking and drug use is abundantly clear in the legal penalties meted out to drunk drivers and illicit drug users. Impairment by alcohol or an illicit drug is more often an exacerbating rather than a mitigating factor in criminal offenses, and in the case of drunk driving is prima facie evidence of guilt. Public opinion and countermeasures have thus been based on the paradox that drug use (addiction, etc.) both is and is not a matter of personal choice.

The science of recovery from drug problems, as summarized in preceding chapters, gives intentional change a prominent role. Most people who recover from drug problems do so on their own, without formal treatment. The stages and processes of such "natural" change are indistinguishable from those that occur with treatment, and are common across the spectrum of problem severity. In this sense, effective interventions facilitate and perhaps speed natural change processes.

There is also evidence that change frequently involves a kind of "click," a decision, commitment, or turnabout. This is reflected both in popular concepts such as "hitting bottom," and in well-documented transformational turning points that are common among people who resolve drug problems. Personal commitment appears to be a final common pathway toward change in drug use (see Principle 4). Processes of intentional self-control have been extensively studied, and could be applied in interventions to prevent and treat drug problems.

In sum, there is every reason to treat the individual drug user as an active participant, a responsible choosing agent, and a collaborator in prevention and treatment interventions. Furthermore, there are myriad opportunities in society to trigger and promote self-change in drug use.

Principle 2. Drug Problems Emerge Gradually and Occur along a Continuum of Severity

No one sets out to become addicted to drugs. It happens gradually, beginning with initial experimentation, moving on to more frequent use, and so on. There is also no clear moment when a person "becomes" dependent or addicted. Instead, dependence emerges over time as the person's life becomes increasingly centered on drug use. The diagnostic criteria for classifying people with "drug abuse" and "drug dependence" represent arbitrary cut points along a gradual continuum. This means that, as with many other conditions, society needs to address a wide array of problem severity, and that interventions appropriate to one region of the continuum may be unhelpful or even counterproductive at another level of development. In general, it is easier to back out of drug use at earlier and less severe stages of problem development.

Principle 3. Once Well Established, Drug Problems Tend to Become Self-Perpetuating

A characteristic of addictive behaviors is that they take on a life of their own, they become "self-organizing" and robust, and once established they become surprisingly resistant to ordinary forces of persuasion, religion, punishment, and self-control. It can be challenging to destabilize such a self-organizing system. Yet addressing just one component of the system is often ineffective.

There are many routes by which problematic drug use can become a stable, self-perpetuating pattern. These are mirrored in part in the risk factors for drug problems (see Principle 7). For some, pharmacological effects are a primary driving force, so it is useful to understand what drug effects a person is seeking. For others, family factors and social networks may be central in establishing and maintaining drug use. This suggests it may be important to understand for each individual what is maintaining the pattern of drug use, and, more importantly, which components need to be addressed in order to produce stable change.

There are clear biological bases for how drug use can become self-perpetuating. Drug use temporarily gratifies basic human needs (e.g., to feel good, to feel better, to alter consciousness). Some drugs hijack the central reinforcement system of the brain by (1) artificially stimulating it and powerfully reinforcing drug use, (2) dysregulating and undermining natural reward systems, and (3) simultaneously evoking stress and aversive states likely to increase hunger for positive reinforcement. These drug effects in themselves can lead to a stable preference for drug use and displacement of natural sources of reinforcement.

One consistent theme is that an initial period of drug abstinence can be helpful in destabilizing dependent drug use. Sometimes such interruption of patterned use occurs as a consequence of drug use (e.g., though incarceration or hospitalization). Antagonist medications and differential reinforcement of nonuse have also been used to produce an initial period of abstinence.

Principle 4. Motivation is Central to Prevention and Intervention

There is abundant evidence that motivational factors (broadly defined) are central in understanding drug use, and also in preventing and reversing drug problems. Earlier onset and progression of use are related to the extent to which children expect positive outcomes, and inversely related to expectancies of negative outcomes of drug use.

Patterns of change also point to motivational factors. People who stop drug use on their own without formal treatment, when later asked how and why they did so, often refer to a choice or a decision point. Life events can instigate a change in drug use. Reduced use or abstinence can also be triggered by relatively brief interventions, the impact of which is hypothesized to be on client motivation for and commitment to change. Transtheoretical research points to a sequence of events or stages through which people pass, starting with increased concern or motivation for change, decisional consideration, commitment, planning, and taking action to change. The decision or commitment to change appears to represent a final common pathway through which change is instigated. Often, once personal commitment has emerged, the individual may require little additional help toward making change.

Taking action also predicts change. Better outcomes follow from attending more sessions or staying longer in treatment, going to more 12-step meetings, adhering to treatment advice, or faithfully taking one's medication. It appears that actively doing *something* toward change may be more important than the particular actions that are taken. The traditional wisdom that "It works if you work it" appears to be true of many different routes to change.

It is clear that motivation for change is malleable, responding to even brief interventions. The idea that there is nothing one can do until a person "hits bottom" is simply mistaken. Positive reinforcement, unilateral intervention through family members, and brief motivational counseling and advice have all been shown to instigate change in seemingly unmotivated individuals. There is no good reason to wait for the person snared in drug problems and dependence to get ready or motivated for change.

Principle 5. Drug Use Responds to Reinforcement

Positive reinforcement is a common theme in addiction science. Preferred drugs are powerful reinforcers, chosen from among available options. Even entrenched dependent drug use is highly responsive to immediate contingent reinforcement. Because stopping drug use simply eliminates one readily available source of positive reinforcement, long-term change typically involves finding competing reinforcers—in essence, developing a rewarding life that does not rely on drug use. A complexity here is that drug use tends to be associated with a foreshortening of time perspective, so that longer term delayed rewards are discounted in value. This is a normal phenomenon in adolescence (one possible reason why adolescence is a period of particular vulnerability to drug problems), as well as a trait on which adults differ. People who more steeply discount delayed rewards are at higher risk for drug use and problems; moreover, drug use exacerbates discounting. Some effective medications reduce the reward value of drug use, which can enhance the appeal of alternative reinforcers. Maintenance medications that successfully compete with preferred drug use offer reinforcement that is longer lasting but less intense than that obtained from drugs of abuse. Providing clear incentives for abstinence often yields rapid reductions in drug uses.

Principle 6. Drug Problems Do Not Occur in Isolation, but as Part of Behavior Clusters

It is well recognized that among adolescents, drug use represents just one part of a much larger cluster of problems such as poor school performance, precocious sexuality, mood problems (e.g., depression, anxiety), and antisocial behavior. The same is true of adults. Drug problems are linked to elevated rates of family discord, violence, health problems, unemployment, poverty and financial problems, homelessness, crime, injury, child behavior problems, child abuse and neglect, disability, and a host of psychological and mood problems. Most people presenting for treatment of substance use disorders have a cluster of life problems and one or more other diagnosable health or mental disorders. This also means that people with drug problems are overrepresented among the clients and patients of agencies that address health and social problems.

Relatedly, interventions that target a broader range of life functioning are more successful in resolving drug problems. Drug use occurs in a context of life problems, and abstinence is often well down on a client's list of priorities. If recovery is promoted by having a more generally rewarding life that does not rely on drug use for reinforcement, it makes little sense to focus solely on drug use in prevention and treatment programs.

Principle 7. There Are Identifiable and Modifiable Risk and Protective Factors for Problem Drug Use

Drug problems are not randomly distributed in the population. There are risk and protective factors that affect the initiation, progression, and maintenance of drug use. This means that it is possible to identify subgroups in society who are at higher risk for drug problems.

The first class that may come to mind are hereditary risk factors. It is clear that heredity contributes to risk for alcohol problems, and evidence is mounting for genetic predispositions for or against other drug use. The clearest of these have to do with the reward value of drugs. Some Asian groups inherit a metabolic abnormality that increases the aversive effects of alcohol, and thereby are at decreased risk for problem drinking. People who are relatively insensitive to the intoxicating and aversive effects of alcohol are at greater risk for alcohol dependence. Being able to "hold your liquor"—to use a drug with relative impunity to its adverse effects—is a risk factor rather than a blessing.

People with more access to nondrug positive reinforcement, stimulating environments, and stress-buffering resources are also at lower risk. One protective factor is having close, high-quality, positive relationships with people who are not themselves involved in drug use or problems. Also protective are social and other coping skills that increase access to reinforcement and modulate stress. Drug use is one response to stress, but also tends to exacerbate stress in the longer run. Escapist reasons for drug use and avoidant styles of coping are both associated with increased risk for drug involvement. Effective prevention and treatment approaches are often those that address coping skills and positive relationships.

Principle 8. Drug Problems Occur within a Family Context

Research also shows the influence of the family context in the prevalence, course, and resolution of drug problems. Parental drug use is,
of course, a risk factor for children's drug use, and is linked to a host
of family problems and more general risk factors. Parents impaired
by drug use are less likely to provide the kind of parenting that reduces their children's risk. Children of drug-impaired parents are, for
example, less likely to develop self-regulation skills, particularly if
parenting is disrupted before the child is age 6, a critical period for
learning self-control. This seems to be particularly true for children
with other developmental risk factors (e.g., difficult temperament or
attention-deficit/hyperactivity disorder). Domestic violence and child
abuse are greatly increased with parental alcohol and other drug
problems.

Conversely, there are protective aspects of family environments
that decrease risk for future drug problems. Factors that delay the first
use of alcohol, tobacco, or other drugs decrease risk. In general, the
later a child starts using these substances (if at all), the lower the risk of
progression. Parental disapproval of drug use is protective. An optimal
parenting style is one that is consistent, supportive, and authoritative
(moderately structured and midway between the extremes of permissive–neglectful and authoritarian–punitive). Parental monitoring of
children's whereabouts, activities, and friends is a particularly important factor. Family involvement in religion and other conventional activities is also a strong protective factor. In adolescence, these family
factors counterbalance the influence of peers. Children particularly
susceptible to adverse peer influence include those who are extroverted, present- (not future-) focused, have low self-esteem and low
grades, use avoidant coping styles, spend more time away from home
(e.g., in part-time work), and tend to be followers. Effective interventions with families have tended to focus on two factors in particular: (1)
strengthening family skills for positive communication and monitoring, and (2) building family reciprocity in exchanging and sharing positive reinforcement.

Principle 9. Drug Problems Are Affected by a Larger Social Context

Beyond the family, the individual's larger social context also strongly
influences the risk, severity, and chronicity of drug problems. There
are large regional differences in the prevalence of drug use and problems. Environments in which drugs are more readily available promote

use, whereas the availability of competing positive reinforcers and activities is protective.

Social modeling can promote or deter use. Cultures in which abstinence is normative and modeled, and in which drug use is stigmatized, tend to have much lower rates of drug use and drug-related problems. On the other hand, criminal sanctions for use are relatively ineffective in suppressing drug use, particularly once it is an established pattern.

Relatedly, norms about drug use have an important impact. Clear norms and modeling of moderation influence drinking rates. However, individuals may and often do misperceive behavioral norms. Youth who overestimate the percentage of peers who smoke or drink are more likely to do so themselves, and to start smoking or drinking at a younger age. Though usually representing a small minority, those who use drugs or drink heavily tend to have a disproportionate impact on peers. Adding one heavy drinker can increase the consumption rate at a table, whereas adding one moderate drinker has little effect. Norm correction—communicating actual behavioral norms for a peer group—can have a deterrent effect on use. Also important is the normative social meaning of drug use, which often has symbolic value. When consciousness-altering drugs become marketable commodities, advertising tends to normalize use and to associate it with attractive and symbolic outcomes.

Having a meaningful role in society is a protective factor, while the loss of a significant role increases risk of drug problems. Unemployment and divorce may precipitate or exacerbate problematic drug use. On the other hand, acquiring new role responsibilities (e.g., through marriage and parenthood) can displace drug use. Social isolation is both a promoter and a consequence of the progression of drug dependence, and social bonding with nonusers can be an antidote.

Principle 10. Relationship Matters

Finally, there is something therapeutic about certain relationships. It makes a difference, for example, who is delivering a treatment for drug problems. When randomly assigned, counselors' clients often differ widely in outcomes even if they are ostensibly delivering the same manual-guided treatment. Counselors who are higher in warmth and accurate empathy have clients who show greater improvement in drug use and problems. As early as the second session, clients' ratings of their working relationship with the counselor are predictive of treatment outcome. Motivation for change seems to emerge in the interpersonal interaction of counselor and client, even in relatively brief spans of counseling.

There is also evidence that randomly assigned clients of some counselors have significantly worse outcomes. Differences among caseload outcomes in drug treatment are sometimes attributable to outstandingly poor results for one particular therapist. A confrontational style that puts clients on the defensive appears to be countertherapeutic.

Implications for Intervention Social Policy

These 10 principles in turn suggest particular directions in designing programs, systems, and social policy to reduce drug use and associated suffering, societal harms and costs. We frame these as 10 broad recommendations for addressing drug problems in society.

Recommendation 1. Intervention Is Not a Specialist Problem but a Broad Social Responsibility That Should Be Shared by Many Public and Private Sectors

For a variety of reasons, the treatment of substance use disorders has been historically segregated into specialist programs, often distanced from mainstream health care services. Although there is widespread acknowledgment of substance dependence as a chronic condition (like hypertension or diabetes), it has not been treated as one. Rather than taking a long-term behavioral health management perspective, treatment has usually been delivered in acute episodes (e.g., 28 days, 12 sessions). These episodes (or patients) have been judged dichotomously as successes or failures based on the recurrence of symptoms after treatment has ended.

We recommend that screening, prevention, and intervention for substance use disorders should be integrated within mainstream health and social services, and more generally should be a shared responsibility among social institutions including schools, sports, employers, religions, and the judicial and correctional systems. This is not a problem to be understood or addressed in isolation.

Treating drug problems in segregated programs has had a range of unintended consequences. Whereas most health professions have long required graduate education, the minimum of even an undergraduate degree is a recent development in the licensure of drug treatment counselors, who are also among the lowest status and most poorly paid health professionals. Segregated specialist treatment has also served to dissuade mainstream health professionals likely to have access to the science base—such as physicians, social workers, and psychologists—from addressing drug problems, and absolved them of responsibility for doing so. Given the high rates of concomitant health, social, and psychological problems among drug-dependent people, treatment should be integrated as much as possible in one-stop health and social service settings that connect people with other services that they need. A further adverse consequence of specialist segregation has been continued stigmatization and an unwarranted mystique that has overemphasized the importance of acute treatment. As with other chronic health problems, the successful resolution of drug problems depends heavily on long-term behavioral self-management.

The same integration is warranted in prevention as well. The major modifiable risk and protective factors (e.g., employment, parental monitoring, and religious involvement) are not specific to drug problems, but influence a broad range of personal and social ills. The prevention of drug problems is therefore not an isolated endeavor, to be delivered through specialist programs targeting only drug use.

> *The major modifiable risk and protective factors are not specific to drug problems, but influence a broad range of personal and social ills.*

Relatedly, it is sensible for (and we think incumbent upon) systems concerned with population health and welfare to be taking the initiative in preventing and addressing drug problems. It is absurd to wait for people to be sufficiently impaired to present for (or be mandated to) specialist services. Mainstream health care has moved toward consistent screening and preventive services for the most common and costly health problems, which surely include those related to drug use. Certain social agents (e.g., child protective services) have social license to take initiative, to inquire, and to take prospective action without waiting for the permission of disaster. Police, schools, and clergy have historically had this kind of access, to make contact and raise concern. The family doctor is also such a time-honored confidant, who can inquire and raise concern as part of her or his normal role. Insurers can and should similarly take the initiative to ensure that drug problems do not fall through the cracks of health care. An instructive example is Humana's recently instituted program whereby higher risk members are assigned a "personal nurse" who checks in periodically by telephone to consult on health concerns and to enhance patient motivation for health behavior change.

There is a legitimate concern and some evidence that if merged into mainstream health and social services, drug problems will simply get lost in chaos and be given low priority. Care should be taken to ensure that this does not happen, and that drug problems receive the attention, services, and priority that are clearly warranted given their enormous impact on public health and welfare. If these are not protected, the system could easily move from bad to worse. The likelihood that effective changes in preventing and intervening with drug problems will reduce both suffering and costs justifies the protection and prioritization of these services.

Recommendation 2. Screen for and Address the Full Range of Drug Problems, and Not Just the Most Severe

A further unfortunate consequence of segregating specialist services has been to focus primary attention and resources on the most severe levels of drug problems and dependence. By the time people find their way into or are persuaded to enter specialist treatment, they have often experienced (and/or inflicted on others) substantial levels of suffering. Furthermore, traditional aspects of specialist treatment may deter less severely impaired people from receiving services (e.g., emphasis on accepting helplessness and identity as "alcoholic," necessity of lifelong abstinence).

Drug problem severity occurs along a smooth continuum, and diagnostic criteria (such as the current distinction between drug *abuse* and drug *dependence*) represent somewhat arbitrary cut points in symptom counts. Drug involvement typically develops through gradually increasing levels of use, consequences, dependence, and variety of drugs. In this sense, prevention and treatment are not distinct interventions, so societal response to drug problems should involve an integrated continuum of care that addresses the full range of problem development. The concept of stepped care is a sensible albeit still largely untested approach suggesting that when one level of care is insufficient, a more intensive level of intervention is warranted and likely to succeed.

Prevention and treatment are not distinct interventions, so societal response to drug problems should involve an integrated continuum of care.

A further argument for a menu and spectrum of services is to permit people to find levels and types of services that they find appropriate and attractive. Poor outcomes are likely to ensue when people's goals are mismatched to program goals. A reasonable and underutilized approach would be to offer brief motivational counseling as a first-line intervention, and then to offer more expensive and intensive services to those who do not respond to this brief intervention.

Recommendation 3. Understand Drug Use and Problems in a Larger Life Context, and Provide Comprehensive Care

Drug problems rarely occur in isolation. In both youth and adults they are typically part of a larger cluster of psychological, medical, family, and/or social problems. These other problems are not necessarily consequences of drug use, resolvable by abstinence. Some may be antecedent risk factors (e.g., child behavior problems, impulsivity, family conflict). Such concomitant problems often need to be addressed, which may or may not alter drug use.

The point is that people presenting with drug problems typically have a range of other problems as well. Often these are of greater concern to the person and to society (e.g., unemployment, crime, violence) than the drug use itself. Furthermore, because drug use may be just one component of a matrix of problems and issues, disrupting only one of those components is unlikely to disrupt this complex self-organizing system (see Bickel & Potenza, Chapter 2, this volume).

Several intervention implications follow from this reality of multiple, interconnected problems. One is that drug use should be understood and addressed in the context of larger personal and social issues. Professionals and systems that address drug problems should therefore be prepared also to screen and provide competent care for common concomitant concerns such as depression and family violence. Prominent among evidence-based treatment approaches for drug dependence are therapies that address broader life problems and skills. Specialist treatment for drug problems has too often focused just on suppressing drug use. Broader attention to clients' life and health problems is warranted. For each individual being treated for drug problems, questions should be asked: What other concerns are there in this person's life? What other problems are in the cluster? For drug-using parents, how are the children doing? Comprehensive care will address this broader range of concerns and connect the person with appropriate resources.

Similarly, prevention efforts should look beyond drug use, making use of scientific knowledge about modifiable risk and preventive factors. Because drug problems are not randomly distributed in the population, it is possible to identify particularly at-risk groups and families for early intervention. People with a family history of drug problems should be counseled that genes are not destiny, but also that greater caution is warranted in their own drug use. Prevention can emphasize connecting individuals and families to protective social systems and resources.

Recommendation 4. Look Beyond the Individual for the Causes of and Solutions to Drug Use and Problems

Many prior interventions for drug problems have been designed to address and to focus on personal pathology, implying that the locus of the problem is within the individual or family. This misses the reality that drug problems are part of a broader self-organizing social system, and the substantial impact of contextual, family, and societal factors in promoting or decreasing risky and harmful use of drugs. Social policy to address drug problems should significantly target societal influences on drug availability and demand.

The United States has particularly relied on judicial and correctional systems to combat drug use. Although criminal sanctions may deter initial use, incarceration is largely ineffective and sometimes counterproductive in suppressing established drug dependence. We support normal accountability and sanctions for offenses committed in relation to drug use, as well as the diversion of nonviolent offenders to evidence-based treatment rather than incarceration.

Because drugs with high abuse potential gratify basic human needs, a societal solution to drug problems is unlikely to be found in deprivation and punishment. Attempts to prevent people from using such drugs are ill-fated without providing access to alternative natural sources of positive reinforcement. Prevention and treatment efforts can address modifiable protective factors, connecting people with personal and social resources that diminish the need for what Aldous Huxley called "artificial paradises."

Recommendation 5. Enhancing Motivation for and Commitment to Change Should Be an Early Goal and Key Component of Intervention

Drug use is a choice from among alternatives. Prevention and treatment efforts should acknowledge and address this aspect of choice. Such efforts are essentially competing with an inherently reinforcing behavior. Change begins with motivation for change. "How to" interventions are unlikely to succeed in the absence of motivation.

This is clear from research on treatment. Brief motivational interventions often trigger change. Other effective strategies enhance positive reinforcement for nonuse, offer a substitution agonist medication, and enhance access to natural sources of positive reinforcement. All of these approaches in effect tip the balance of motivation away from problem drug use.

Prevention programs can also target motivation, promoting reinforcing alternatives and undermining common motivations for drug use. In a campus-wide prevention program at the University of New Mexico, self-regulation theory was used as a conceptual basis to construct an interlocking set of interventions to impact student motivation and choice regarding drug use, producing significant population changes relative to a control campus. Much is known about how to impact human motivation and commitment to change beyond simplistic advice to "just say no." This science can be used to craft effective intervention approaches.

Recommendation 6. Changing a Well-Established Pattern of Drug Use Usually Begins by Interrupting the Pattern to Produce an Initial Period of Abstinence

Once drug dependence is established, it becomes self-perpetuating. A period of interruption helps to destabilize this self-organizing patterns and to jump-start change. An initial period of abstinence can be fostered, for example, by contingent reinforcement, residential care, or medication. This is an important pathway out of dependence, as the longer abstinence continues, the more stable it becomes. A question, then, is how to help each individual to interrupt the cycle and experience a period of sobriety. Choice and motivation are important components of this, as external enforced abstinence tends to be less effective than periods of abstinence where the individual has choice. For example, the concept of "sobriety sampling" from the community reinforcement approach involves negotiating a specific period of time to try out abstinence. Contingency management approaches involve choosing abstinence in order to gain access to other reinforcers.

Recommendation 7. Enhance Positive Reinforcement for Nonuse and Enrich Access to Alternative Sources of Positive Reinforcement

Stopping drug use simply removes one source of reinforcement. It is predictable that if a person, family, or group does not have reliable alternative sources of positive reinforcement, drug use will continue to be an attractive choice. It makes sense, therefore, to organize prevention and treatment efforts around helping people to develop meaningful and rewarding lives. If a drug-free life is not fun and rewarding, it is unlikely to be stable.

People who have become drug-dependent are often cut off from other sources of reinforcement and social support for sobriety. A significant task for them is to establish or reestablish contact with social networks that favor sobriety, and to sample and gain access to nondrug sources of reinforcement. Fulfilling employment and a range of social role responsibilities can be important sources of reinforcement that are incompatible with drug problems. Connection or reconnection with spiritual/religious communities is another promising avenue. Involvement in 12-step groups is yet another reliable, free, and readily available source of social support for sobriety. In essence, the goal is to develop a rewarding drug-free life that competes successfully with the allure of the positive and negative reinforcement that drugs can provide.

Recommendation 8. Diminish the Rewarding Aspects of Drug Use

Conversely, it makes sense to reduce the reinforcing value of drug use. One effective means for doing so is through pharmacotherapies. Naltrexone, for example, effectively blocks mu opioid receptors and thereby removes the incentive for using drugs that act through these receptors. Naltrexone also appears to decrease the reinforcing value of alcohol. A partial agonist like buprenorphine occupies receptors while also providing more modest levels of the sought-after drug effect. Disulfiram provides an incentive to avoid drinking because it produces aversive illness when alcohol is consumed. These and other medications undermine the pharmacological incentives for drug taking by blocking, replacing, or offsetting drug effects. The principal problem in their therapeutic use has been medication compliance: people often refuse them, or discontinue use when they choose to use drugs. Longer acting and implantable preparations can partially address this problem.

Pharmacological reinforcement is only part of the picture. Drug use is exquisitely responsive to monetary and social reinforcement. Peers are obviously influential in norms and modeling regarding drug use. Families often fall into adaptive behavior patterns that inadvertently reinforce continuing drug use. In treating an individual, it is important to consider what reinforcement the person is receiving for drug use, beyond the pharmacological incentives of the drug itself. With proper support and coaching, families can learn to reinforce behavior incompatible with drug use, and most of the time can engage an initially unmotivated loved one in treatment. Conditions that protect people from the natural negative consequences of their own drug use can be removed. Prevention programs targeting a subgroup or community are also well advised to address factors that create positive incentives for drug use. Successful interventions are not those that make a person's life more miserable, but rather those that offer a more rewarding alternative.

Successful interventions are not those that make a person's life more miserable, but rather those that offer a more rewarding alternative.

Recommendation 9. Make Services Easily Accessible, Affordable, Welcoming, Helpful, Potent, Rapid, and Attractive

As the pervasiveness and longevity of drug problems in human history attest, people do that which is rewarding and attractive to them. In order to encourage people to make use of services that address drug problems, then, those services should be easy to access, affordable, welcoming, and perceived as helpful. Unfortunately, this has often not been the case for drug intervention services in the United States. Common obstacles include waiting lists, stigma, geographic inaccessibility, cost, restricted hours, and limited program goals that do not match the individual's priorities.

All of these obstacles can be addressed in redesigning service systems. Evening and weekend hours of service are particularly attractive for this population, as well as for families and those with daytime employment (stores that want to sell their wares don't usually close on evenings and weekends). Addressing drug problems within the context of existing accessible networks of health care and social services can decrease the stigma associated with specialist programs, with the further advantage of avoiding "not in my backyard" opposition to locating services in readily accessible areas. Financial barriers to help seeking can be removed by social commitment to funding of services on demand. Waiting lists are a substantial barrier that can also be removed. Given adequate funding, at least brief initial consultation can be made available with little or no delay, and often a little effective counseling can go a long way.

Intake systems should also be welcoming and attractive. Beyond waiting lists, it has been common to require people to go through several levels of screening, questioning, and assessment before even seeing a health care professional. Our recommendation is to begin professional consultation with the very first visit. This means seeing a health professional at the outset, and keeping questions in the initial consultation to the absolutely necessary minimum. Half an hour of listening, letting people tell their story and express their concerns and goals, is a good start before asking questions and completing the forms needed for administrative purposes.

Other aspects of attractiveness have to do with the mindset for services. Programs and health professionals are there to meet the needs of clients, not vice versa. The high rate of attrition in the earliest stages of treatment underscores the reality that people will not persist in seeking help when they perceive a mismatch with their own perceptions and priorities. Services should take into account, respect, and address the client's own goals, needs, priorities, and values. Offer a menu of alternative services and goals from which people can choose what best meets their needs and preferences. Express clearly that there is no one effective approach for all affected individuals and make a commitment to keep working with the person until you find what works and his or her goals are met. An unsuccessful outcome is a failure of treatment, not the person, and warrants trying a different approach.

Recommendation 10. Use Evidence-Based Approaches

Finally, concentrate prevention and treatment services on those approaches with the best evidence of efficacy. Although it is not yet established that implementing evidence-based practices will substantially improve outcomes, it is folly to persist in paying for interventions that are ineffective. Current services are replete with these. All treatment is not effective, and there are large differences in outcomes depending on the services provided. Some "prevention" programs have increased rather than decreased the drug use they were intended to address. Some forms of treatment are ineffective or harmful. It is long overdue for science, rather than opinion and ideology, to shape interventions for drug problems.

It is no simple matter to persuade clinicians to change established practices. Learning a new treatment approach requires more than reading a book or attending a workshop. Training that actually changes practice involves ongoing supervision and coaching, as well as support from administrative officials and funding sources. We believe that effective supervision cannot be done unless the supervisor observes (usually via audiotape) what practitioners are actually doing in practice behind closed doors. Learning a new complex skill rarely occurs without feedback on actual practice, yet certification or licensure on the basis of demonstrated competence in delivering interventions with proven effectiveness is absent in the current treatment system. Who would want to have surgery performed by a physician who had only read about the procedure, and not been trained to do it, let alone observed and supervised while actually doing it?

The person who has the most influence on changing services is often the one who hires new staff. It is far easier to hire people at the outset who have the requisite skills and will provide evidence-based services than to persuade and reeducate clinicians to change their practice behavior. Attention should also be given in hiring to the qualities of practitioners (e.g., accurate empathy, competence to deliver a range of evidence-based interventions) that are associated with better outcomes. One of the largest determinants of how clients will fare in treatment is the clinician to whom they are entrusted.

Better still is a system that monitors the ongoing outcome of services, providing timely, accurate, and reliable feedback to treatment providers, managers, and funding sources as well as to affected individuals and their families. "Evidence-based" treatment methods do not have the same effect in all programs or with all populations. Some systems have tied funding to demonstrated outcomes. When outcome goals are clearly specified, an individual, family, or institution can often find effective means to achieve them. Regular and timely feedback on outcome also provides a means whereby clinicians and systems can improve the effectiveness of their practice. It further serves to protect the public from staff, programs, or treatments with outstandingly poor outcomes.

As a closing piece of advice, we do not recommend ossifying practice into a list of "approved" evidence-based treatments. A central purpose of this book and the conference that led to it was to step back from current practices, and to ask what to do if we were starting over from the scientific practices and principles that have emerged from research to date. A short list of approved interventions would stifle creativity and limit services to the practices of the past. While interventions with a strong evidence base are a good starting point, a creative service system will also encourage innovation to accomplish specified goals and to monitor outcomes to know which practices do, in fact, promote the achievement of those goals.

Suggested Readings

Diaz, R. M., & Fruhauf, A. G. (1991). The origins and development of self-regulation: A developmental model on the risk for addictive behaviours. In N. Heather, W. R. Miller, & J. Greeley (Eds.), *Self-control and the addictive behaviours* (pp. 83–106). Sydney: Maxwell Macmillan.

Fletcher, A. M. (2001). *Sober for good: New solutions for drinking problems–Advice from those who have succeeded*. Boston: Houghton Mifflin.

Forcehimes, A. (2004). De profundis: Spiritual transformations in Alcoholics Anonymous. *Journal of Clinical Psychology, 60*, 503–517.

Glaser, F. B. (1993). Matchless?: Alcoholics Anonymous and the matching hypothesis. In B. S. McCrady & W. R. Miller (Eds.), *Research on Alcoholics Anonymous: Opportunities and alternatives* (pp. 379–395). New Brunswick, NJ: Rutgers Center of Alcohol Studies.

Glasser, W. (1998). *Choice theory: A new psychology of personal freedom*. New York: HarperCollins.

Huxley, A. (2004). *The doors of perception and Heaven and hell*. New York: Perennial Classics.

Meyers, R. J., & Smith, J. E. (1995). *Clinical guide to alcohol treatment: The community reinforcement approach*. New York: Guilford Press.

Miller, W. R., Toscova, R. T., Miller, J. H., & Sanchez, V. (2000). A theory-based motivational approach for reducing alcohol/drug problems in college. *Health Education and Behavior, 27*, 744–759.

Vuchinich, R. E., & Heather, N. (Eds.). (2003). *Choice, behavioural economics and addiction*. New York: Pergamon Press.

Index

AA (Alcoholics Anonymous), 258, 260, 270–271, 280–281
Abstinence/failure dichotomy, 213–215
Acamprosate, 75
Activation of brain stress systems, 37–38
Addiction
  biological contributions to, 47–48
  brain reward system in, 31–32, 36–37, 42–44
  characteristics of, 25
  dopamine and, 33–34, 245–246
  evolutionary contributions to, 9–12
  gamma-aminobutyric acid and, 35
  as impulse control disorder, 225–226
  as lifestyle, 209
  mechanism, singular, for, 8–9
  neuropharmacology of, 39–42
  stages of, 25–26
  "street culture" of, 213
  vulnerability to, 39–40, 48–49
ADHD (attention-deficit/hyperactivity disorder), 57
Adherence
  to change efforts, 143
  to pharmacotherapy, 251–252
  to treatment, 280
Admissions criteria, 212, 279–280
Adolescence
  comorbid disorders in, 127–131
  early use in, 84–85
  "GO!" and "STOP!" framework and, 49–50
  peer influences in, 104–105
  risk factors for substance abuse in, 57
  socialization of substance use and, 184–186
  treatment system for, review of, 288–289

Adoption studies, 66, 68–69
Agonist drug, 146, 241, 242–243
Al-Anon program, 139, 268–269
Alcohol
  as commodity, 208–209
  dopamine and, 33
  pharmacotherapy and, 243–246, 283–284
Alcoholics Anonymous (AA), 210, 258, 269, 270–271, 280–281
Alcohol-metabolizing genes, 71–72
Allele, 62–63
Allostatic view of neuropharmacology of addiction, 40–42
Ambivalence, 147
Animal models of drug abuse and dependence
  brain stimulation reward, 27–28
  craving, 30–31
  escalation of intake, 28–29
  intravenous drug self-administration, 27
  motivational effects of withdrawal, 29–30
  overview of, 25–27
  place preference, 28
Antagonist drug, 241
Anticonvulsants, 244
Antidepressants, 248
Antisocial personality disorder, 117
Assessment
  of adolescents with comorbid disorders, 127–128
  of motivation, 135
Association analyses, 67–68, 72–73
Atomoxetine (Strattera), 57–58

313

Attention and motivation for change,
145
Attention-deficit/hyperactivity disorder
(ADHD), 57, 100

Baclofen, 53, 55, 75, 248
Behavior
broad perspectives on, 6–7
drug problems as clusters of, 298–299
drug use as, 294–296
motivation inferred from, 136
Behavioral economics or behavioral
choice theory, 183
Behavioral therapies
background and overview of, 223–225
brief and motivational models, 227–
228
contingency management models,
228–229
dissemination of effective, 234–236
effectiveness of, 226–227
fundamental principles of, 225–226
for improving impulse control, 231–
232
pharmacotherapy and, 252–254
for reducing drive, 232–234
social learning, skills training, and
cognitive-behavioral models, 229–
230
social support, social network, and
family models, 230–231
Behavioral undercontrol, 99
Benzodiazepine treatment, 243–244
Bidirectional models of comorbidity,
121–122
Birth cohort effects, 107–108
Bonding, 184–185, 186, 187, 195
Brain
heredity and, 48–49
as modular system, 9–11
See also "GO!" and "STOP!" framework
Brain imaging, 50–58
Brain inhibitory system, 47
Brain reward system
in addiction, 31–32, 36–37, 42–44
deficits in, 226
"GO!" system and, 47
imaging and, 50–56
Brain stimulation reward, 27–28
Brain stress systems, activation of, 37–38
Brief intervention
efficacy of, 227–228
motivation and, 146, 148
natural change and, 92

Buprenorphine, 214, 247, 283
Bupropion, 242, 250

CACTUS discussions, 5, 6
Catchment area approach, 162
Certification programs for counselors,
282, 289
Change
family impact on, 173–174
influencing motivation for, 144–147
instigation to, 147–149
natural language and, 135–136, 138,
149
obstacles to, 141–142
predicting, 142–144
tasks and stages of, 83–84
See also Motivation; Natural change
Childhood psychopathology, 100
Choice aspect of drug use, 294–296
Chromosomes, 62
Chronic health problem, disorders as,
213–215
Clonidine, 242
Close relationships
adults and, 190–191
definition of, 166–167
reciprocal nature of, 169–170
remission, relapse, and, 191
robust principles of, 197–198
treatment models and, 230–231
youth and, 187–190
See also Family
Cocaine
brain response to stimulant and, 53–54
frontal regions of brain and, 56–57
low D dopamine receptors and, 51–52
Cocaine Anonymous, 270
Cognitive-behavioral models of
treatment, 229–230
Cognitive functioning, 101–102
Collaboration model, 125
College environment, 190
Committing language, 135–136, 138, 149
Commodity, alcohol or drug as, 208–209
Common factor models of comorbidity,
121
Community systems approach to
treatment, 161–164
Comorbidity
in adolescents, 127–131
in adults compared to youths, 128
bidirectional models of, 121–122
common factor models of, 121
consequences of, 116–117, 129

natural change and, 85–86
prevalence of, 116, 128–129
secondary psychopathology models of, 117–119
secondary substance abuse models of, 119–121
systemic approaches to, 122–127
Competence and interaction, 12–14
Complex trait, disease, or disorder, 66
Compliance. *See* Adherence
Concordance, 69
Conditioning, classical and operant, 225–226
Conduct disorder, 57, 100
Confrontation strategies, 145, 210–211
Consequences
of comorbid disorders, 116–117, 129
epidemiological data about differences in, 156–157
Consultation model, 125
Consumption, epidemiological data about differences in, 154–156
Contemplation stage, 140
Contingencies, social, for use, 142
Contingency management, 16, 228–229
Continuing care, 278, 281
Coping responses of family, 171
Corticotropin-releasing factor (CRF), 37–38
Counselor effects, 137–138, 148, 281–282, 301–302
Counteradaptation, 40–41
Couple therapy, 173–174
Craving, animal models of, 30–31
Criminalization, 211–212
Croix Bleue and Croix d'Or, 258, 260
Cue-induced reinstatement, 39
Cues for drug use, brain response to, 54–56
Cultural competence, 267–268
Culturally tailored compared to culturally specific interventions, 159

Delay discounting, 11–12
Dependence, characteristics of, 25
Depression, 118
Desipramine, 248
Detoxification/stabilization phase of treatment, 277
Developmental perspectives on risk
environmental factors, 103–106
general model of, 106–110
overview of, 97–98

personal factors, 98–102
social policy factors, 112–113
Deviance proneness model of risk, 106–107
Discounting curve, 11, 298
Disulfiram, 244, 248, 252, 283, 284
DNA, 62
Domestic violence, 103, 175
Dopamine
in addiction, 33–34
alcoholism and, 245–246
brain imaging studies and, 50–51
low D dopamine receptors, 51–53
stimulants and, 248
Dopaminergic "partial agonists," 55–56
Drive reduction, 232–234
Drug-induced reinstatement, 39
Drugs of abuse, brain response to, 53–54

Economics of treatment, 213
Elasticity of demand, 13
Emergent properties, 15–16
Empathy, accurate, 137–138
Endocannabinoids, 35–36
Endophenotype, 64
Engaged coping, 171
Enlightenment strategies, 144
Environment
genetic vulnerability and, 52, 65
risk factors in, 103–106
See also Gene–environment interaction study; Social contexts
Escalation of drug intake, 28–29
Ethnic differences
in consequences, 156–157
in consumption, 154–156
implications of, 160–164
Linkage studies, 66–67, 70–71
in onset of use, 85, 109–110
overview of, 153–154
in prevention effectiveness, 159–160
in treatment effectiveness, 157–158
Ethnographic approach
benefits of, 216–217
overview of, 201–205
political economy and, 215–216
prevention and treatment and, 210–215
symbolic mediation and, 205–209
Evolutionary contributions to addiction, 9–12
Expectancies, alcohol-related, 101
Extended amygdala, 38

False consensus effect, 140
Family
    in change process and treatment
        success, 173–174, 187
    definition of, 166–167
    in development and maintenance of
        disorders, 170–172, 300
    interaction in, 103–104
    motivation to change and, 172–173
    as protective factor, 170
    socialization of substance use in, 184–
        187
    as social system, 167–168
    violence in, 103, 175, 178
Family intervention
    effective preventive, 175–176
    motivation and, 139
Family involvement
    appropriateness of, 178–179
    in problem recognition and help
        seeking, 176–177
    in treatment, 177–178, 230–231
Family study, 66
Fieldwork in ethnographic research, 202
Five-factor model of personality, 99–100
Format of book, 4–5
Friends. See Close relationships; Peer
    influences
Frontal regions of brain, 56
Funding for treatment, 286, 289, 293–
    294

Gabapentin, 75
Gamma-aminobutyric acid (GABA)
    in addiction, 35
    baclofen and, 53
    benzodiazepines and, 243
    genetic association studies and, 73
    topiramate and, 246
Gateway hypothesis, 187
Geeking, 203
Gender
    consequences and, 156–157
    consumption and, 154–156
    implications of, 160–164
    natural change and, 85
    overview of, 153–154
    prevention effectiveness and, 159–160
    substance use patterns and, 108–109
    treatment effectiveness and, 157–158
Gene–environment interaction study, 68,
    111–112
General dysphoria theory, 119–120
Genetic association studies, 67–68, 72–73

Genetic factors
    environment and, 52
    ethnicity and, 109–110
    evidence for, 110–112
    vulnerability to addiction and, 39–40,
        48–49, 64, 97–98
Genotype, 63
Global context, 215–216
Goals, mismatch in, 210–211
"GO!" and "STOP!" framework
    adolescence and, 49–50
    brain imaging and, 50–58
    heredity and, 48–49
    overview of, 46–48
Guided self-change intervention, 92

Haya people, 206–207
Heredity, 48–49. See also Genetic factors
Hyperbolic curve, 11

Impulse control disorder, addiction as,
    225–226
Indirect agonist drug, 241
Inpatient treatment, 223–224, 279
Instigation to change, 147–149
Integrated treatment model, 123–124,
    125, 131
Interaction and competence, 12–14
Interpersonal motivation, 137–140
Intertemporal substitution, 13–14, 17, 18
Intervention system
    comprehensive care and, 304–305
    indictments of, 275–276
    review of, 4, 286–290, 293–294
    as shared responsibility, 302–304
    starting over from scratch to create, 3–
        4
    See also Treatment
Interviewing
    ethnographic, 211
    motivational, 138–139, 146
Intracranial self-stimulation (ICSS), 27–28
Intrapersonal motivation, 135–137
Intravenous drug self-administration, 27,
    28–29

Life course pattern, 82–83
Limbic system, 10
Linkage studies, 66–67, 70–71

Marijuana and pharmacotherapy, 249
Matching law, 17
Matching patient and treatment, 250,
    285–286

Mechanism, singular, for addiction, 8–9
Medications
    for ADHD, 57–58
    behavioral therapies and, 233
    dopamine-blocking, 52–53
    effective, and process of addiction, 20
    over-the-counter, 254
    to reduce brain response to drug cues,
        55–56
    See also Pharmacotherapy; *specific
        medications*
Memantine, 75
Mendelian trait or disease, 66
Mesocorticolimbic dopamine system, 32,
    33–34
Methadone, 246–247, 283
Minimal intervention, 92
Modeling
    influence of, 301
    intervention and treatment and, 196
    neighborhood, 193–194
    parental, 185
    peer, 188, 190
    school, 188–189
    spouse, 186–187
    work, 192
Modules, 10–11, 13, 14, 16
Monitoring, 184–185, 193, 194, 195
Mothers Against Drunk Driving, 145
Motivation
    allostatic model of, 41–42
    as contextual, 140–142
    enhancing, 306
    family factors in, 172–173
    importance of, 297–298
    influencing, 144–147
    as interpersonal, 137–140
    as intrapersonal, 135–137
    intrinsic vs. extrinsic, 93
    overview of, 134
    predicting change and, 142–144
Motivational effects of drug withdrawal,
    29–30
Motivational interviewing, 138–139, 146
Motivational models of treatment, 227–
    228
Multidimensional family therapy, 131
Multisystemic therapy, 131
Mu opioid receptor, 35, 40, 71

Naltrexone
    alcoholism and, 240, 244–245, 284
    cognitive-behavioral therapy and, 253–
        254

    description of, 74
    opiates and, 247–248, 251, 283
Narcotics Anonymous, 269–270, 280–281
Narrowing of behavioral repertoire, 17–
    18
Natural change
    onset of problematic use and, 84–86
    overview of, 81–83
    process of intentional behavior change
        and, 88–94
    substance abuse careers and, 86–88
Natural language and change, 135–136,
    138, 149
Needle-sharing myth, 203
Negative affectivity, 99
Negative reinforcement, 145
Neighborhoods, 193–195, 198
Neuroadaptation and allostasis, 41–42
Neurocognitive functioning, 226
Neuromodulator, definition of, 36
Neuropeptide Y (NPY), 38
Neuropharmacology
    of addiction, 39–42
    of intoxication, 31–36
    of motivational effects of dependence,
        36–38
    of relapse, 38–39
Neurotransmitters, genes and, 72–73
Nicotine, 33, 241–243, 254
Norms
    influence of, 301
    motivation and, 140–141
    of neighborhood, 193–194
    at school, 188–189
    at work, 192
Nortriptyline, 242

Ondansetron, 75
Onset of problematic use and natural
    change, 84–86
Opiates and pharmacotherapy, 246–248,
    283
Opioid peptides, 34–35
Opponent process theory, 40–41
Order for free process, 14–15
Origins of addiction, 9–12

Parallel or simultaneous model of
    treatment, 130–131
Parental monitoring, 185
Partial agonist drug, 55–56, 241, 242–
    243
Pattern, interrupting, 307
Peer cluster theory, 188

Peer influences
    adults and, 190–191
    intervention and treatment and, 196
    remission, relapse, and, 191
    robust principles of, 197–198
    youth and, 104–105, 187–190
Penetrance, incomplete, 65
Personality disorders, 117, 118–119
Personal risk factors, 98–102
Pharmacodynamics, 64–65
Pharmacogenetics, 74–76
Pharmacokinetics, 65
Pharmacotherapy
    adherence and, 251–252
    alcohol and, 243–246, 283–284
    behavioral therapies and, 233, 252–
        254
    combination, 249
    marijuana and, 249
    nicotine and, 241–243, 254
    opiates and, 246–248, 283
    patient–treatment matching, 250
    role of, 240–241
    stimulants and, 248–249, 284
    without long-term dependence, 250–251
    See also Medications;
        Neuropharmacology; specific
        medications
Phenocopy, 64
Phenotype, 63
Place aversion, 30
Place preference, 28
Political economics, 215–216
Polymorphism, 63
Positive reinforcement. See Reinforcement
Precontemplation stage, 140
Prevalence of comorbid disorders, 116,
    128–129
Prevention
    of adolescent substance disorders,
        129–130
    effectiveness of, 159
    family intervention and, 175–176
    motivation and, 297–298
    religion and, 262–263
    social contexts and, 195–196
    spiritual mutual help organizations
        and, 264
Probands, 71
Protective factors
    family as, 170, 300
    overview of, 299
    religious affiliation as, 261–262
Protective genetic effect, 63–64, 71–72

Proteins and genetic code, 62
Protocols, 13
Psychiatric disorders, comorbidity of
    bidirectional models of, 121–122
    common factor models of, 121
    prevalence and consequences of, 115–
        117
    secondary psychopathology models of,
        117–119
    secondary substance abuse models of,
        119–121
    systemic approaches to, 122–127
Psychoactive substances
    as commodities, 208–209
    as symbolic mediators, 206–208
    use of, 205–206
Public health and safety approach to
    treatment, 161–164
Punishment, 145

Quadrant model, 124–126
Quality of counseling relationship, 143,
    301–302
Quantitative flexibility, 10–11
Questions
    about addiction, 8, 18–19
    in field of neurobiology of addiction,
        42–43

Racial differences
    in consequences, 156–157
    in consumption, 154–156
    implications of, 160–164
    overview of, 153–154
    in prevention effectiveness, 159–160
    in treatment effectiveness, 157–158
Recovery, 262–263, 268–272. See also
        Natural change
Rehabilitation, 277–278
Reinforcement, 20, 146–147, 298, 307
Relapse
    contact with using friends and, 174
    factors in, 30–31
    friends, peer groups, and, 191
    neuropharmacology of, 39
Religion
    abstinence and, 267
    cultural competence training and,
        267–268
    importance of, 271–272
    overview of, 257–258
    prevention policy and, 262–263
    protective effects of, 261–262
    social science and, 260–261

in treatment, 264–268
treatment outcome and, 266–267
view of substance use, 259
Rewarding aspects of drug use,
    diminishing, 308
Risk factors
    ADHD and conduct disorder as, 57,
        100
    environmental, 103–106
    overview of, 299
    personal, 98–102
Robust principles
    of behavioral interventions, 236–237
    of brain imaging studies, 58–59
    of comorbid disorders, 132
    description of, 4–5
    in developmental perspectives, 113
    of ethnographic approach, 217–218
    of family involvement, 179–180
    of genetics, 76
    intervention system and, 290–291
    of motivation, 149–150
    of natural change, 94–95
    of neurobiology of addiction, 44
    of pharmacotherapy, 254–255
    regarding racial/ethnic/gender
        differences, 164
    of religion and spirituality, 272–273
    self-organizing system and, 19–20
    of social contexts, 196–199
Role transitions, 186

Schizophrenia, 117–118
School norms, 189
Science-based principles, 5
Screening issues, 304
Secondary psychopathology models of
    comorbidity, 117–119
Secondary psychosocial effects model,
    120–121
Secondary substance abuse models of
    comorbidity, 119–121
Secular trends, 107–108
Selected readings, 5
Selective serotonin reuptake inhibitors
    (SSRIs), 246, 250
Selegiline, 242
Self-change, 81–82, 89. *See also* Natural
    change
Self-efficacy, 143
Self-medication, 119, 215–216
Self-organizing system
    addiction as, 9
    characteristics of, 15–16

definition of, 14–15
development of, 16–18
looking for causes and solutions in,
    305–306
robust principles and, 19–20
Self-perpetuation of problems, 296–297,
    307
Self-regulation theory, 141, 306
Sensitization theory, 41
Significant others. *See* Close
    relationships; Family; Peer
    influences
Silo approach to community services, 161
Skills training, 229–230
Social contexts
    friends and peer groups, 187–191
    intervention and prevention programs,
        195–196
    neighborhoods, 193–195
    overview of, 182, 300–301
    theoretical perspectives on, 182–184
    work, 191–193
    See also Family; Peer influences
Social control theory, 182–183
Social investment, 177–178
Social learning theory, 183, 229–230
Social network, 167–170, 176–178
Social network model of treatment, 230–
    231
Social policy factors, 112–113
Social policy implications
    accessibility of treatment, 308–309
    causes and solutions, looking for, 305–
        306
    evidence-based approaches, using,
        309–311
    intervention as shared responsibility,
        302–304
    life context and comprehensive care,
        304–305
    motivation, enhancing, 306
    pattern, interrupting, 307
    positive reinforcement, enhancing, 307
    rewarding aspects, diminishing, 308
    screening issues, 304
Social stigma, 86, 90, 211
Social support, 105–106
Societal change, history of, 7
Spiritual mutual help organizations
    definition of, 258
    as initiators and maintainers of
        recovery, 268–272
    prevention and, 264
    view of substance use by, 259–260

Spouse modeling, 186–187
SSRIs (selective serotonin reuptake
    inhibitors), 246, 250
Stigma, 86, 90, 211
Stimulants and pharmacotherapy, 248–
    249, 284
"Street culture" of addiction, 213
Stress
    of neighborhood, 194
    relapse and, 30, 31, 39
    work-related, 193
Stress and coping theory, 183
Substance dependence, characteristics of,
    25
Substitute, 13
Supersensitivity model, 120
Symbolic mediation and psychoactive
    substances, 205–209
Synaptic sites, 27

Temperament, 98–100
Temperance movement, 257, 262
Temporal horizon, shortening of, 17, 18
Terminology
    ethnographic documentation of, 203
    genetics, 62–68
    overview of, 5
THC, 35–36
Therapist effects, 137–138, 148, 281–282,
    301–302
Therapist experience, 212–213, 282, 289
"Think tank" conference, 4
Tiagabine, 248
Tolerant coping, 171
Topiramate, 75, 245–246
"Toxic" family, 178–179
Transductive mechanisms, 27
Treatment
    accessibility of, 308–309
    for adolescents, review of, 289
    for adults, review of, 286–288
    barriers to linkage, engagement, and
        outcome, 210–215
    brief intervention, 92, 146, 148, 227–228
    for comorbid disorders, 122–127, 130–
        131

culturally tailored vs. culturally
    specific, 159
economics of, 213
effectiveness of, 157–158
evidence-based, 310–311
family impact on success of, 173–174,
    187
family/social network approaches to,
    176–178, 230–231
length of and compliance with, 280
matching patient and, 250, 285–286
motivational models of, 227–228
motivation and, 297–298
natural recovery and, 90–92
parallel or simultaneous model of,
    130–131
phases of, 276–278
provision of specialized services and,
    284–285
public health and safety approach to,
    161–164
religious and spiritual, 265–268
setting of, 279–280
social contexts and, 195–196
See also Behavioral therapies;
    Intervention system;
    Pharmacotherapy
"Troublesome use" title, 5
Twin studies, 66–67, 69–70
12–step organizations, 258, 259–260,
    270–271

Unilateral family therapy, 139, 176–177

Vaccines, 243, 248–249, 251
Victim impact panels, 145
Violence in family, 103, 175, 178

Waiting lists, 212
Withdrawal, motivational effects of, 29–
    30
Withdrawal coping, 171
Work, 191–193

Youth. See Adolescence